The Sexualization of
Girls and Girlhood

The Sexualization of Girls and Girlhood

Causes, Consequences, and Resistance

EDITED BY EILEEN L. ZURBRIGGEN
and
TOMI-ANN ROBERTS

OXFORD
UNIVERSITY PRESS

OXFORD
UNIVERSITY PRESS

Oxford University Press is a department of the University of Oxford. It furthers the University's objective of excellence in research, scholarship, and education by publishing worldwide.

Oxford   New York
Auckland   Cape Town   Dar es Salaam   Hong Kong   Karachi
Kuala Lumpur   Madrid   Melbourne   Mexico City   Nairobi
New Delhi   Shanghai   Taipei   Toronto

With offices in
Argentina   Austria   Brazil   Chile   Czech Republic   France   Greece
Guatemala   Hungary   Italy   Japan   Poland   Portugal   Singapore
South Korea   Switzerland   Thailand   Turkey   Ukraine   Vietnam

Oxford is a registered trademark of Oxford University Press in the UK and certain other countries.

Published in the United States of America by
Oxford University Press
198 Madison Avenue, New York, NY 10016

© Oxford University Press 2013

Library of Congress Cataloging-in-Publication Data
The sexualization of girls and girlhood/edited by Eileen L. Zurbriggen, Tomi-Ann Roberts.
p. cm.
Includes bibliographical references and index.
ISBN 978–0–19–973165–7
1. Young women—Sexual behavior—United States. 2. Girls—United States. 3. Girls in popular culture—United States. I. Zurbriggen, Eileen L. II. Roberts, Tomi-Ann.

HQ27.5.S494 2012
613.9′55—dc23
2011050568

CONTENTS

PART V. RESISTANCE, ACTIVISM,
AND ALTERNATIVES

CONTRIBUTORS

Laina Y. Bay-Cheng, MSW, PhD
University at Buffalo, SUNY
Buffalo, New York

Elizabeth A. Daniels, PhD
Oregon State University Cascades
Bend, Oregon

Kyla Day, PhD
University of Michigan Substance
  Abuse Research Center
Ann Arbor, Michigan

Marina Epstein, PhD
University of Washington
Seattle, Washington

Melissa Farley, PhD
Prostitution Research & Education
San Francisco, California

Nicole M. Fava, MSW
University at Buffalo, SUNY
Buffalo, New York

Janet Shibley Hyde, PhD
University of Wisconsin–Madison
Madison, Wisconsin

Ingrid Johnston-Robledo, PhD
State University of New York at
  Fredonia
Fredonia, New York

Sharon Lamb, EdD
University of Massachusetts, Boston
Boston, Massachusetts

Nicole M. LaVoi, PhD
The Tucker Center for Research on
  Girls & Women in Sport
University of Minnesota
Minneapolis, Minnesota

Jennifer A. Livingston, PhD
Research Institute on Addictions
University at Buffalo, SUNY
Buffalo, New York

Sarah K. Murnen, PhD
Kenyon College
Gambier, Ohio

Jennifer L. Petersen, PhD
University of Wisconsin–Whitewater
Whitewater, Wisconsin

Natalie J. Purcell, PhD
University of California at Santa Cruz
Santa Cruz, California

Rocio Rivadeneyra, PhD
Illinois State University
Normal, Illinois

Tomi-Ann Roberts, PhD
Colorado College
Colorado Springs, Colorado

Linda Smolak, PhD
Kenyon College
Gambier, Ohio

Margaret L. Stubbs, PhD
Chatham University
Pittsburgh, Pennsylvania

Khia Thomas, PhD
Broward College
Ft. Lauderdale, Florida

Elisabeth Morgan Thompson, PhD
Frances McClelland Institute for
    Children, Youth and Families
University of Arizona
Tucson, Arizona

Marika Tiggemann, PhD
Flinders University
Adelaide, South Australia

Deborah L. Tolman, EdD
Hunter College School of Social Work
    and CUNY Graduate Center
New York, New York

L. Monique Ward, PhD
University of Michigan
Ann Arbor, Michigan

Eileen L. Zurbriggen, PhD
University of California at Santa Cruz
Santa Cruz, California

PART ONE

WHAT IS SEXUALIZATION?

Scope of the Problem and Theoretical Foundations

The Problem of Sexualization

What Is It and How Does It Happen?

TOMI-ANN ROBERTS AND EILEEN L. ZURBRIGGEN

Our culture is saturated with sexuality. One look at the newsstand will convince the skeptic that sex is a key part of capitalist consumer culture; sexually appealing bodies are used to sell just about anything. But, as Karen Horney indicated decades ago, sexualized bodies are far more often female than male. And, increasingly, alarm bells have sounded about the imposition of sexuality upon younger and younger female bodies. The sexualization of girls is argued to be a broad and increasing problem, with consequences not only for girls themselves, but for all of us.

Public concern for the sexualization of young girls was most famously aroused over a decade ago in the aftermath of the JonBenét Ramsey murder. The American public was shocked by the sexualized photos of a 6-year-old "beauty queen" and other girls in children's beauty contests, wearing fake teeth, hair extensions, and makeup, encouraged to sashay and flirt onstage (Cookson, 2001). At the time, public concern was over the effects of such sexualization on the individual girls themselves, as well as over the presence of pedophiles in our midst who might be stimulated by them. Today, journalists, child advocacy organizations, parents, and psychologists have recognized that the sexualization of girls and girlhood is a problem that extends far beyond beauty pageants.

In 2005, the American Psychological Association established a Task Force on the Sexualization of Girls, and, in 2007, it published a report summarizing psychological theory, research, and clinical experience addressing this mental health concern (American Psychological Association [APA], 2007). Among the recommendations made in that report was a call for more and better research documenting the prevalence of the sexualization of girls and girlhood in the culture, examining the far-reaching consequences of this sexualization, and providing theoretically grounded hope for healthier alternatives. This book is a follow-up to the Task Force Report and is our effort to heed that call for continuing the scholarly conversation.

Although public concern is arguably a good thing if we believe that girls ought not to be sexualized, we are troubled by an increasing looseness around the definition and scope of the problem. Like a lot of psychological concepts that make their way into the public vernacular, the idea of "sexualization" is one that has taken on an "I know it when I see it" quality, and this may help account for the proliferation of titles on bookstore shelves such as *Don't Dress Your Daughter Like a Skank*, and *The Lolita Effect*. In this chapter, and throughout this book, we intend to clarify the scope of the problem of the sexualization of girls and carefully define what we mean (and what we do *not* mean) by the term "sexualization" from a theoretically rigorous and psychological research-based perspective.

Defining Sexualization

For the Task Force, and for us, there are several components to sexualization, and these set it distinctly apart from healthy sexuality. According to the Sexuality Information and Education Council of the United States (SIECUS) (2004), healthy sexuality is an important component of the physical and mental health of youth and adults. Healthy sexuality (when it is experienced or portrayed) is characterized by intimacy, bonding, and shared pleasure, and it involves mutual respect between consenting partners. In contrast, sexualization occurs when:

A person's value is determined only or primarily by sexual appeal or behavior, to the exclusion of other characteristics.

Sexuality is inappropriately imposed upon a person.

A person is held to a standard that equates a narrow definition of attractiveness with "being sexy."

A person is sexually objectified; made into a tool for others' sexual use and pleasure, rather than treated as a person with the capacity for independent action and decision making.

All four of the conditions need not be present to constitute sexualization; any one is an indication. Let us consider each of these four components more carefully with some illustration.

Valued Primarily or Only for Sex Appeal

The first way in which sexualization can occur is when sexual appeal is the most valued characteristic of a girl or young woman, to the exclusion of other qualities.

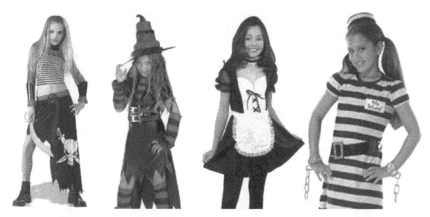

Figure 1.1 Girls' Halloween costumes from the Lillian Vernon online catalog at
www.lillianvernon.com. For reference to these costumes and a discussion about
the sexualization of girls' Halloween costumes, see Matthew Philips' article in
Newsweek's online blog The Daily Beast: *"Eye Candy: Little girls' Halloween costumes
are looking more like they were designed by Victoria's Secret every year. Are we prudes or
is this practically kiddie porn?"* (*Newsweek*, 10/29/2007 Web exclusive: http://www.
newsweek.com/id/62474.)

It is easy to see that "sexy" has become synonymous with feminine in the
media and advertising. In this catalog entry of the selection of girls' Halloween
costumes (Figure 1.1), we see that the "character" being depicted takes a back
seat to a sexy presentation. In sports journalism, for example, research has shown
that female athletes are often targets of sexualized treatment, in ways that imply
that their sex appeal is more important than their athletic achievements (Fink
& Kensicki, 2002). Shugart (2003) examined the print and television coverage
of the 1999 U.S. women's soccer team and found that most coverage redefined
"female strength…as male pleasure" (p. 27). The magazine cover image of Jennie
Finch (Figure 1.2) certainly emphasizes that her value is primarily her sex appeal.
Besides the nod to her athleticism via the plastic whiffle ball and bat, there is
nothing here to indicate that she is, in fact, a gold and silver Olympic medalist
softball player. Instead, the focus is on her breasts, her hair, and a denim mini-
skirt that she appears to be just about to slip out of. Moreover, posing her with a
whiffle ball and bat trivializes and minimizes her accomplishments. Whiffle ball
is a game played by children or at picnics, rather than for Olympic gold, and you
certainly can't pitch a fast ball with a whiffle ball.

Ariel Levy (2005) and others argue that, increasingly, feminine sexuality is
being "pornografized," that is, presented to girls and women by MTV, in song
lyrics, and enacted by them in "Girls Gone Wild" videos, in ways that emphasize service to boys and men, voyeurism, and performance. In other words,
stripping equals sexy, and sexy equals feminine. Indeed, this tawdry, cartoon-
ish, performative version of feminine sexuality has become so prevalent that

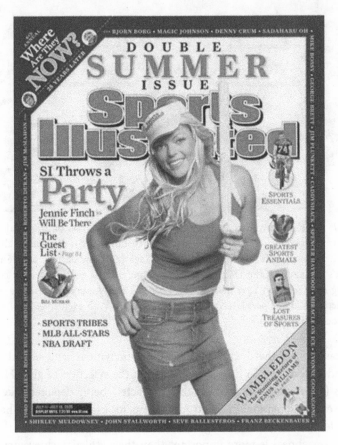

Figure 1.2 Magazine cover (2005, July 11) featuring softball player Jennie Finch. *Sports Illustrated* 103(2). From the *Sports Illustrated* Vault at: http://sportsillustrated. cnn.com/vault/cover/featured/10055/index.htm

it no longer seems noteworthy. What was once regarded as a *type* of sexual expression, Levy (2005) writes, is now viewed *as* feminine sexuality. And, furthermore, as Pollet and Hurwitz (2004) point out, this "mass-marketed ideal of female sexiness derived from stripper culture is being sold to an ever younger set" (p. 21). In their article in *The Nation*, they discuss some of the toys marketed to girls, including a pole dance kit, that reinforce this notion that, even at 6 or 7 years old, girls' primary value comes from their sex appeal.

Inappropriate Imposition of Sexuality

The second way in which we see sexualization occurring is when a person is inappropriately imbued with sexuality. This appears to happen most frequently in two ways. First, a young girl can be portrayed or treated as having adult

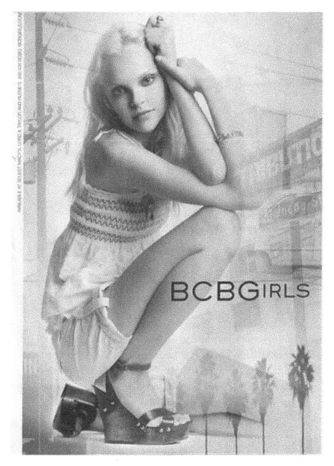

Figure 1.3 An advertisement for BCBGirls shoes, http://www.bcbg.com/

sexuality. Or, second, an adult woman can be portrayed or treated as being girlish yet sexy. The media present the public with both this "trickle-up" and "trickle-down" framework on girls and women (Cook & Kaiser, 2004). In these two advertisements, we can see this phenomenon clearly. The first (Figure 1.3) depicts a young girl with adult makeup and platform shoes, and the second (Figure 1.4) presents an adult woman posing in a kittenish way, licking a lollipop.

Other evidence for trickle-up includes the launching of new magazines *Cosmo Girl* and *Elle Girl* in 2001, and *Teen Vogue* in 2003. These magazines "downsize" the sexualizing message of their adult version publications, but the gist remains the same: the "body project" involved in attaining just the right sexy appearance. Lamb and Brown (2006) point out a parallel process in retail, with stores like *Abercrombie Kids* or *Limited, Too* (now *Justice*) presenting

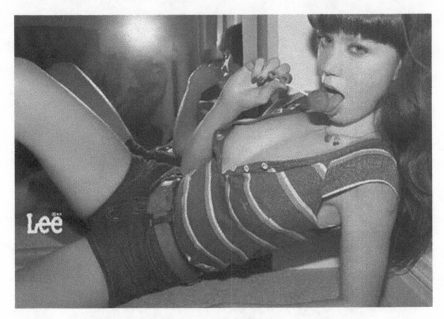

Figure 1.4 A Lee Jeans' advertisement for its "Lolita" campaign from Spring-Summer 2006, which was approved by the Advertising Standards Board in Australia. For information about the advertisement and the debate over the image, see Kenneth Nguyen's article in *The Age* online: *"Lee's Lolita OK, board rules"* (*The Age*, 10/04/2006: http://www.theage.com.au/news/national/lees-lolita-ok/2006/10/04/1159641365538.html)

adult-style sexy versions of camisoles, underwear, and emblazoned tee shirts to a tween population defined as 7 to 17 (Lamb & Brown, 2006). The trickle-down, or "youthification" side of the equation includes sexual portrayals of adult women as young girls (Kilbourne, 1999). In ads like that in Figure 1.4, women often are shown in kids'-style clothing (short shorts) or schoolgirl uniforms and licking lollipops or popsicles, or wearing scaled-up versions of children's clothing styles, like baby-doll dresses and tops, knee socks, and Mary Janes, marketed as adult women's wear, thus leading some critics to denounce "pedophilic fashion" (Menkes, 1994).

Narrow Definition of Attractive Sexiness

A third way in which sexualization can occur is through holding girls to a standard of physical attractiveness that is narrowly defined and, some would argue, almost impossible to attain (Wolf, 1991). This standard is invariably equated with sexiness. The cover for *Cosmo Girl* magazine shown in Figure 1.5 provides an illustrative example of the instructions delivered to girls on how to look sexy and win boys' attention.

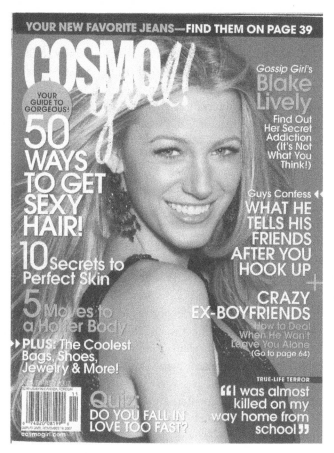

Figure 1.5 Cosmogirl! Magazine cover (November 2007) featuring Blake Lively. The magazine folded in 2008 but currently maintains a blog: http://www.seventeen.com/cosmogirl/

Groesz, Levine, and Murnen (2002) showed that the media tend to depict a narrowly defined idea of feminine beauty, characterized by "flawless skin, a thin waist, long legs and well-developed breasts" (p. 2). Computer retouching and other techniques for enhancing these images only serve to increase the gap between them and the reality of the average girl's or young woman's appearance (Kilbourne, 1999).

Garner, Sterk, and Adams (1998) examined the social and cultural norms for sex and sexual relationships in magazines popular among 12- to 24-year-old females. They argued that such magazines serve as training manuals for teens and that these manuals limit girls' sexuality within very narrowly defined heterosexual norms and practices. The rhetoric of sexual etiquette in teen magazines encourages girls to engage in beautifying practices in order to be "sexy," thus subordinating themselves to boys' desires.

It is important to note that the number of teen-focused magazines has increased dramatically in recent years, from five in 1990, to 19 in 2000, and research shows that 15- to 18-year-olds spend an average of 13 minutes per day reading magazines (Roberts, Foehr, & Rideout, 2005; Teen Market Profile, 2005). Sixty-six percent of 11- to 18-year-olds report regularly reading such magazines. Furthermore, new fashion-oriented magazines directed at *pre*-teens are launching (e.g., *Barbie* and *Total Girl*). Clark and Tiggemann (2007) found that reading these appearance-focused magazines was related to investment in appearance, body dissatisfaction, and dieting behaviors among 9- to 12-year-old girls.

Sexual Objectification

The final characteristic of sexualization has been the most widely studied to date. Sexual objectification refers to the practice of regarding or treating another person merely as an instrument (object) for another's sexual pleasure, with insufficient regard for the person's other human qualities (Bartky, 1990). Sexual objectification occurs both in interpersonal encounters as well as in cultural depictions, in which the body is portrayed purely as a decorative object, viewed as capable of representing the entire person, and/or "dismembered" (body parts are excluded or obscured). Ample research has demonstrated that sexual objectification of the female body is particularly prominent in advertising and that such treatment has increased over time (e.g., Baker, 2005; Lindner, 2004; Reichert & Carpenter, 2004).

Advertisers and marketers are usually careful not to sexually objectify young girls directly, but, as we saw in the previous section, they have ways of blurring the line between child and adult, often through the use of youthful or

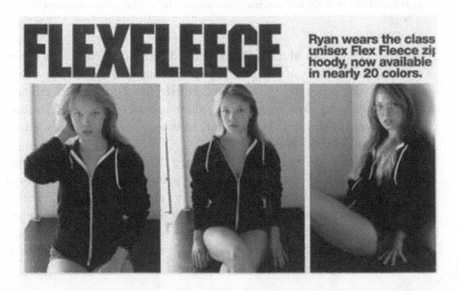

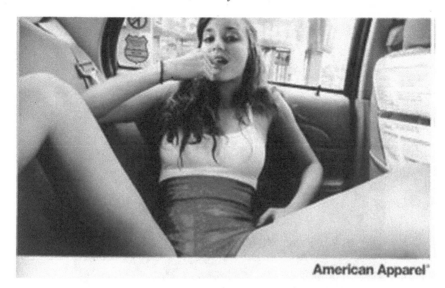

Figures 1.6 and 1.7 Advertisements from American Apparel, http://www.americanapparel.net/

"barely legal" adolescents or the implication of a surreptitiously candid photo shoot, as in these American Apparel ads (Figures 1.6 and 1.7).

Is the Sexualization of Girls on the Rise?

The questions of whether younger and younger girls are being depicted in sexualized ways in media or whether the sexualization of girls is increasing over time remain largely unexplored. However, the evolution of the following advertising campaign certainly gives us pause. In Figure 1.8 is the first advertisement for Christian Dior's fragrance "Addict," from 2002. In Figure 1.9 is "Addict 2," their advertisement in 2005.

Both ads are examples of sexual objectification: the focus is on body parts as opposed to the whole person, the image is there for the viewer's pleasure. However, the second ad is clearly intended to depict a much younger person; the face is very young, the body prepubescent. Her age is exaggerated with the use of the color pink, her little girl underwear, her pout, and the way that she is playing with her hair. Another example that suggests an increase in sexualization is the reinvention of the popular "troll" dolls from the 1970s to today (Figures 1.10 and 1.11).

Today's *Trollz* are hip teenagers with miniskirts, bare midriffs, and magical "belly gems." The name change from the letter "s" to "z," along with the introduction of five sexy characters here is clearly a nod to the wildly

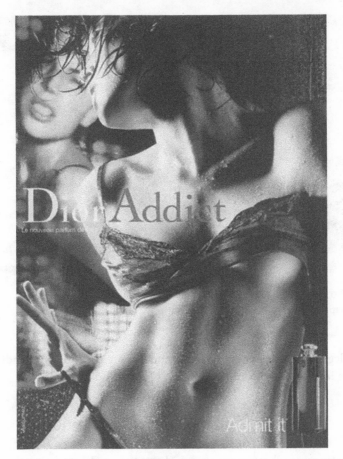

Figure 1.8 An advertisement for Christian Dior Addict fragrance. Image can be found at http://www.footluxe.com/2011/06/perfume-collection-review-for-christian-dior-addict-fragrance-for-women/

popular *Bratz* dolls, a line of toys beloved by 6- to 12-year-old girls, but widely criticized by mothers and child advocacy groups for their sexualized appearance (LaFerla, 2003).

Only one study has examined changes over time in the sexualization of girls and girlhood. O'Donohue, Gold, and McKay (1997) analyzed advertisements in popular magazines such as *Newsweek* and *Ladies Home Journal* over a 40-year period. They found that advertisements depicting children in sexual ways increased significantly over time, and that 85% of such ads depicted girls. Often, these images of sexualized girls were found alongside sexualized adult women, in matching "downsized" outfits or mimicking a seductive pose.

Clearly, more research is needed to document the frequency of sexualization of girls and to examine carefully whether this treatment is

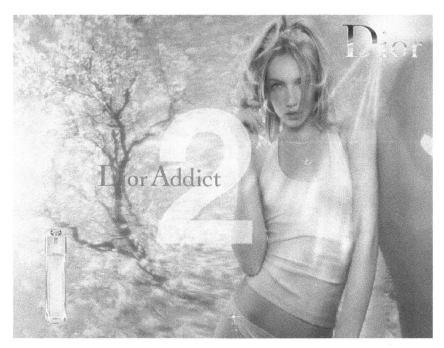

Figure 1.9 An advertisement for Christian Dior Addict 2 fragrance. Image can be found at http://www.footluxe.com/2011/06/perfume-collection-review-for-christia n-dior-addict-2-for-women/

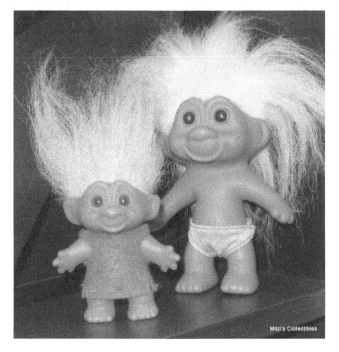

Figure 1.10 Troll dolls from the 1970s.

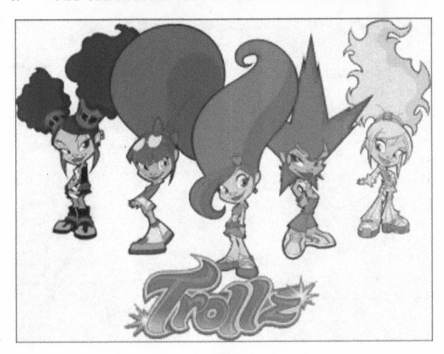

Figure 1.11 Trollz dolls in the animated series created by DiC Entertainment. For more information and images on the sexualization of dolls and toys, including the Trollz dolls, see Linda Dahlstrom and Kavita Varma-White's article on MSNBC's *Today's* Parenting website: *"Hot-to-trot ponies? Dolls that wax? Toys get tarted up: Racy new toys and revamped favorites scandalize parents"* (Today.com, 3/07/2011, http:// today.msnbc.msn.com/id/41895570/ns/today-parenting_and_family/t/hot-to-trot-po nies-dolls-wax-toys-get-tarted/)

increasing, as so many cultural commentators suspect. It is our hope that both the APA Task Force Report and this volume, by clarifying what is and what isn't sexualization, will provide useful operationalizations for such investigations. That is, we do not believe it is sufficient to simply say that girls have "gone skank" or to confound sexualization with sexuality more broadly defined or even with gender role stereotyping. It is time we investigate this particular public health concern using a more scholarly, rigorous approach.

The Three Spheres of Sexualization

The Task Force Report (APA, 2007) provided evidence that sexualization happens in three interrelated spheres: a sociocultural one, an interpersonal one, and also an intrapersonal one, as girls internalize the sexualized messages around them and fashion themselves as sexy. This volume includes reports of newer research on the prevalence of sexualization in all three spheres, as well as the consequences across the spheres for girls themselves and for society as a whole.

Cultural Sexualization

The media and other cultural contributions to the sexualization of girls have been studied the most extensively of the three spheres of influence. Indeed, children spend more time with entertainment media than they do with any other activity except school and sleeping (Roberts et al., 2005) and so the concern about the messages being delivered to girls via these cultural agents is rightfully placed. Throughout U.S. culture and across virtually every media form (prime-time television, commercials, music videos, magazines, video games, song lyrics), women and girls are depicted in sexualized ways (e.g., Gow, 1996; Grauerholz & King, 1997; Krassas, Blauwkamp, & Wesselink, 2003; Linn, 2004, 2005; Ward, 1995). And girls are major consumers of media, receiving these sexualized messages for at least 6.5 hours every day on their various media devices: television, Internet, iPod, and cell phone (Nielsen Media Research, 1998; Roberts et al., 2005).

Contributors to this volume provide increasingly nuanced research exploring cultural contributions to the sexualization of girls, as well as discussions of the damage done to the culture at large when girls are sexualized, with chapters by Ward and colleagues examining the sexualized content of black music videos (2013, Chapter 3, this volume), Daniels and LaVoi investigating the sexualization of female athletes (2013, Chapter 4, this volume), and Tolman theorizing about the consequences of this cultural phenomenon extending beyond girls themselves to boys, men, and adult women (2013, Chapter 5, this volume).

Interpersonal Sexualization

Although it is easy to point fingers at the media, they are, of course, not the only perpetrators of sexualization. Girls' interpersonal relationships with their parents, siblings, peers, and teachers also contribute to this phenomenon. Because the people in girls' lives are themselves influenced by the cultural messages that sexualize girls and girlhood, they may contribute to sexualizing girls when they convey their support for these ideas, whether consciously or unconsciously, overtly or covertly. Fathers may, for example, nod approvingly when their daughters enact a "sexy dance" during dress-up. Mothers have been shown to routinely engage in "fat talk" about their own bodies and the bodies of their daughters, creating an environment in some homes of excessive concern over physical appearance

(Nichter, 2000). Furthermore, we must acknowledge that sexual harassment, abuse, assault, and trafficking are extreme forms of sexualization, and a shocking percentage of girls experience these forms, often at the hands of trusted adults or peers.

In this volume, we expand the conversation around the interpersonal contributions to the sexualization of girls, with chapters by Petersen and Hyde addressing the problem of sexual harassment by peers (2013, Chapter 6, this volume), Thompson providing evidence for the sexualization of sexual-minority girls and young women, along with consequences for this understudied group (2013, Chapter 7, this volume), Purcell and Zurbriggen examining the relationship between sexualization and sexual violence (2013, Chapter 8, this volume), and Farley exploring the horrors of prostitution and trafficking as extreme exemplars of sexualization (2013, Chapter 9, this volume).

Self-Sexualization

To imagine that girls are passive recipients of the cultural and interpersonal messages about sexualization that surround them is to ignore girls' own agency. Many a parent bemoans their 6-year-old's love of *Bratz* dolls or their pre-teen daughter's selection of low-cut tank top, but it is often extremely difficult to get girls to make less sexualizing choices. They are savvy consumers and recognize the many social advantages that come when they "buy into" their own sexualization. In this way, we see that girls themselves are active agents and often self-sexualize. The motivations for and consequences of this process are now being studied by psychologists.

Girls sexualize themselves in all of the ways we have discussed—when they think of themselves mostly or entirely in terms of their sexy appearance, when they equate their sexiness with a narrow standard of attractiveness, and when they engage in age-inappropriate sexuality. However, researchers have focused most extensively on *self-objectification*, or the tendency of girls and women to view and treat themselves and their own bodies as objects of others' desires, to take, in other words, a third-person perspective on their physical selves (Fredrickson & Roberts, 1997). Self-objectification, demonstrated to be common among girls as young as 9–12 (Clark & Tiggemann, 2006; 2007), carries a host of emotional, cognitive, and behavioral consequences.

Several contributors focus on self-sexualization. Roberts (2013, Chapter 2, this volume) offers theoretical perspectives on how girls translate the cultural and interpersonal messages of sexualization into their self-concepts, Tiggemann (2013, Chapter 10, this volume) examines pre-teen and teen girls' appearance and body image concerns, Stubbs and Johnston-Robledo (2013, Chapter 11, this volume) explore how the cultural context of sexualization complicates the impact of menarche on girls' emerging sexual self-concepts, and Murnen and Smolak (2013, Chapter 12, this volume) take an in-depth look at both the perceived rewards and the costs for girls and women of internalizing a sexualized perspective of themselves.

Even So, Reason for Hope

Despite the undeniable evidence for the widespread sexualization of girls and girlhood, and despite the sobering data we now have on the consequences of such treatment not only for girls themselves, but for all of us, we have hope. First, there are indications that negative outcomes are neither inevitable nor universal. Many girls, and many of those who support girls, resist cultural characterizations of them as sexual objects. And they do so in myriad ways. Second, the overwhelmingly positive response to the APA Task Force report made us realize that parents, educators, and girls are eager for information and ideas for combating sexualization. In that report, we gave a number of suggestions for positive alternatives and approaches to counteracting the influence of sexualization, including working through schools, the family, and with girls themselves.

In this volume, we offer three chapters that provide evidence for existing forces of resistance and suggestions for the future. Lamb (2013, Chapter 14, this volume) examines popular frameworks on girls' and young women's sexuality and offers a healthy alternative for creating "good sexual citizens." She asks that parents and sex educators help enable adolescents to think about relationships in terms of fairness and compassion and apply principles of justice and caring to all relationships, particularly sexual relationships. Based on their work in focus groups with girls, Bay-Cheng, Livingston, and Fava (2013, Chapter 13, this volume) recommend the cultivation of safe spaces in which adolescent girls are free to engage in open, candid discussion and debates with one another and with adults to construct their own individual views of sexuality and sexual decision making. Finally, Zurbriggen and Roberts (2013, Chapter 15, this volume) make some suggestions for parents, teachers, and children, based on the work throughout this volume, for fighting back against the cultural sexualization of girls.

A Commencement

The APA Task Force Report (2007) described study after study that found ample evidence for the widespread sexualization of girls, from media and merchandizers to parents increasingly encouraging the maintenance of a sexy, attractive physical appearance as the top goal for their daughters, buying them size 7 thong underwear or tiny T-shirts with slogans like, "Wink, wink" or "Booty call," or even paying for plastic surgery for their pre-teens to help them reach that goal. And, perhaps most sobering, girls come to view and treat *themselves* as sexual objects, internalizing the idea that their bodies are valuable primarily for how sexually appealing they are to others. Why shouldn't they? The most successful models of femininity around them are sexed-up.

Does this matter? Yes. We believe that the sexualizing of girls and of girlishness in grown women functions to keep them *in their place*. This treatment has been linked to three of the most common mental health problems in girls and women: low self-esteem, eating disorders, and depression. Studies show that girls and young women who internalize a sexually objectified view of themselves throw a ball less effectively, fail to use proper birth control if they have sex, are more likely to take up smoking, and have trouble concentrating on their school work. These are concerning consequences indeed. Parents, teachers, and child advocates rightly want more for our girls. They deserve better. In our work publicizing and circulating the Task Force report, we found that it touched a chord in nearly everyone that we spoke to. We believe there is a very real hunger for more information on this problem, as well as for suggestions on how to combat it. This book is intended to meet this need by presenting the best, most rigorous empirical data, combined with theoretically based analyses of possible effects that have not yet been thoroughly researched and a thorough discussion of empirically derived suggestions for resistance and change. We hope this volume will be of value to researchers, teachers, and health care providers, to girls themselves, and to all of us who love, care for, and mentor them.

References

American Psychological Association, Task Force on the Sexualization of Girls. (2007). *Report of the APA Task Force on the Sexualization of Girls*. Washington, DC: American Psychological Association. Retrieved from www.apa.org/pi/wpo/sexualization.html

Baker, C. N. (2005). Images of women's sexuality in advertisements: A content analysis of black- and white-oriented women's and men's magazines. *Sex Roles, 52*, 13–27.

Bartky, S. L. (1990). *Femininity and domination: Studies in the phenomenology of oppression*. New York: Routledge.

Bay-Cheng, L. Y., Livingston, J. A., & Fava, N. M. (2013). "Not always a clear path": Making space for peers, adults, and complexity in adolescent girls' sexual development. In E. L. Zurbriggen & T.- A. Roberts (Eds.), *The sexualization of girls and girlhood: Causes, consequences, and resistance* (Chapter 13). New York: Oxford University Press.

Clark, L., & Tiggemann, M. (2006). Appearance culture in nine- to 12-year-old girls: Media and peer influences on body dissatisfaction. *Social Development, 15*, 628–643.

Clark, L., & Tiggemann, M. (2007). Sociocultural influences and body image in 9 to 12 year old girls; The role of appearance schemas. *Journal of Child and Adolescent Psychology, 36,* 76–86.

Cook, D. T., & Kaiser, S. B. (2004). Betwixt and be tween: Age ambiguity and the sexualization of the female consuming subject. *Journal of Consumer Culture, 4,* 203–227.

Cookson, S. (Writer, Director). (2001). Living dolls: The making of a child beauty queen. In L. Otto (Producer) *American undercover* [HBO documentary]. New York: Home Box Office.

Daniels, E. A., & LaVoi, N. M. (2013). Athletics as solution and problem: Sport participation for girls and the sexualization of female athletes. In E. L. Zurbriggen & T.- A. Roberts (Eds.), *The sexualization of girls and girlhood: Causes, consequences, and resistance* (Chapter 4). New York: Oxford University Press.

Farley, M. (2013). Prostitution: An extreme form of girls' sexualization. In E. L. Zurbriggen & T.- A. Roberts (Eds.), *The sexualization of girls and girlhood: Causes, consequences, and resistance* (Chapter 9). New York: Oxford University Press.

Fink, J. S., & Kensicki, L. J. (2002). An imperceptible difference: Visual and textual constructions of femininity in *Sports Illustrated* and *Sports Illustrated for Women. Mass Communication & Society, 5,* 317–339.

Fredrickson, B. F., & Roberts, T.- A. (1997). Objectification theory: Toward understanding women's lived experience and mental health risks. *Psychology of Women Quarterly, 21,* 173–206.

Garner, A. Sterk, H. M., & Adams, S. (1998). Narrative analysis of sexual etiquette in teenage magazines. *Journal of Communication, 48,* 59–78.

Gow, J. (1996). Reconsidering gender roles on MTV: Depictions in the most popular music videos of the early 1990s. *Communication Reports, 9,* 151–161.

Grauerholz, E., & King, A. (1997). Primetime sexual harassment. *Violence Against Women, 3,* 129–148.

Groesz, L. M., Levine, M. P., & Murnen, S. K. (2002). The effect of experimental presentation of thin media images on body satisfaction: A meta-analytic review. *International Journal of Eating Disorders, 31,* 1–16.

Kilbourne, J. (1999). *Deadly persuasion: Why women and girls must fight the addictive power of advertising.* New York: Free Press.

Krassas, N. R., Blauwkamp, J. M., & Wesselink, P. (2003). "Master your Johnson": Sexual rhetoric in *Maxim* and *Stuff* magazines. *Sexuality & Culture, 7,* 98–119.

LaFerla, R. (2003, October 26). Underdressed and hot: Dolls moms don't love. *The New York Times,* Section 9, p. 1.

Lamb, S. (2013). Toward a healthy sexuality for girls and young women: A critique of desire. In E. L. Zurbriggen & T.- A. Roberts (Eds.), *The sexualization of girls and girlhood: Causes, consequences, and resistance* (Chapter 14). New York: Oxford University Press.

Lamb, S., & Brown, L. M. (2006). *Packaging girlhood: Rescuing our daughters from marketers' schemes.* New York: St. Martin's Press.

Levy, A. (2005). *Female chauvinist pigs: Women and the rise of raunch culture.* New York: Free Press.

Lindner, K. (2004). Images of women in general interest and fashion advertisements from 1955 to 2002. *Sex Roles, 51,* 409–421.

Linn, S. (2004). *Consuming kids: The hostile takeover of childhood.* New York: The New Press.

Linn, S. (2005). The commercialization of childhood. In S. Olfman (Ed.), *Childhood lost: How American culture is failing our kids* (pp. 107–121). Westport, CT: Praeger.

Menkes, S. (1994, March 27). Runways: Robbing the cradle. *The New York Times,* p. A1.

Murnen, S. K., & Smolak, L. (2013). "I'd rather be a famous fashion model than a famous scientist": The rewards and costs of internalizing sexualization. In E. L. Zurbriggen &

T.- A. Roberts (Eds.), *The sexualization of girls and girlhood: Causes, consequences, and resistance* (Chapter 12). New York: Oxford University Press.

Nichter, M. (2000). *Fat talk: What girls and their parents say about dieting.* Cambridge, MA: Harvard University Press.

Nielsen Media Research. (1998). *1998 report on television.* New York: Author.

O'Donohue, W., Gold, S. R., & McKay, J. S. (1997). Children as sexual objects: Historical and gender trends in magazines. *Sexual Abuse: Journal of Research & Treatment, 9*(4) 291–301.

Petersen, J. L., & Hyde, J. S. (2013). Sexual harassment by peers. In E. L. Zurbriggen & T.- A. Roberts (Eds.), *The sexualization of girls and girlhood: Causes, consequences, and resistance* (Chapter 6). New York: Oxford University Press.

Pollet, A., & Hurwitz, P. (2004). Strip til you drop. *The Nation* (Jan 12/19), 20–21, 24–25.

Purcell, N. J., & Zurbriggen, E. L. (2013). The sexualization of girls and gendered violence: Mapping the connections. In E. L. Zurbriggen & T.- A. Roberts (Eds.), *The sexualization of girls and girlhood: Causes, consequences, and resistance* (Chapter 8). New York: Oxford University Press.

Reichert, T., & Carpenter, C. (2004). An update on sex in magazine advertising: 1983 to 2003. *Journalism and Mass Communication Quarterly, 81,* 823–837.

Roberts D. F., Foehr U. G., & Rideout V. J. (2005). *Generation M: Media in the lives of 8 – 18 year olds.* Menlo Park, CA: The Henry J Kaiser Family Foundation Report.

Roberts, T-. A. (2013). She's so pretty, she looks just like a Bratz doll!": Theoretical foundations for understanding girls' and women's self-objectification. In E. L. Zurbriggen & T.- A. Roberts (Eds.), *The sexualization of girls and girlhood: Causes, consequences, and resistance* (Chapter 2). New York: Oxford University Press.

Sexuality Information and Education Council of the United States. (2004). *Guidelines for comprehensive sexuality education: Kindergarten—12th grade* (3rd ed.). New York. Retrieved February 20, 2010 from www.siecus.org/pubs/guidelines/guidelines.pdf

Shugart, H. A. (2003). She shoots, she scores: Mediated constructions of contemporary female athletes in coverage of the 1999 US women's soccer team. *Western Journal of Communication, 67,* 1–31.

Stubbs, M. L., & Johnston-Robledo, I. (2013). Kiddy thongs and menstrual pads: The sexualization of girls and early menstrual life. In E. L. Zurbriggen & T.- A. Roberts (Eds.), *The sexualization of girls and girlhood: Causes, consequences, and resistance* (Chapter 11). New York: Oxford University Press.

Teen Market Profile. (2005). New York: Mediamark Research. Retrieved February 22, 2010 from www.magazine.org/content/files/teenprofile04.pdf

Thompson, E. M. (2013). "If you're hot, i'm bi": Implications of sexualization for sexual-minority girls. In E. L. Zurbriggen & T.- A. Roberts (Eds.), *The sexualization of girls and girlhood: Causes, consequences, and resistance* (Chapter 7). New York: Oxford University Press.

Tiggemann, M. (2013). Teens, pre-teens, and body image. In E. L. Zurbriggen & T.- A. Roberts (Eds.), *The sexualization of girls and girlhood: Causes, consequences, and resistance* (Chapter 10). New York: Oxford University Press.

Tolman, D. L. (2013). It's bad for us too: How the sexualization of girls impacts the sexuality of boys, men, and women. In E. L. Zurbriggen & T.- A. Roberts (Eds.), *The sexualization of girls and girlhood: Causes, consequences, and resistance* (Chapter 5). New York: Oxford University Press.

Ward, L. M. (1995). Talking about sex: Common themes about sexuality in the prime-time television programs children and adolescents view most. *Journal of Youth & Adolescence, 24,* 595–615.

Ward, L. M., Rivadeneyra, R., Thomas, K., Day, K., & Epstein, M. (2013). A woman's worth: Analyzing the sexual objectification of black women in music videos. In E. L.

Zurbriggen & T.- A. Roberts (Eds.), *The sexualization of girls and girlhood: Causes, consequences, and resistance* (Chapter 3). New York: Oxford University Press.

Wolf, N. (1991). *The beauty myth: How images of beauty are used against women.* New York: Anchor Books.

Zurbriggen, E. L., & Roberts, T.- A. (2013). Fighting sexualization: What parents, teachers, communities, and kids can do. In E. L. Zurbriggen & T.- A. Roberts (Eds.), *The sexualization of girls and girlhood: Causes, consequences, and resistance* (Chapter 15). New York: Oxford University Press.

2

"She's So Pretty, She Looks Just Like a Bratz Doll!"

Theoretical Foundations for Understanding Girls' and Women's Self-Objectification

TOMI-ANN ROBERTS

A number of years ago, when my younger daughter was 7, we spent some time in Berlin, Germany. One day, on the street car, I noticed we had entered an area where prostituted women solicit openly, and my daughter was positively entranced. More shocking to me than their presence on the street (we were in Berlin, after all) was my daughter's careful scrutiny of and obvious enchantment with these women, who wore mini skirts, thigh-high vinyl boots, bleached-blonde hair, and over-the-top make-up. "Look, Mommy!" she cried, "They're so pretty! They look just like Bratz dolls!"

In this chapter, I present a number of theoretical perspectives on how girls and women come to adopt a sexually objectified perspective of themselves, how it is that the culture "out there" gets "in here." My daughter's response to the women in Berlin highlights several important features of any attempt to get a grip on girls' and young women's incorporation of a sexualized femininity into their own self-concepts. First, girls and women are not passive recipients of cultural messages. They are active agents, making choices about what cultural models to attend to and fashion themselves after. Second, "pretty" is an essential feature of positively valenced femininity. Third, "pretty" is associated today with "sexy," and this sexualized version of pretty is one that even 7-year-olds are clearly cognizant of and wish, therefore, to be.

Two general classes of theories exist to explain how media and cultural messages about sexualization, as well as interpersonal sexualized treatment, get translated and incorporated into the self, and, in turn, influence the physical and mental health of girls and women: psychological and sociocultural. I review these theories, each of which provides a unique contribution to our understanding of how my daughter—and many girls and women—come to a sexualized understanding of "good" femininity and of themselves. Psychological theories emphasize girls' development and women's interactions with others and how these experiences shape their identity. Sociocultural theories illuminate how the cultural milieu in which girls and women exist provides the scripts for appropriate femininity. I then present *objectification theory* (Fredrickson & Roberts, 1997) as a unifying theory that I believe provides the best framework for understanding girls' and women's development within a sexually objectifying culture, and which adds the intrapsychic phenomenon of *self*-objectification to our understanding.

Psychological Theories

Psychology has offered several theoretical perspectives on gender development that are helpful in understanding how girls develop into women within a given familial and societal framework on gender stereotypes. What constitutes appropriate, culturally acceptable femininity changes over time, and Wolf (1991) has argued that, whereas femininity was associated with domesticity a generation ago, it is now associated with beauty and physical attractiveness.

Socialization

Social learning theory (e.g., Bussey & Bandura, 1999) and gender schema theory (Bem, 1985) both provide explanations for the learning of culturally appropriate gender roles via reinforcement from others, modeling, observational learning, and through the construction of cognitive schemas. Within these perspectives, girls learn about the female role and strive to enact its expectations because doing so brings rewards and because being consistent with expectations is itself rewarding. These theories help us see that girls' understanding of appropriate femininity is not "natural" or innate but is acquired through a developmental process whereby girls draw information from the adults and peers, real and fictional, around them. For example, when parents purchase clothing and praise their daughters for being pretty or even "sexy," this teaches the idea that appropriate femininity involves appearing attractive to others. In addition, girls observe adult women receiving rewards (in the form of attention, approval, or even money) in their immediate environment or the media when they are presented in a manner that emphasizes their physical attractiveness as their most important value. They also likely observe punishments in the forms of exclusion, derision, and rejection when women do not do so.

Pannell (2008) conducted a study of child beauty pageants and found support for social learning theory's tenets. The very young pageant contestants received lavish reinforcement in the form of praise or treats not only from their mothers, but from pageant personnel and even strangers for their successful enactment of "beautiful" (which included heavy makeup, hair extensions, and flirty sashaying for the judges). The girls also received punishment, mostly from their mothers, for behaving less like adult women pageant contestants and more like the children they actually were (e.g., having temper tantrums or refusing to cooperate with choreographed moves). Thus, these girls learned a hypersexualized femininity.

Cognitive Development and Identity Formation

The cognitive developmental framework for understanding gender development places less importance on external rewards and punishments and more on girls' own active strivings to understand the world and their role in it. Once girls have the cognitive capacity to understand their gender, and once they learn that gender is a constant feature of who they are, girls come to value behaviors, objects, and attitudes that are consistent with the label "girl" or "feminine" (Warin, 2000). They want to wear the clothes, play with the toys, and enact the behaviors characterized as "girly." Indeed, Maccoby (1980) showed how children exaggerate gender roles and stereotypes beyond what we would predict from their direct observation of actual adult models around them. That is, this psychological developmental theory adds the important element of girls' willing socialization of themselves into the feminine role (Crawford & Unger, 2000). If Bratz dolls and child-sized tees with slogans like "Future Hottie" are the available emblems of femininity, then girls will want them, because associating with these items helps them solidify their membership in their valued gender category.

Once girls reach adolescence, the developmental stage during which Erikson (1950) argued that individuals strive to form an identity, a crisis appears for many. Strassburger and Wilson (2002) argue that preadolescents and adolescents are like actors as they experiment with different features of their newly forming identities and try on different social "masks." This plasticity may make girls especially susceptible to cultural messages about appropriate femininity, which increasingly emphasize attractiveness as their most important value (Jackson, 1992). Importantly, the attractiveness standard emphasized by Western culture (thin, smooth-skinned, large-breasted, heterosexual, white) cannot be attained by the majority of girls and women, which undoubtedly leads to repeated feelings of failure, probably particularly for nonmajority girls whose demographics are very different from those featured in the media (see Chapter 3 in this volume for more information about the unique challenges that African American girls face). So, perhaps not coincidentally, just at the time that girls begin to construct their identity, they begin to suffer losses in self-esteem. Ample research has documented this loss in self-esteem for girls in adolescence (e.g., Harter, 1998; Major, Barr, & Zubek, 1999), and perceived physical attractiveness is closely linked to self-esteem (Polce-Lynch, Myers, & Kilmartin, 1998). For these reasons, adolescent girls may be particularly vulnerable to cultural messages that promise them popularity, effectiveness, and social acceptance through the right products and "look." Furthermore, it may be that their vulnerability to these interpersonal and cultural messages contributes to drops in self-esteem.

Psychodynamics

Psychodynamic theories focus on the development of girls within the family constellation to help understand the roots of women's body-esteem. Early theories of the etiology of eating disorders among women, for example, locate the problem in early psychosexual development (Bruch, 1973) or dysfunctional family systems (Boskind-Lodahl & White, 1978). The idea is that disturbed parent–child interactions lead to "ego deficiencies" in the girl, who becomes unaware of her own internal needs.

Psychodynamic work pointing the finger at "parental seduction" in the form of overstimulation or boundary crossing (e.g., Greenberg, 2001) helps illuminate the development of dysfunctional sexual self-image in some women. These problematic parent–child interactions are argued to create guilt and conflict, which later have a negative impact on sexual relationships in adulthood. Research on trauma shows that early introduction of adult sexual material or behavior in the lives of young girls can cause lifelong struggles with their sexuality and ability to form satisfying intimate relationships (Herman, 1992; Scharff & Scharff, 1994). Often, the girl develops a hypersexualized view of herself, engages in risky sexual behavior, and hence retraumatizes herself (Rachman, Kennedy, & Yard, 2005).

Psychodynamic perspectives can help illuminate the problematic perspective some girls and women have with respect to their bodily selves, but may not go far enough to help us understand the "normative discontent" that the majority of adolescent and adult women—even those from functional family backgrounds—appear to feel about their attractiveness. Social learning and cognitive developmental theories help us understand girls' development within a culture that often associates "good femininity" with physical attractiveness, and specifically sexiness, but they do not do enough to clarify the mechanisms involved in the interface between psychological states and social or cultural pressures. Therefore, I now turn to several theories that attempt to make sense of the ways such cultural pressures come to influence girls' and women's self-image.

Sociocultural Theories

The fields of communication studies, sociology, and social psychology offer several theories that shed light on the importance of the sociocultural context in which we develop and interact. Girls and young women learn what is considered appropriate femininity not only from their direct interactions with actual others, but also through interfacing with media and other cultural products.

Social Comparison and the Looking-Glass Self

Foundational to understanding why and how the culture "out there" can get "in here" is the human drive to compare ourselves to others. Mead (1934) argued that the self "takes the role of the other," and social comparison theory (Festinger, 1954), developed out of this view, postulated that individuals are driven to look outside themselves to evaluate their own opinions and abilities. Looking outside oneself can involve examining physical reality or comparing to other people, and, according to the theory, we are motivated to do so because we believe the images portrayed by others are desirable, obtainable, and realistic.

Social comparison processes are known to be at work with respect to girls' and women's evaluations of their bodies and attractiveness (e.g., Morrison, Kalin, & Morrison, 2004). Importantly, these comparisons are typically "upward." That is, girls and women tend to compare to others whom they deem more attractive than they themselves are (Morrison et al., 2004; Wheeler & Miyake, 1992). This most certainly sets the stage for media models of nearly impossible, often sexualized, attractiveness to appear to be reasonable and achievable for girls.

A related sociological concept is the "looking-glass self" (Cooley, 1902) wherein identity is the result of learning to see ourselves as others do. According to Yeung and Martin (2003), the looking-glass self has three main components. First, we imagine how we must appear to others. Second, we imagine the judgment of that appearance. And finally, we develop our self through the judgments of others. One relatively straightforward illustration of the power of looking-glass reflected appraisals on bodily self-image is the finding that in cultures where thinness is valued, such as in the United States, heavy people are significantly less happy than they are in cultures where obesity is accepted and afforded high status, such as in some African countries (Pinhey, Rubinstein, & Colfax, 1997). In other words, holding constant physical or psychological qualities, it is likely that girls' and women's perceptions of the *value* that others place on a sexy, attractive appearance plays an important role in their satisfaction with their own appearance.

Cultivation Theory

An important theory in communication studies is cultivation theory (Gerbner & Gross, 1976; Gerbner, Gross, Morgan, & Signorielli, & Shanahan1994), which proposes that mass media present a vivid but unreal reality. As individuals consume more and more media, they come to cultivate or adopt beliefs about the actual world that coincide with this mediated world. That is, the more media consumption, the more the consumer believes that the content promoted by media is realistic.

Cultivation theorists emphasize the impact of media on attitudes, including general beliefs about the world, rather than on individuals' personalities or particular behaviors. Several studies provide support for the fundamentals of cultivation theory with respect to girls' and women's attitudes about physical appearance. For example, the more young women consume mainstream media content, the more strongly they endorse sex-role stereotypes that characterize women as sex objects (Ward, 2002; Ward & Rivadeneyra, 1999). Zurbriggen and Morgan (2006) found that higher reality-television viewing rates among young women were associated with stronger beliefs in the importance of physical appearance. Perhaps most alarming, high school students who consumed more mainstream media attributed greater importance to sexiness and beauty in judging women than did students who consumed less (Ward, 2004; Ward, Hansbrough, & Walker, 2005).

Furthermore, studies also show that the impact of exposure goes deeper than attitudes about appearance generally, with higher consumption of appearance-oriented media correlating with actual lower levels of body esteem among consumers of those media forms. *Appearance-oriented media* is typically defined as television shows, music videos, magazines, and advertising that present women as thin and attractive, and often sexualized (that is, provocatively or scantily dressed). Higher rates of consumption of such media have been shown to predict lower satisfaction with one's own appearance in adult women (Stice & Whittenton, 2002), adolescents (Borzekowski, Robinson, & Killen, 2000; Tiggemann & Pickering, 1996), preadolescents (Harrison, 2000; Jones, Vigfusdottir, & Lee, 2004), and, shockingly, even girls like my daughter at the time of my opening example: as young as 5 to 8 years old (Dohnt & Tiggemann, 2006).

One prominent criticism of cultivation theory, however, is that it offers a purely additive model. That is, the more media one is exposed to, the more one begins to consider the messages and images promoted by media as realistic. Hesse-Biber and her colleagues (Hesse-Biber, Howling, Leavy, & Lovejoy, 2004; Hesse-Biber, Leavy, Quinn, & Zoino, 2006) argue that while cultural exposure is an important component of our understanding of girls' and women's body image, it does not account for our agency and therefore for the diversity of responses to cultural messages. Indeed, not all girls and women suffer from poor body image, not even all consumers of appearance-oriented mass media and marketing suffer, and different periods in the lifespan are characterized more and less by body image concerns.

Uses and Gratifications Theory

Levine and Smolak (1996) argue that mass media's impact on self-image is dependent on personal motivations and the ways we select the media content to which we wish to expose ourselves. Uses and gratification theory (Katz, Blumler, & Gurevitch, 1973) thus suggests that the consumer's level of involvement with media must be considered. This approach emphasizes the importance of understanding the relationship of individuals to mass media, as opposed to emphasizing media's content only. There are clearly a variety of purposes for which consumers use media and a variety of different gratifications they derive from their consumption.

Research on the relationship between media consumption and eating disorders among women, for example, has shown that eating-disordered patients point to models in fashion magazines as a primary source of motivation for their drive for thinness (Levine & Smolak, 1996). In other words, these young women selected fashion magazines as their source of gratification, and doing so provided them with models that motivated their desire to lose weight. Other work in this area shows that dissatisfaction with one's body in the first place intensifies the dissatisfaction brought about by exposure to media images of idealized women's bodies (Posovac, Posovac, & Posovac, 1998). Applying this framework to sexualized self-image, we might predict that it is not only exposure to sexually objectified media content that impacts girls' and women's self-image, but rather that their prior dispositions and motivations for consuming particular media forms must also be taken into account.

Sociocultural theories, then, help us understand the importance of the cultural context in which girls grow and women interact. Because all humans are driven by social comparison and looking-glass reflected appraisals to seek and incorporate others' standards into our own self-attitudes, girls and women are primed to turn to the media and mass marketing for information about how to be. When they consume appearance-focused media, girls and women suffer consequences to their bodily self-image. However, such theories lack a specific focus on the sexualized content of cultural and interpersonal messages. Objectification theory offers a unifying approach that borrows features of both psychological and sociocultural theories to understanding girls and women's development and lived experience within a sexually objectifying culture. It is to this framework that I now turn.

Objectification Theory

My colleague Barbara Fredrickson and I proposed objectification theory as a comprehensive framework for understanding how the cultural milieu of the sexual objectification of female bodies provides a kind of instructional backdrop for women's development across the lifespan (Fredrickson & Roberts, 1997). Bartky (1990) defined sexual objectification as occurring whenever a person's sexual parts or functions are separated out from her person, when her body parts are regarded as representing her, or when her entire self is identified with her body. Girls and women encounter this treatment second-hand, through media and marketers' representations (Kilbourne & Jhally, 2000), as well as in actual interpersonal encounters (Swim, Hyers, Cohen, & Ferguson, 2001). We argued that girls and women are coaxed through social and cultural experiences of sexual objectification to treat them*selves* as objects to be gazed at and evaluated based on physical appearance, an effect we termed "self-objectification" (Fredrickson & Roberts, 1997).

Self-objectification involves adopting a third-person perspective on the physical self and is manifested by a chronic attention to the body's outward appearance. That is, girls and women who self-objectify are expected to habitually monitor their bodies so as to ensure that they meet cultural standards of attractiveness. Furthermore, McKinley and Hyde (1996) argue that an important component of the sexually objectifying culture is the belief that one can control how well one's body conforms to the standards of attractiveness (think about all the products marketed to girls and women to enable that conformity). Thus, the cognitive resources and effort required of self-objectification are theorized to fragment consciousness, and hence disrupt other, concurrent activities. Indeed, several studies have shown that inducing young women to be aware of their body's appearance as opposed to its health and functioning leads to poorer performance in a number of domains, including math (Fredrickson, Roberts, Noll, Quinn, & Twenge, 1998), color-naming (Quinn, Kallen, Twenge, & Fredrickson, 2006), and even throwing a softball effectively (Fredrickson & Harrison, 2005).

Objectification theory posits several negative emotional and experiential consequences of self-objectification, including increased body shame resulting from the comparison of one's own body against the cultural standard of physical attractiveness and perceiving oneself as failing, appearance anxiety resulting from anticipating evaluations of one's body, lowered awareness of internal bodily states resulting from competing attention to the body's outward appearance, and reduced "flow" or intrinsic motivation. These emotional consequences are then theorized to compound to predispose girls and women to particular mental health consequences: depressive symptoms, eating disorders, and sexual dysfunction. Finally, the theory proposes a developmental trajectory, with the experiential consequences and mental health risks of self-objectification changing over the life course: intensifying in early adolescence, and lessening in later middle age, in step with observable changes in the female body (Fredrickson & Roberts, 1997).

Moradi and Huang (2008) reviewed the accumulation of both experimental and correlational evidence supporting the tenets of objectification theory. Among the many studies conducted in the decade since the theory was published are those showing that self-objectification leads to increased body shame (e.g., Fredrickson et al., 1998; Quinn, Kallen, & Cathey, 2006), which in turn predicts eating disturbances (e.g., Forbes, Jobe, & Revak, 2006), poor self-esteem (e.g., Aubrey, 2006), and increased depressive symptoms (e.g., Miner-Rubino, Twenge, & Fredrickson, 2002). Self-objectification also leads to appearance anxiety (e.g., Calogero, 2004) and other negative emotions, such as self-disgust (Roberts & Gettman, 2004). Higher self-objectification is related to poorer attitudes about one's own body functions, such as menstruation and lactation, and sexuality (e.g., Impett, Schooler, & Tolman, 2006; Johnston-Robledo, Wares, Fricker, & Pasek, 2007; Roberts, 2004). Moradi and Huang (2008) also reviewed the evidence linking actual experiences of sexual objectification, whether mediated or interpersonal, to negative outcomes. The evidence suggests that self-objectification, body surveillance, and internalization of cultural beauty standards mediate the links between sexually objectifying experiences "out there" and mental health risk factors in girls and women, such as eating disorders.

In a fascinating, if disheartening, qualitative study, Brumberg (1997) examined the ways adolescent girls described their self-improvement goals in their diaries over the past 100 years. The change over time was clear. Whereas girls of yesteryear focused on improving their manners or their study habits, in the most recent 20 years, girls' focus has become almost exclusively their "body projects," that is, enhancement of their physical appearance. Slater and Tiggemann (2002) showed that girls as young as 12 years old self-objectify; they place significantly greater emphasis on their body's appearance than on its competence, health, or well-being. Other evidence shows that even younger girls are already dissatisfied with their bodies, and especially their weight (Phares, Steinberg, & Thompson, 2004).

Objectification theory's concept of self-objectification provides an intrapsychic contribution to our understanding of the sexualization of girls. During their early years of gender socialization, perhaps through reinforcements, as social learning theorists would argue, or even through trauma, as psychodynamic theorists would argue, girls learn to internalize a sexually objectified view of their bodies. Once they have done so, much as cognitive developmental psychologists would predict, they set about the work of solidifying their identity as a physically attractive female. The media step in to supply increasingly impossible standards of sexy attractiveness to which they can aspire, and marketers sell them the products that promise to help them meet the standard (Lamb & Brown, 2007).

Importantly, self-objectification provides the motivational fuel for the body project in which girls and women themselves are engaged. This means that our efforts to counter the sexualization of girls have to include education about this pernicious self-view. In addition to our efforts to combat the sexually objectifying culture "out there," we need to educate our girls about the perils of self-objectification "in here." It won't be easy. Girls and women self-objectify because it's rewarding to do so. Ample evidence exists that females deemed physically attractive reap economic, interpersonal, and educational benefits over their less attractive peers (Fredrickson & Roberts, 1997). However, research on objectification theory has now provided us with ample evidence that self-objectification carries significant emotional, behavioral, and health costs. So, in addition to holding marketers accountable for feeding our daughters toys like Bratz dolls, we must also provide our girls with alternative ways of feeling successful and, yes, beautiful.

Conclusion

When Abigail Breslin's character, the 8-year-old Olive, does her "Super Freak" erotic dance for the beauty pageant in the movie *Little Miss Sunshine*, we're meant to recognize the hypocrisy of a culture that says it's good fun to parade our young daughters in false eyelashes, makeup, and perms before pageant judges, but it's decidedly *not* okay to have them dance suggestively for us at that pageant. Did we? The point of that movie, and of my daughter's mistaking a lady of the evening in Berlin for a child's toy, is that there is something pernicious about the saturation of sexualized girls and girlhood in our culture. Perhaps we haven't been paying careful enough attention. Are we being trained to perceive sexualized girls as "seductive?" Compared to women, men consistently perceive a greater degree of sexual intent in women's behavior (e.g., Abbey, 1982; Abbey, Zawacki, & McAuslan, 2000; Farris, Treat, Vicken, & McFall, 2008). We shouldn't be surprised if young girls who are made to look like adult women evoke similar responses.

My daughter stopped playing with Bratz dolls by age 12, and promptly plugged into her iPod. I recall once hearing her sing the *Pussycat Dolls* lyric, "Don't ya wish your girlfriend was a freak like me? Don't ya wish your girlfriend was raw like me?" I doubt she knew then what it means to be a "freak" any more than little Olive did, doing her erotic dance. But I do. And a lifetime of exposure to countless media forms, marketers, peers, and even adults with the same message—that our girls' most valuable asset is their sex appeal—is undeniably damaging. This chapter was my attempt to shed some light on how these forces in the culture make their way into our daughters' and our own heads. There is much work still to be done. Let's continue to do that work, because we all want more for our daughters, and for all girls.

References

Abbey, A. (1982). Sex differences in attributions for friendly behavior: Do males misperceive females' friendliness? *Journal of Personality and Social Psychology, 4*, 830–838.

Abbey, A., Zawacki, T., & McAuslan, P. (2000). Alcohol's effects on sexual perception. *Journal of Studies on Alcohol, 61*, 688–697.

Aubrey, J. S. (2006). Exposure to sexually objectifying media and body self-perceptions among college women: An examination of the selective exposure hypothesis and the role of moderating variables. *Sex Roles, 55*, 159–172.

Bartky, S. L. (1990). *Femininity and domination: Studies in the phenomenology of oppression.* New York: Routledge.

Bem, S. L. (1985). Androgyny and gender schema theory: A conceptual and empirical integration. In Theo B. Sonderegger (Ed.), *Nebraska symposium on motivation, 1984: Psychology and gender* (pp. 179–226). Lincoln: University of Nebraska Press.

Borzekowski, D. L., Robinson, T. N., & Killen, J. D. (2000). Does the camera add 10 pounds? Media use, perceived importance of appearance, and weight concerns among teenage girls. *Journal of Adolescent Health, 26*, 36–41.

Boskind-Lodahl, M., & White, W. C. (1978). The definition and treatment of bulimarexia in college women: A pilot study. *Journal of the American College Health Association, 27*, 84–97.

Bruch, H. (1973). *Eating disorders: Obesity, anorexia and the person within.* New York: Basic Books.

Brumberg, J. J. (1997). *The body project: An intimate history of American girls.* New York: Vintage.

Bussey, K., & Bandura, A. (1999). Social cognitive theory and gender development and differentiation. *Psychological Review, 106*, 676–713.

Calogero, R. M. (2004). A test of objectification theory: The effect of the male gaze on appearance concerns in college women. *Psychology of Women Quarterly, 28*, 16–21.

Cooley, C. H. (1902). *Human nature and the social order.* New York: Scribner's.

Crawford, M., & Unger, R. (2000). *Women and gender: A feminist psychology.* Boston: McGraw Hill.

Dohnt, H., & Tiggemann, M. (2006). The contribution of peer and media influences to the development of body satisfaction and self-esteem in young girls: A prospective study. *Developmental Psychology, 42*, 929–936.

Erikson, E. (1950). *Childhood and society.* New York: Norton.

Farris, C., Treat, T. A., Vicken, R. J., & McFall, R. M. (2008). Sexual coercion and the misperception of sexual intent. *Clinical Psychology Review, 28*, 8–66.

Festinger, L. (1954). A theory of social comparison processes. *Human Relations, 7*(2), 117–140.

Forbes, G. B., Jobe, R. L., & Revak, J. A. (2006). Relationships between dissatisfaction with specific body characteristics and the Sociocultural Attitudes Toward Appearance Questionnaire-3 and Objectified Body Consciousness Scale. *Body Image, 3*, 295–300.

Fredrickson, B. L., & Harrison, K. (2005). Throwing like a girl: Self-objectification predicts adolescent girls' motor performance. *Journal of Sport & Social Issues, 29*, 79–101.

Fredrickson, B. L., & Roberts, T. -A. (1997). Objectification theory: Toward understanding women's lived experiences and mental health risks. *Psychology of Women Quarterly, 21,* 173–206.

Fredrickson, B. L., Roberts, T, -A., Noll, S. M., Quinn, D. M., & Twenge, J. M. (1998). That swimsuit becomes you: Sex differences in self-objectification, restrained eating, and math performance. *Journal of Personality and Social Psychology, 75,* 269–284.

Gerbner, G., & Gross, L. (1976). Living with television: The violence profile. *Journal of Communication, 26,* 172–199.

Gerbner, G., Gross, L., Morgan, M., Signorielli, N., & Shanahan, J. (1994). Growing up with television: The cultivation perspective. In J. Bryant, & D. Zillman (Eds.), *Media effects: Advances in theory and research* (pp. 61–90). Hillsdale, NJ: Lawrence Erlbaum Associates.

Greenberg, J. (2001). The ambiguity of seduction in the development of Freud's thinking. *Contemporary Psychoanalysis, 37,* 417–426.

Harrison, K. (2000). Television viewing, fat stereotyping, body shape standards, and eating disorder symptomatology in grade school children. *Communication Research, 27,* 617–640.

Harter, S. (1998). The development of self-representations. In W. Damon, & N. Eisenberg (Eds.), *Handbook of child psychology: Vol. 3: Social, emotional, and personality development* (5th ed., pp. 553–618). Hoboken, NJ: Wiley.

Herman, J. L. (1992). *Trauma and recovery: The aftermath of violence—from domestic abuse to political terror.* New York: Basic Books.

Hesse-Biber, S. N., Howling, S. A., Leavy, P., & Lovejoy, M. (2004). Racial identity and the development of body image issues among African-American adolescent girls. *The Qualitative Report, 9,* 49–79.

Hesse-Biber, S. N., Leavy, P., Quinn, C. E., & Zoino, J. (2006). The mass marketing of disordered eating and eating disorders: The social psychology of women, thinness and culture. *Women's Studies International Forum, 29,* 208–224.

Impett, E. A., Schooler, D., & Tolman, D. L. (2006). To be seen and not heard: Femininity ideology and adolescent girls' sexual health. *Archives of Sexual Behavior, 35,* 131–144.

Jackson, L. A. (1992). *Physical appearance and gender: Sociobiological and sociocultural perspectives.* Albany, NY: State University of New York Press.

Johnston-Robledo, I., Wares, S., Fricker, J., & Pasek, L. (2007). Indecent exposure: Self-objectification and young women's attitudes toward breastfeeding. *Sex Roles, 56,* 429–437.

Jones, D. C., Vigfusdottir, T. H., & Lee, Y. (2004). Body image and the appearance culture among adolescent girls and boys: An examination of friend conversations, peer criticism, appearance magazines, and the internalization of appearance ideals. *Journal of Adolescent Research, 19,* 323–339.

Katz, E., Blumler, J. G., & Gurevitch, M. (1973). Uses and gratification research. *Public Opinion Quarterly, 37,* 509–523.

Kilbourne, J. (Producer), Jhally, S. (Director). (2000). *Killing us softly 3: Advertising images of women* [videorecording]. (Available from Media Education Foundation)

Lamb, S. & Brown, L.M. (2007). *Packaging girlhood: Rescuing our daughters from marketers' schemes.* New York: St. Martin's Press.

Levine, M. P., & Smolak, L. (1996). Media as a context for the development of disordered eating. In L. Smolak, M. P. Levine, & R. Striegel-Moore (Eds.), *The developmental psychopathology of eating disorders—Implications for research, prevention, and treatment* (pp. 235–257). Mahwah, NJ: Lawrence Erlbaum Associates.

Maccoby, E. E. (1980). *Social development: Psychological growth and the parent-child relationship.* New York: Harcourt, Brace, Jovanovich.

Major, B., Barr, L., & Zubek, J. (1999). Gender and self-esteem: A meta-analysis. In W. Swann, J. H. Langlois, & L. Gilbert (Eds.), *Sexism and stereotypes in modern society:*

The gender science of Janet Taylor Spence. Washington, DC: American Psychological Association.

McKinley, N. M., & Hyde, J. S. (1996). The Objectified Body Consciousness Scale: Development and validation. *Psychology of Women Quarterly, 20,* 181–215.

Mead, G. H. (1934). *Mind, self, and society.* Chicago: University of Chicago Press.

Miner-Rubino, K., Twenge, J. M., & Fredrickson, B. L. (2002). Trait self-objectification in women: Affective and personality correlates. *Journal of Research in Personality, 36,* 147–172.

Moradi, B. & Huang, Y.P. (2008). Objectification theory and psychology of women: A decade of advances and future directions. *Psychology of Women Quarterly, 32,* 377–398.

Morrison, T. G., Kalin, R., & Morrison, M. A. (2004). Body–image evaluation and body–image investment among adolescents: A test of sociocultural and social comparison theories. *Adolescence, 39,* 571–593.

Pannell, S. C. (2008). Mothers and daughters: The creation and contestation of beauty and femininity. *Dissertation Abstracts International Section A: Humanities and Social Sciences, 68*(12-A), 5220.

Phares, V., Steinberg, A. R., & Thompson, J. K. (2004). Gender differences in peer and parental influences: Body image disturbance, self-worth and psychological functioning in preadolescent children. *Journal of Youth and Adolescence, 33,* 421–429.

Pinhey, T. K., Rubinstein, D. H., & Colfax, R. S. (1997). Overweight and happiness: The reflected self appraisal hypothesis reconsidered. *Social Science Quarterly, 78,* 747–755.

Polce-Lynch, M., Myers, B. J., & Kilmartin, C. T. (1998). Gender and age patterns in emotional expression, body image and self-esteem: A qualitative analysis. *Sex Roles, 38,* 1025–1048.

Posovac, H. D., Posovac, S. S., & Posovac, E. J. (1998). Exposure to media images of female attractiveness and concern with body weight among young women. *Sex Roles, 38,* 187–201.

Quinn, D. M., Kallen, R. W., & Cathey, C. (2006). Body on my mind: The lingering effect of state self-objectification. *Sex Roles, 55,* 869–874.

Quinn, D. M., Kallen, R. W., Twenge, J. M., & Fredrickson, B. L. (2006). The disruptive effect of self-objectification on performance. *Psychology of Women Quarterly, 30,* 59–64.

Rachman, A. W. M., Kennedy, R., & Yard, M. (2005). The role of childhood sexual seduction in the development of an erotic transference: Perversion in the psychoanalytic situation. *International Forum of Psychoanalysis, 14,* 183–187.

Roberts, T. -A. (2004). Female trouble: The menstrual self-evaluation scale and women's self-objectification. *Psychology of Women Quarterly, 28,* 22–26.

Roberts, T. -A., & Gettman, J. Y. (2004). Mere exposure: Gender differences in the negative effects of priming a state of self-objectification. *Sex Roles, 51,* 17–27.

Scharff, J. S., & Scharff, D. E. (1994). *Object relations therapy of physical and sexual trauma.* Northvale, NJ: Jaason Aronson.

Slater, A., & Tiggemann, M. (2002). A test of objectification theory in adolescent girls. *Sex Roles, 46,* 343–349.

Strassburger, V. C., & Wilson, B. J. (2002). *Children, adolescents and the media.* Thousand Oaks, CA: Sage.

Stice, E., & Whitenton, K. (2002). Risk factors for body dissatisfaction in adolescent girls: A longitudinal investigation. *Developmental Psychology, 38,* 669–678.

Swim, J. K., Hyers, L. L., Cohen, L. L., & Ferguson, M. J. (2001). Everyday sexism: Evidence for its incidence, nature, and psychological impact from three daily diary studies. *Journal of Social Issues, 57,* 31–53.

Tiggemann, M., & Pickering, A. S. (1996). Role of television in adolescent women's body dissatisfaction and drive for thinness. *International Journal of Eating Disorders, 20,* 199–203.

Ward, L. M. (2002). Does television exposure affect emerging adults' attitudes and assumptions about sexual relationships? Correlational and experimental confirmation. *Journal of Youth and Adolescence, 31*, 1–15.

Ward, L. M. (2004, March). *The sexy/cool ideal: Contributions of media use to adolescents' gender and sexual schema.* Poster/paper presented at the biennial meeting of the Society for Research on Adolescence, Baltimore, Maryland.

Ward, L. M., Hansbrough, E., & Walker, E. (2005). Contributions of music video exposure to black adolescents' gender and sexual schemas. *Journal of Adolescent Research, 20*, 143–166.

Ward, L. M., & Rivadeneyra, R. (1999). Contributions of entertainment television to adolescents' sexual attitudes and expectations: The role of viewing amount versus viewer involvement. *Journal of Sex Research, 36,* 237–249.

Warin, J. (2000). The attainment of self-consistency through gender in young children. *Sex Roles, 42*, 209–232.

Wheeler, L. & Miyake, K. (1992). Social comparison in everyday life, *Journal of Personality and Social Psychology, 62*, 760–773.

Wolf, N. (1991). *The beauty myth: How images of beauty are used against women.* New York: Anchor Books.

Yeung, K., & Martin, J. L. (2003). The looking glass self: An empirical test and elaboration. *Social Forces, 81*, 843–879.

Zurbriggen, E. L., & Morgan, E. M. (2006). Who wants to marry a millionaire? Reality dating television programs, attitudes toward sex, and sexual behaviors. *Sex Roles, 54*, 1–17.

CULTURAL CONTRIBUTIONS AND CONSEQUENCES

3

A Woman's Worth

Analyzing the Sexual Objectification of Black Women in Music Videos

L. MONIQUE WARD, ROCIO RIVADENEYRA, KHIA THOMAS,
KYLA DAY, AND MARINA EPSTEIN

Girls can acquire lessons about society's gender role expectations from a number of sources, including family members, teachers, and friends. Prominent among them is television, whose appealing visual images and dynamic character portrayals offer girls numerous examples of what it means to be a woman. American youth watch an average of 3–4 hours of TV each day, with higher rates among black and Latino youth (Roberts, Foehr, & Rideout, 2005). Unfortunately, analyses indicate that the bulk of portrayals available construct rather narrow and stereotypical views of the sexes (for review, see Signorielli, 2001). The dominant roles for women on TV are nurturing mother, single career woman, and anonymous sexual object, with little mixing of the three. Especially prominent are portrayals of women as sexual objects (e.g., Gow, 1996; Lin, 1998), whose role is to look sexy and attract attention. Findings indicate that across all media, women are judged and valued by their looks, and women's bodies and faces are frequently presented as objects of beauty and adornment for others' viewing pleasure (for review, see American Psychological Association [APA], 2007; Durham, 2008).

One arena where images of sexually objectified women are especially prevalent is the world of music videos. Music videos represent an important area of study, both because of their popularity with younger viewers (Ashby & Rich, 2005) and because love and sex predominate as themes (Andsager & Roe, 1999; Arnett, 2002). As a visual, storytelling format with little time to devote to deep characterizations, music videos often *rely* on short-cuts and stereotypes, working to convey their points with a quick image or gender-role cue (Andsager & Roe, 1999). Moreover, for years, this genre has been reported to be more gender segregated and male-dominated than other genres, with reports that between 56% and 84% of the artists and/or leads in the videos are men (Gow, 1996; Seidman, 1992; Sommers-Flanagan, Sommers-Flanagan, & Davis, 1993), as are 90% of directors (Andsager & Roe, 1999). Researchers comment that because the music industry is dominated by men, it most frequently reflects the desires of this group, leading some to refer to music videos as "representations of adolescent male fantasies" (Jhally, 1995).

What we seek to do here is to take a closer look at the nature and impact of the portrayal of women in music videos, focusing, in particular, on sexually objectifying images. How frequently do objectifying images occur? What messages about femininity do these images convey to girls? What is their demonstrated impact on girls and young women? Given the current popularity of rap and hip-hop music, we focus our attention on their portrayals of African American women. We address these issues via four pathways. First, we summarize findings from existing research concerning the nature of gender portrayals in music videos. Second, we turn our attention to African American artists and summarize findings about the images of black women in music videos. Third, we present new data from an analysis we conducted of the sexual content in black music videos, providing both quantitative and thematic analyses. Finally, we summarize findings about the demonstrated impact of music video exposure on young viewers' gender beliefs and body image concerns.

Existing Findings About the Portrayal of Women in Music Videos

What images do these video fantasies present about femininity? Initial content analyses that studied music videos from the 1980s and 1990s indicated that the treatment of women was predominantly stereotypical and sexist, in terms of appearance, social roles, and personality attributes (Andsager & Roe, 1999; Seidman, 1992, 1999; Vincent, Davis, & Boruszkowski, 1987). Portrayals most often followed stereotypical gender norms, with women depicted as affectionate, dependent, fearful, and nurturing (Seidman, 1992, 1999), and seldom shown in professional roles (Alexander, 1999; Andsager & Roe, 1999; Seidman, 1992). The most salient aspect of depictions of femininity in these music videos was their focus on women as "decorative objects" designed solely to please and entice men, with an emphasis almost exclusively on their physical appearance and sexual appeal (e.g., Gow, 1996; Vincent, 1989; Vincent et al., 1987). For example, 57% of the videos analyzed in one study were seen to portray women in a condescending, less-than-human manner, and another 17.1% were seen to depict women in very traditional, "keep her in her place" roles

(Vincent et al., 1987). Within these portrayals, a consistent finding was that women more frequently than men are presented in provocative and revealing clothing (e.g., Andsager & Roe, 1999; Vincent, 1989; Vincent et al., 1987). For example, in the 182 videos analyzed by Seidman (1992), 37% of women wore revealing clothing compared to 4.2% of men.

Moreover, evidence drawn from five recent content analyses indicates that these patterns have continued into the new millennium. First, analyses show more sexual behaviors by female characters and artists than by male characters and artists (King, Laake, & Bernard, 2006; Wallis, 2011). Second, analyses that have looked specifically for the sexual objectification of women note high levels. Frisby and Aubrey (2012) analyzed four indicators of sexual objectification in a set of R & B, pop, and country music videos by female artists. Overall, 71% of the videos contained at least one of the indicators of sexual objectification. Indeed, in their analysis of sexual objectification in 147 videos representing top Billboard songs, Aubrey and Frisby (2011) noted that, in comparison to male artists, female artists revealed significantly more body parts, were more likely to be coded as attractive (72.5% vs. 31.3%), and were more likely to engage in sexually suggestive dance (31.4% vs. 4.2%). A final trend that has continued into the new millennium is that researchers continue to find that, in music videos, women are more likely than men to be dressed provocatively and are less likely to be in neutral attire (Aubrey & Frisby, 2011; King et al., 2006; Turner, 2011; Wallis, 2011).

Understanding the Role of Race: Black Women in Music Videos

Given the prominence of rap and hip-hop in American music, we were curious about the portrayal of women in black music videos, which likely make up a notable proportion of the current rotation. Indeed, evidence suggests that sexual content may be especially high in rap/hip-hop videos, which typically feature black artists. In one of the earlier analyses, Jones (1997) analyzed the prevalence of violent and sexual imagery in 203 videos of diverse genres drawn from four cable channels. For eight of the 11 sexual behaviors coded (e.g., fondling, simulated intercourse, "hot" pants), levels were *highest* in the hip-hop or rap videos. For example, 58.3% of the hip-hop videos were coded as featuring women dancing sexually, compared to 7.8% of rock videos. Similarly, 41.7% of hip-hop videos featured women in "hot pants" versus 5.9% of rock videos.

Current analyses indicate that this pattern continues today, with several recent studies finding that levels of sexual content and sexual objectification are especially high in rap, R & B, and hip-hop videos (e.g., Aubrey & Frisby,

2011; Frisby & Aubrey, 2012). For example, in their analysis of 411 music videos drawn from four cable channels, King, Laake, and Bernard (2006) found that both sexual attire and sexual behavior were more prevalent among women on Black Entertainment Television (BET) than among women on MTV and country channels. Turner (2011) analyzed 120 videos from five channels for the presence of each of 18 sexual behaviors. Sexual content of some kind occurred in 58.5% of all videos, but this rate varied significantly by genre. The highest prevalence rates were for mixed rap and R & B videos (82.9%) and R & B videos (78.9%), and the lowest rates were for country (35.6%) and rock (36.8%) videos. In addition, the mean number of sexual acts in African American videos (9.45) was significantly higher than the mean in white videos (3.04). Moreover, black artists and characters were significantly more likely than whites to appear in provocative clothing (36.3% vs. 22.7%). These findings indicate that African American music videos are more sexualized than white music videos both in terms of provocative clothing and frequency of depictions of sexual behavior. At the same time, data show that black youth consume more media than youth of other ethnic groups, suggesting that their exposure to such imagery is likely to be the highest of all youth. In a national survey of more than 2,000 youth (Roberts et al., 2005), black youth were found to spend substantially more daily time (5 hours: 53 minutes) with screen media (TV/videos/DVDs) than either Latino (4:37) or white (3:47) youth.

In addition to these studies that compared across genres, other analyses have focused more directly on the content of rap and hip-hop videos and provide further context for these findings. Conrad, Dixon, and Zhang (2009) analyzed overall themes and gender portrayals in 108 rap music videos drawn from the 2005 year-end reviews of the top videos on MTV, VH-1, and BET. Findings indicated that female characters were more likely than male characters to appear in videos in which controversial themes, such as misogyny and materialism, dominated. Indeed, whereas male characters were likely to be associated with a variety of themes, female characters were confined mainly to videos centered on misogyny. Focusing on appearance issues, Zhang, Dixon, and Conrad (2010) analyzed the body size of women in the same set of rap videos, investigating both the presence of the thin-ideal, and variation in body size across video themes. Across the videos, 47.1% were coded as placing a high emphasis on materialism, and 45.2% as placing a high emphasis on sex. "Thin" female characters, those with a body size score of a 1, 2, or 3 on a 9-point scale, made up 51% of the female characters. This is much higher than the 24% estimated in the population. As expected, the body size of the female characters varied as a function of the video theme. Women in videos that were high in sex or materialism were more likely to have smaller body sizes. Conversely, women in videos high in political awareness were more likely to have larger body sizes.

In addition to these data-driven, empirical analyses of the portrayal of black women in music videos, others have taken a more conceptual approach, offering theoretical analyses of the salient themes and likely impressions left. The consensus emerging from these analyses is that the sexual objectification of black women is rampant in black music videos. In her analysis of 56 popular music videos featuring black female artists, Emerson (2002) concluded that music videos reflect an overall image of black women as "decorative eye candy" rather than as multidimensional beings, and emphasize the sexual availability of women's bodies for men's sexual desires. In a similar vein, Stephens and Phillips (2003) discussed how historical stereotypes of black women are perpetuated today in the sexual scripts of black womanhood dominating hip-hop culture and music videos, including portrayals of the insatiable sexual Freak, the materialistic Gold Digger, the glamorous but high-maintenance Diva, and the violent Gangster Bitch. In their analysis, they found that most black female artists have one characteristic in common: sexuality and sexual appeal are central to defining who these women are. In video representations of this dynamic, "women are less likely to be depicted as individuals; rather they serve as backdrops with a focus on select body parts for male consumption" (Stephens & Few, 2007, p. 60). In her essay analyzing the existing research in the field, West (2009) concludes, "Just like their enslaved ancestors, contemporary black women's bodies are accessible, exchangeable, and expendable on the new cyber-auction block" (p. 91).

Emerging from these quantitative and qualitative studies, then, is the notion that portrayals of black women in current music videos center heavily on their sexuality and sexual objectification. However, because the data-driven studies that analyzed black music videos (i.e., Conrad et al., 2009; Zhang et al., 2010) did not focus on sexuality, we do not have a sense of the breadth of imagery portrayed about black women's sexuality and romantic relationships. Are objectifying portrayals the most prevalent types of sexual images of black women, or are romantic or nurturing images equally prevalent? Similarly, because the conceptual and qualitative analyses frequently focused on a select subset of videos, it is unclear if their themes apply more broadly across popular videos. To address these concerns, we combined the two approaches and conducted a numbers-driven analysis of the sexual content of top music videos *and* a broader conceptual analysis of their salient themes. Our first goal was to investigate the range of sexual imagery presented, drawing on coding schemes used in previous analyses. As part of this analysis, we also investigated more closely the nature of objectifying images, conducting both counts of objectifying camera cuts and analyses of the levels of dress and undress. Borrowing from Sommers-Flannagan et al. (1993), we defined objectification as, "instances in which the camera focuses in on an isolated body part. Any portrayals of a person being primarily one body part or a set of body parts rather than a whole, complete human" (p. 747). Our second goal was to look more closely at two specific themes conveyed about heterosexual courtship: adversarial relations and materialism. Our third goal was to examine the gendered context of music videos, to look broadly at what women are shown doing. Finally, we sought to conduct a more conceptual analysis of the videos and of their salient messages about black women's sexuality.

New Data: Content Analysis Methods

We took as our sample 70 videos featured in a New Year's Eve year-end review on BET of the top videos of 2000. This included videos ranked No. 55 to No. 1, as well as 15 videos nominated in special categories (e.g., Most Overplayed Song, Sexiest Comeback). Each video was coded for the presence (yes/no) of 18 specific sexual behaviors (e.g., kissing, self-touching, women dancing sexually, implied intercourse) compiled from previous research. Each video was also coded for the visual presence (yes/no) of two courtship themes: (a) adversarial sexual relations, which included images of infidelity, fighting, arguments, and deception; and (b) a focus on material wealth, which included images highlighting wealth and status, such as driving an expensive car (e.g., Rolls Royce), showing off expensive jewelry, and throwing money around. Forty videos were coded by the lead author Ward, 21 by co-author Rivadeneyra, and 9 by both of us, with an average interrater agreement of 89%. Videos typically averaged approximately 3–4 minutes in length.

We also coded the levels of dress/undress of each outfit of each female and male main character. Clothing was evaluated on a 1–4 scale, with 1 representing neutral/nonsexy (e.g., jeans and t-shirt), 2 signifying somewhat alluring (e.g., women in tight skirts or shorts; men with tank tops), 3 signifying alluring (e.g., women in lingerie or bathing suits; men with no shirts); and 4 representing implied nudity. We also recorded the highest level of undress of supporting characters.

Finally, in looking at what women and men do, we recorded all actions other than singing engaged in by all male and female characters and performers appearing on the screen. We kept a running list, and tabulated and combined items later. Only data about the women are reported here.

Prevalence of Sexual Content in the Videos Analyzed

Of the 70 videos analyzed, 59 or 84.3% were coded as containing sexual imagery of some kind. This means that only 11 of the videos did *not* have

Table 3.1 **Prevalence of Sexual Behaviors Across Videos (percentage of videos)**

Sexual Behavior	Overall (70 videos)	Male Artists (43 videos)	Female Artists (16 videos)	Mixed Artists (11 videos)
Sexual objectification	58.6	62.8	43.8	63.7
Women dancing sexually	57.1	60.5	43.8	63.6
Fondling-self	45.7	41.9	50.0	54.5
Fondling-others	45.7	44.2	50.0	45.4
Kissing	34.2	30.2	43.8	36.4
Hugging	28.6	23.8	43.8	27.3
Holding hands	22.9	16.3	37.5	27.3
Men dancing sexually	21.4	18.6	18.8	36.4
Multiple partners	17.1	20.9	6.25	18.2
Implied intercourse	5.7	9.3	0	0
Male chasing female	4.3	4.7	6.25	0
Voyeurism	4.3	2.3	6.25	9.1
Implied oral sex	1.4	2.3	0	0
Sadomasochism	1.4	2.3	0	0
Female chasing male	1.4	0	0	9.1
Heavy petting	1.4	2.3	0	0
Prostitution	0	0	0	0
Bondage	0	0	0	0

sexual imagery. The distribution of particular types of sexual images varied by the sex of the performer. The rates of occurrence for each of the 18 sexual behaviors examined are listed in Table 3.1. The two most prevalent behaviors overall were sexual objectification and women dancing sexually. Of the 70 videos coded, sexual objectifying images appeared in 58.6%, and women were shown dancing sexually in 57.1%. Among the 43 videos featuring male artists, which made up the bulk of the sample, these numbers were even higher, hitting 62.8% and 60.5%, respectively. Sexual objectification, which could be of women or men, was nearly always of women. Of the 27 videos by male artists coded as containing sexual objectification, 25 featured objectification of women, one featured the objectification of men, and one featured objectification of both sexes. Although objectification was also very common in videos by female artists, it did not lead the list of sexual images. Instead, more romantic/

relational sexual behaviors were equally or more prevalent among female artists, behaviors such as fondling others, hugging, and kissing. Looking at the full set of results, overall, we see that women's bodies dancing and moving in a sexual way, and being sexually objectified, were the most common ways in which the sexuality of black women was featured in these music videos.

Depth of Sexually Objectifying Images

To explore more closely the intensity of sexual objectification, we conducted a deeper analysis of all of the videos that had received this code. Of the 70 videos, 41 had been noted to feature sexual objectification of some kind. However, a yes/no code does not reflect frequency of occurrence because a video containing one quick objectifying image is scored the same (yes) as one featuring 17 individual shots of women's buttocks. We therefore analyzed these 41 videos again, counting each individual instance or cut to an objectifying image. Included in our analysis were the following four images: a shot focusing on a woman's breasts, a shot focusing on a woman's buttocks, a shot focusing on a woman's crotch, or a shot focusing on a full body jiggle with partial/or no focus on the face. One coder was trained on these components, and viewed each of the 41 videos several times to get an accurate count.

Results indicate that 31 of the 41 videos (75.6%) featured a shot focusing solely on a woman's breasts. Such a shot appeared anywhere from 1 to 14 times ($M = 3.87$) within a given video within this subset. Even more prevalent were shots focusing on a woman's buttocks, which were featured in 37 of the 41 videos (90.2%) coded as containing objectification. Such a shot appeared from 1 to 19 times within a given video within this subset ($M = 5.57$). We also found that 34 of the 41 videos (82.9%) featured a "crotch shot," which appeared from 1 to 17 times within an individual video ($M = 4.38$). Finally, 31 of the 41 videos (75.6%) featured a full body jiggle. This was a very common occurrence, appearing up to 18 times within an individual video within this subset, with a mean of 8.03 times per video. A richer impression of the density of objectifying images can be obtained when these counts are put together, for most of the 41 videos contained instances of each of these objectifying images. For example, video No. 29 on the countdown, entitled "What Chu Like" by Da Brat and Tyrese, contained 6 breast shots, 11 buttock shots, 4 crotch shots, and 9 full body jiggles. Exceeding these levels was video No. 4, entitled "Shake it Fast" by Mystikal, which contained 11 breast shots, 17 buttock shots, 17 crotch shots, and 15 full body jiggles. Thus, although each of the 41 videos was coded "yes" for containing sexual

Table 3.2 **Levels of Dress and Undress of Main and Supporting Characters**

	Dress of Main Characters		Highest level of Dress/ Undress	
	Male (N = 344 outfits)	Female (N = 147 outfits)	Male Supporting	Female Supporting
None present			9.3%	10.0%
Neutral/nonsexy	**64.4%**	29.3%	**37.2%**	12.9%
Mildly provocative	25.8%	**44.2%**	32.6%	24.3%
Provocative (lingerie, swimsuit)	7.5%	23.8%	20.9%	**38.6%**
Nudity/implied nudity	2.4%	2.7%	0	14.3%

Note: The highest percentage in each column is bolded.

objectification, a closer analysis revealed that such images were abundant and frequent within an individual video.

Objectification via Clothing

A second manner by which sexual objectification was assessed was by the level of dress or undress of the individuals appearing in the videos. Although some characters wore the same type of clothing throughout the video, many characters changed clothes from scene to scene. Each outfit was scored for each main character. For the supporting characters, because of their sheer numbers, we did not score each character. Instead, we noted the most provocative level of dress appearing across all supporting characters across the entire video. The final percentages are provided in Table 3.2. Male main characters/performers were seen in 334 different outfits, 64% of which were rated as neutral/nonsexy, which were generally jeans/slacks and shirts or suits. Female main characters wore a total of 147 different outfits, 29% of which were neutral/nonsexy clothes. Of the rest, 44% of outfits were mildly provocative, typically tank dresses, shorts, or tight skirts, and 24% were provocative clothing, such as lingerie. Overall, 71% of female main character clothing was provocative/mildly provocative, versus 35.6% for male characters.

This pattern of women's appearing more frequently in provocative clothing was also apparent for supporting characters. The most typical clothing of the male supporting characters was neutral or mildly provocative. None of the supporting men were nude. Among the supporting women, 38.6% were dressed provocatively, in lingerie or swimsuits, the dominant clothing type for supporting women, and 14.3% were nude/nudity implied. Thus, corroborating existing analyses, black women in these music videos were more provocatively dressed than men. Women were shown in swimsuits and lingerie at nearly the same rate that men were shown in regular, casual dress.

One-Dimensional Portrayals: Little Diversity in What Women Do

To provide a fuller picture of women's portrayals in these videos, and to provide some context for the sexual content, we also documented all actions that all adult women (and men) were shown doing on screen, other than singing. For any given video, this often resulted in a listing of several specific activities. For example, for video No. 33, the following female actions were listed: stripping in a club, walking with men, drinking, dancing at club, spraying champagne at a woman, getting sprayed with champagne, and swinging around a pole. For video No. 31, the following female actions were listed: riding in a car, walking on a beach, dancing. Emerging from these data were 160 different behaviors by women appearing in the music videos. As listed in Table 3.3, the most frequent activity, with 45 occurrences, and appearing in 64.3% of the videos was dancing/jiggling. Women were shown dancing in a club, on a street, at home, on a platform, and at a number of locations. The second most common activity was walking/strutting, with 38 occurrences, and appearing in 54.3% of the videos. Other common behaviors were lying down (on a bed, couch, beach, or stage), sitting, getting wet, and riding in a car. For many of these behaviors, women were quite passive; these behaviors involved women just being there to be looked at, as was the case with much of the dancing and strutting. There was little personal agency featured.

As a secondary component of this analysis, we also kept track of when characters in the videos were shown working and what kind of work they were shown doing. For the male characters, this list was quite extensive, for men were depicted in 21 different jobs, the most frequent of which were police officer (eight occurrences), security guard/body guard (four occurrences), and food service/chef (three occurrences). Among the women, female characters were shown engaged in only nine different occupations, less than half the diversity of career depictions for men. Moreover, the most common occupational depiction for women was stripper (six occurrences), followed by reporter (five occurrences). Rounding out the limited group of female career images was police officer, casting agent, clerk, florist, maid, nurse, and restaurant worker—which each occurred once or twice.

Thus, from these analyses, we see a very limited world for women in these videos. They are most commonly shown dancing sexually, wearing alluring clothing, and serving as sexual objects. The activities they engage in are typically very passive, those that highlight that they are there to be looked at.

Table 3.3 **Most Prevalent Actions and Behaviors by Women Appearing in the Videos**

Rank	Activity	Percentage of videos
1	Dancing/jiggling	64.3
2	Walking/strutting	54.3
3	Laying down alone	24.3
	Moving items (dropping/placing)	24.3
5	Getting wet (bathing, playing in water)	20.0
	Sitting inside (on couch, chairs, bed)	20.0
	Talking/whispering	20.0
8	Riding/bouncing in car	17.1
9	Beautifying/primping	15.7
	Sitting outside	15.7
	Using a telephone or pager	15.7
12	Driving a car	14.3
	Performing domestic duties (preparing food, ironing)	14.3
14	Caretaking/nurturing (e.g., holding children, checking on sick)	12.9
	Opening doors, curtains, or windows	12.9

Indeed, of *all* possible occupations they could be shown doing, the lead one was stripper.

The Nature of Courtship: Exploring Themes of Adversarial Relations, Power, and Status

Expanding traditional assessments of media sexual imagery, we also examined the prevalence of two specific courtship themes: adversarial relations and materialism. We found that 28.6% of videos featured adversarial relations, typically depicting competition or infidelity. This theme was especially prevalent in videos by female artists (43.8%), appearing almost twice as frequently as it did in videos by male artists (27.9%). In terms of depictions of wealth and status, we saw examples of this in 48.6% of videos overall. This theme was more prevalent in videos by male artists than in videos by female artists (51.2% vs. 37.5%), which is a likely consequence of the importance of financial success to traditional definitions of masculinity. Emerging was a somewhat disturbing

view of heterosexual relations, whereby 51% of videos by male artists emphasized wealth and status symbols, and 44% of videos by female artists featured
adversarial relations.

A Closer Look at Female Images and Male–Female Relations via Qualitative and Thematic Analysis

To investigate more in-depth the dominant messages about black femininity
and black women's bodies appearing in these videos, our final analysis was a
qualitative and thematic analysis of the music video imagery. Five members of
the research team (four black women and one white woman, all aged 23–39)
met multiple times as a group to analyze and discuss each of the 70 music
videos over the course of several weeks. Together, we watched one video at
a time and took notes (independently) on the themes, messages, and images.
We then discussed that video as a group and recorded our observations. Once
each of the 70 videos had been reviewed in this way, each member of the
research team created a list from her notes of the dominant themes across
the 70 videos. These individual lists were compiled into one master list, with
redundancies removed. What we offer here is a profile of some of the prominent themes about black women, their sexuality, and their sexual relationships
emerging from this analysis.

Overview of Findings from Thematic Analysis

Our analysis revealed a rather dismal portrayal of black women's sexuality.
Although the majority of videos followed a specific storyline, some had none
at all, focusing instead only on men's ogling and fondling women's bodies or
on faceless body parts. Moreover, although sex was featured as something serious or important enough for men to constantly pursue, women were *seldom*
taken seriously as equitable partners; instead, women's chief value was their
sexuality or physical attributes. In the section that follows, we review these
themes in more detail, citing the dominant images and messages depicted in
the videos.

"I'm Objectified and Loving It"

One of the salient impressions emerging from our research discussions was
that sexually objectifying images were dominant, so much so that they seemed
almost normative, and women were seldom shown objecting to this treatment.
Such objectification took many forms. Frequently, women were seen in groups,
dancing and seeking the attention of male artists or featured male characters.

These women often appeared faceless, with the camera zooming in on specific body parts, such as jiggling breasts or gyrating buttocks as women danced. In another form of objectification, women's body parts served as stand-ins for other objects. For example, in the video "You Owe Me" by rapper Nas, women's legs were used as tripods to frame shots of another featured artist. A woman's abdomen was used as a golf tee in Ja Rule's "Between Me and You." Black women's bodies were also used more globally as scenery and decoration to adorn men's arms, houses, and expensive cars. Rather than acting as autonomous characters, these women appeared lifeless and were actually posed similar to statues in some videos, such as "You Owe Me."

As additional support of the premise that women are insignificant and replaceable objects, not real people, men featured in the videos frequently would not even acknowledge existence of the women around them. For example, one of the major scenes in Trick Daddy's "Shut Up" featured the lens of the camera pointed squarely toward a woman's behind as she danced provocatively. While Trick Daddy is rapping, the woman's arms are wrapped around his waist, trying to get his attention. Never once does the rapper divert his visual attention toward her face. Instead, in one shot, he is seen fondling her buttocks while still rapping directly to the camera. Later in the video, another featured rapper takes center stage, rapping into the camera, with two women physically pulling on his shirt, jockeying for his attention. They do not get it. The message conveyed is that women are inconsequential and must vie with other women to get (or keep) a man's attention.

At the same time, several videos showed women waiting to be "chosen" from among the throngs of beautiful women. Ja Rule's "Between Me and You" pictured the rapper with no less than 10 women crowded around him at a time. Whether lined up in formation around the hot tub, side by side in bikinis to gain entry to his mansion, or standing along the walls, the women were almost always scantily clad—many with simulated nudity—and presumably at his sexual beck-and-call. Rather than actively choosing their partners, women, instead, were waiting to be chosen from among the vast numbers of others waiting with them. Many scenes highlighted a lack of power and agency on the part of women, often resembling the dynamics of a brothel. The message was that women are sexually accessible to whatever man deems them worthy of attention.

Overall, when sexual situations were presented in music video imagery, there was the distinct impression that sex occurs exclusively for men's benefit. For example, Ludacris' "What's Your Fantasy" was dedicated to the ways in which a woman should enact a man's sexual fantasies. Featuring multiple phallic symbols (women with popsicles, lollipops, ice cream cones, bananas), there was a noticeable lack of consideration of women's fantasies, which is interesting considering the title of the song is "What's *your* fantasy" (not *my* fantasy). Apparently, the only fantasies being acted out are men's fantasies.

Interestingly, there was not one video in which women appeared upset or vocalized their displeasure with sexual objectification—whether in videos led by male or female artists. Instead, much of the imagery suggested that these women were willing participants in their own sexual objectification. For example, in the Hot Boys' video "I Need A Hot Girl," as the track chants "Do your thing, bitch," we see women acting out the words to the song, shaking their behinds in the camera lens. Some videos featured female singers rapping or singing along during the chorus, thereby offering their implicit agreement with the content and images. In addition, women were often seen touching and fondling themselves for the camera's gaze. In several videos, such as in "Between Me and You," women are seen lying on beaches and lawns, fondling and stroking their breasts for the camera. Even videos with female artists advance these notions of self-sexual objectification. For example, Lil' Kim's "No Matter What People Say" showed her and several female dancers in choreographed routines making provocative hand gestures towards their crotches and behinds.

Flipping the Script or Playing into the Same Old Stereotypes?

Although the majority of videos featured images of a male-dominated universe, there were several female artists who attempted to tell a different story. Black female artists often touted "flipping the script" and taking control of their own bodies and lives to counter testosterone-driven themes of men's dominance in and outside of the bedroom. Black female artists often projected control over their sexuality, describing how they wanted to be treated or what kind of man they desired. For example, Da Brat's "What 'Chu Like," advanced notions of women's rights to sexual pleasure. She focused on what she has to offer sexually, what kind of partner she likes, and on what a partner could do to please her. Although this is a different message than those presented in male-oriented videos, nevertheless, some of the imagery, such as men's fondling women's behinds, seemed to undercut such proclamations of sexual power. Similarly, Toni Braxton's "He Wasn't Man Enough For Me" advanced the idea of a black female cartoon superhero. Although this image led the audience to believe the video's message would center on ways in which women could garner power, the character unzipped her costume while men stopped and ogled, portraying this as a form of "female power." It therefore became clear that the chief power this character possessed was sexual.

Indeed, despite these assertions of power and agency, more often than not, these videos played into the same patriarchal story. Women who appeared to be in control were not. Some women who portrayed themselves as powerful, like female rapper Lil' Kim in "No Matter What People Say," could also be seen crawling on runways or on the floor toward a man, an action not engaged in by the men in the video. Crawling is typically perceived as a submissive and demeaning position even when under the guise of being sexy. Male dominance and control were also shown in this video as rapper Puff Daddy walked around telling the women to "dance" for his benefit and that of other male spectators. Again, we saw a lack of agency on behalf of women, even among female artists attempting to present alternate images of women.

Is Sex All There Is to Relationships?

Although some love ballads were part of the sample and often featured the only images of black women and men in committed relationships, the perspective on "love" in these videos was often very limited, typically centering on women's physical appearance. Often contrary to most of the songs' lyrics, the imagery emphasized an appreciation for the sexual appeal of a woman rather than her personality or any substantive value she adds to the quality of the relationship. When men sang about women, what they loved and missed about them, the focus was almost exclusively on sex and women's bodies. When characters were clearly in committed relationships, they were almost exclusively seen being sexual with one another. For example, Joe's "Treat Her Like A Lady" was a cautionary tale for men to show attention and appreciation to their partners. Even though the lyrics spoke about performing nice gestures, asking, "When is the last time you bought her roses or bought her a card to tell her how you feel," the actual imagery showed the woman being "appreciated" only in the bedroom. Across videos, few couples were seen outside of the bedroom or in nonsexual situations (e.g., eating dinner, visiting with family), suggesting that sex is all there is to relationships.

"What Is a Woman Worth?"

A final theme emerging from our discussions was that, in the world of music videos, women exist as a form of currency, a convenient display of a man's status and power, right alongside his cars, clothes, and cash. In these music videos, women were depicted as abundant and interchangeable; obtaining more women was never a problem for a man of wealth and status. Wealthy men seemed to be able to "afford" these trophy women, who seemed to be unlimited in their quantity and readily available to the highest bidder to be used at his disposal. For example, in his "Big Pimping" video, rapper Jay-Z promoted an image of attainment of the "American Dream" via international travel, unlimited amounts of cash, and crowds of sexually available women. The video showed men dousing women with expensive champagne and pulling off women's bikini tops. The women never protested or complained—after all, this is a man's world and his ultimate definition of success.

This confounding of women and money as the capital by which a man gains status and a woman gains value was prevalent in the videos we observed. In fact, many of the videos consistently paired women and expensive goods in the same camera shot. Although this pairing objectified women and reduced them to materials goods, it did something similar to men, indicating that a man's only utility is his material wealth and ability to keep a woman on his arm.

In being valued for their bodies by the men in the videos, women were then seen to "capitalize" on this objectification and trade on sexuality to enhance their own status. Whereas men were seen to "take care of women" with material things, women seemed to gladly accept this trade, for in doing so, in this music video world, these "chosen" women gained power over the other women. However, given that women were interchangeable, this power was often limited and short-lived. As soon as a woman is no longer desired, she is quickly discarded and replaced. This false sense of power seemed to keep the women in the music videos prepared to fight for a place behind a man, using whatever sexually appealing qualities they possessed.

Finally, women were found to be indebted to men, owing sexual favors for the material things men had provided. This dangerous message was often seen once a man had given a woman a valuable item (e.g., jewelry, a car). Sex was the *expected* and *accepted* currency of exchange. The message was that if a man gave a woman something, then she *must* repay him with sex. One video entitled "You Owe Me" by Nas articulated this recurrent message very well, with lyrics describing this quasi-prostitute/pimp relationship that is portrayed as normal in rap culture. Lyrics included statements such as, "I gave you ... you know what you owe me." This particular video theme seemed to suggest that women should be satisfied with whatever they get from the men, and they should not demand or expect anything else. Here, it seemed to place women in need of the objectification of men in order to survive.

Existing Findings of the Effects of This Content on Gender Ideologies and Sexual Stereotypes

How might exposure to this narrow portrait of femininity shape the developing belief systems of girls and young women? Does repeated viewing of this limited range of roles and behaviors lead girls' perceptions of femininity to be equally constrained? Several studies have attempted to investigate this issue, with some researchers testing contributions of music video exposure to gender beliefs and others exploring contributions to body image and appearance concerns. We summarize the key findings here, including survey or correlational data, as well as experimental data.

Correlational Evidence

One set of studies has used survey data to examine whether the amount of time students regularly spend watching music videos relates to their attitudes toward women. Here, findings across several studies indicate that more frequent exposure to or involvement with music videos is associated with more stereotypical attitudes toward gender roles (Ward, 2002), more adversarial attitudes toward male–female relationships (Bryant, 2008), a stronger acceptance of women as sexual objects (Hust & Lei, 2008; Ward, 2002), and more accepting attitudes toward sexual harassment (Strouse, Goodwin, & Roscoe, 1994) and date rape (Kaestle, Halpern, & Brown, 2007). These findings have emerged among studies testing seventh- and eighth-grade girls and boys, older teens, and undergraduates. A related set of studies has examined the consequences of exposure to videos that are particularly sexual or misogynistic. Zhang, Miller, and Harrison (2008) reported that among undergraduates, frequent viewing of *sexual* music videos was a significant predictor of support for a sexual double standard, and was a stronger and more consistent predictor than was overall television viewing. Among a sample of black undergraduates (79% female), Conrad, Dixon, and Zhang (2007) found that students who reported more regular exposure to *misogynistic* music videos (as rated by a team of students) also reported a stronger identification with the characters in the videos and a greater acceptance of the degradation of women in the videos. Thus, across several studies, more frequent exposure to music videos, especially to the more sexual or misogynistic ones, has been linked with students' holding more stereotypical or misogynistic attitudes toward women.

Experimental Evidence

Another set of studies has used experimental paradigms to test how the attitudes of students exposed to specific types of imagery compare to the attitudes of students without this exposure. Findings here are equally compelling. Across several studies (e.g., Kalof, 1999), young people exposed to sexually objectifying images of women from mainstream music videos were found to be significantly more accepting of objectifying notions about women, stereotypical gender roles, teen dating violence, and adversarial beliefs about relationships than were those without this exposure. For example, Johnson, Adams, Ashburn, and Reed (1995) examined effects of exposure to nonviolent rap music videos on black adolescents' acceptance of teen dating violence. Thirty black girls and 30 black boys aged 11–16 were assigned to view either eight nonviolent rap videos containing images of women in sexually subordinate roles or no videos. They all then read a vignette that involved teen dating violence and rated the appropriateness of the male's actions. Girls exposed to the videos showed greater acceptance of the man's violent behavior than did girls not exposed; boys' attitudes were not affected. The reverse pattern emerged in an experiment by Kistler and Lee (2010), in which undergraduate men, but not women, exposed to five objectifying music videos offered more support for sexual objectification, rape myths, and traditional gender attitudes than did students exposed to less sexual videos. Additionally, Aubrey, Hopper, and Mbure (2011), who tested *only* undergraduate men, reported that those men exposed to three sexually objectifiying music videos expressed greater acceptance of adversarial sexual beliefs, interpersonal violence, and sexual harassment than did men without this exposure.

In one of the few studies to use both correlational and experimental methods, Ward, Hansbrough, and Walker (2005) examined the impact of music video exposure on black adolescents' endorsement of gender and sexual stereotypes. Results indicated that more frequent viewing of music videos was associated with holding more stereotypical gender role attitudes and with attributing greater importance to superficial qualities (e.g., being attractive, cool, sexy) in one's feminine ideals. Moreover, students assigned to view four sexist and sexual music videos offered stronger endorsement of sexual stereotypes (e.g., "Using her body and looks is the best way for a woman to attract a man") and of the importance of superficial qualities for women than did students who had viewed four nonsexist videos.

Finally, evidence indicates that laboratory exposure to sexual or objectifying music videos can alter viewers' impressions of real-world people observed in similar contexts, often making neutral behavior appear more sexualized, and making actions that fit stereotypical gender schemas seem more favorable (e.g., Hansen & Hansen, 1988; Hansen & Krygowski, 1994). For example, Hansen and Hansen (1988) reported that whereas students who had watched three nonsexist music videos later perceived a man's hitting on a female colleague to be akin to sexual harassment, students who had viewed stereotypic music videos perceived his sexual advances as appropriate, and thought less favorably of her if she rejected him. Gan, Zillmann, and Mitrook (1997) examined how exposure to images of black women in music videos affects white undergraduates' perceptions of attractive black and white women encountered later. For this study, 55 white male and female students first rated their ideals (e.g., a person they would love to be dating) on 30 attributes. They then viewed either four music videos by black artists that focused on devoted love, four videos that focused on sexual enticement, or no videos. For the final task, they rated pictures of six women (three black, three white) on multiple attributes. Results indicate that type of video exposure was inconsequential for the white women rated. However, the neutral black women evaluated were judged less "good" (e.g., qualities like attractive, caring, sexy, and romantic), more "bad" (e.g., qualities like obscene, vulgar, sluttish, sleazy, reckless), and further from the ideal by those who had just viewed the sexualized images compared to students who had seen either the devoted love videos or no videos. Exposure to sexual videos appears to have fostered perceptions of stronger negative traits and diminished positive traits in black women, in general. Thus, findings from both survey and experimental work reveal connections between music video exposure and students' beliefs about women, gender roles, and sexual relationships.

Existing Findings of the Effects of This Content on Body Image and Appearance Concerns

Effects of exposure to the narrow images of women in music videos also extend to women's body image concerns. Here, findings suggest that exposure to the very narrow portrayal of women in music videos is associated with girls' and young women's feeling less satisfied with their own bodies. Data drawn from surveys of regular media use indicate contributions for both younger and older adolescents. Surveying the media use of 837 ninth-grade girls, Borzekowski et al. (2000) found that more frequent music video viewing was related to greater perceptions of the importance of appearance and greater weight concerns. Tiggemann and Pickering (1996), who surveyed 94 adolescent girls, reported that frequent music video viewing predicted a stronger drive for thinness. In their survey of 522 black girls aged 14–18, Peterson, Wingood, DiClemente, Harrington, and Davies (2007) found that girls who perceived more portrayals of sexual stereotypes in rap music videos reported watching more hours of videos each week and also reported a more negative body image than did girls who perceived fewer sexual stereotypes in rap music videos. Drawing on data from 195 13-year-old girls, Grabe and Hyde (2009) demonstrated that more frequent music video viewing predicted greater body surveillance, which was linked with lower body esteem and higher levels of depressive symptoms.

Yet, emerging evidence also indicates that effects for black youth are not universal and may vary based on their connections to the content and their existing identities. More specifically, Gordon (2008), testing a sample of 176 black high school girls, found that stronger identification with music artists rated by researchers to be *more objectifying* (e.g., Lil Kim) was associated with greater support of the importance of appearance for women. Conversely, stronger identification with music artists rated to be *less objectifying* was associated with less support of these notions. Zhang, Dixon, and Conrad (2009) examined how ethnic identity may moderate the effects of exposure to thin images. Researchers surveyed 111 black female undergraduates, assessing their ethnic identity, body image perceptions, and regular viewing of 30 popular rap music videos. Researchers also evaluated the mean body sizes of the women in these videos. No global effects of viewing the video ideals emerged; instead, effects varied by the strength of students' ethnic identity. Among black women with a weaker ethnic identity, greater regular viewing of rap videos featuring thin women was associated with higher body dissatisfaction, increased drive for thinness, and increased bulimic tendencies. Conversely, among black women with a stronger ethnic identity, greater regular exposure to thin black women in rap videos was associated with lower body dissatisfaction, a lower drive for thinness, and few bulimic tendencies.

Additional evidence of the impact of music videos on girls' body image can be drawn from experimental data. Testing 84 undergraduate women attending a university in Australia, Tiggemann and Slater (2004) found that those women who had viewed six music video clips emphasizing female thinness and attractiveness later reported feeling fatter, less physically attractive, less confident, and less satisfied with their bodies than did women who had viewed clips that did not focus on female thinness and attractiveness. Similar results were obtained by Bell, Lawton, and Dittmar (2007), whose participants were 87 girls (95% white) attending an all-girl high school in England. Here, girls who had viewed three music videos featuring thin, all-girl bands (e.g., The Pussycat Dolls) reported larger postexposure increases in body dissatisfaction than girls who had only heard the songs or than girls who had studied a list of words.

Thus, existing data demonstrate many potential consequences of repeated exposure to music videos, including greater appearance concerns and body dissatisfaction, more traditional gender role attitudes, and a stronger acceptance of objectifying notions about women, sexual harassment, dating violence, rape myths, and beliefs that romantic relationships are adversarial. These outcomes have emerged using both survey and experimental methods, for black and white students, and among pre-teens, adolescent girls, and undergraduate women.

Implications of These Images on the Lives of Black Youth

It can be argued that these are just fictional images, that seeing sexy women is just a part of life. Yet, as existing data show, repeated exposure to these limited portrayals of black and white women does appear to contribute to how girls and young women conceptualize femininity, sexual roles, and expected behavior in relationships with men. The implications of these norms and beliefs are all too apparent when analyses are done of how young people evaluate dating violence. Squires, Kohn-Wood, Chavous, and Carter (2006) assessed these notions in focus groups with 35 black high school students. After viewing and discussing images of femininity and sexual violence in hip-hop and in music videos, participants read and discussed a vignette about the date rape of a hip-hop fan. What emerged from these sessions were multiple indications that the youth seemed to blame women more than men for the violence. Women, through their character or behavior, were commonly considered to be at least equally, if not mostly, responsible for their abusive relationships with men. Girls and boys had a low opinion of most women in the world of hip-hop, referring to them as "ho's," "nasty," and inappropriately dressed. These perceptions of women in hip-hop appeared to extend to their evaluations of real women. When discussing the real-life rape of the hip-hop fan, the majority of teen participants argued that women could bring such abuse upon themselves through the exercise of poor judgment or "nasty" behavior, such as dancing or dressing provocatively. Although there is no direct proof that hip-hop music and videos caused youth to have these views, the authors concluded that these youth "have learned somewhere that certain women are "nasty" and that certain women "choose" to be abused, and also that abusive men are the products of their environment, but abused women are products of their (faulty) choices" (p. 733).

Conclusion

Since rap and hip-hop music videos were introduced in the 1980s, they have become one of the more popular music genres among young people. Despite the declines experienced in the music recording industry, music videos have remained a powerful source in representing identities (Balaji, 2009) and are increasingly more accessible to youth via iPods and the Internet. Analyses indicate that one of the more prevalent images in this genre viewed heavily by young girls and boys is the sexual objectification of women. This finding has emerged in videos analyzed from the 1980s to today, and dominated our analysis of images of black women in music videos. Moreover, the videos we analyzed are already 12 years old, and there is indication that current videos may be even *more* sexual and graphic, especially with popular songs such as Young Money's "Every Girl," which references his wanting to "F— every girl in the world." Although these videos are fictional and perhaps fantasies, they are not wholly harmless. Evidence indicates that repeated exposure to music videos is linked to several negative outcomes, including greater appearance concerns and body dissatisfaction, more stereotypical gender role attitudes, and a stronger acceptance of objectifying notions about women, sexual harassment, dating violence, and beliefs that romantic relationships are adversarial.

Repeatedly, the message emerging is that a woman's worth comes not from her brains or her heart but from her beauty and sexual appeal.

References

Alexander, S. (1999). The gender role paradox in youth culture: An analysis of women in music videos. *Michigan Sociological Review, 13,* 46–64.

American Psychological Association. (2007). *Report of the APA task force on the sexualization of girls.* Washington, DC: American Psychological Association.

Andsager, J. L., & Roe, K. (1999). Country music video in country's year of the woman. *Journal of Communication, 49,* 69–82.

Arnett, J. J. (2002). The sounds of sex: Sex in teens' music and music videos. In J. D. Brown, J. R. Steele, & K. Walsh-Childers (Eds.), *Sexual teens, sexual media: Investigating media's influence on adolescence sexuality* (pp. 253–264). Mahwah, NJ: Lawrence Erlbaum Associates.

Ashby, S., & Rich, M. (2005). Video killed the radio star: The effects of music videos on adolescent health. *Adolescent Medicine, 16,* 371–393.

Aubrey, J. S., & Frisby, C. M. (2011). Sexual objectification in music videos: A content analysis comparing gender and genre. *Mass Communication & Society, 14,* 475–501.

Aubrey, J. S., Hopper, K. M., & Mbure, W. (2011). Check that body! The effects of sexually objectifying music videos on college men's sexual beliefs. *Journal of Broadcasting & Electronic Media, 55,* 360–379.

Balaji, M. (2009). Owning Black masculinity: The intersection of cultural commodification and self-construction in rap music videos. *Communication, Culture, & Critique, 2,* 21–38.

Bell, B. T., Lawton, R., & Dittmar, H. (2007). The impact of thin models in music videos on adolescent girls' body dissatisfaction. *Body Image, 4,* 137–145.

Borzekowski, D. L. G., Robinson, T. N., & Killen, J. D. (2000). Does the camera add 10 pounds? Media use, perceived importance of appearance, and weight concerns among teenage girls. *Journal of Adolescent Health, 26,* 36–41.

Bryant, Y. (2008). Relationships between exposure to rap music videos and attitudes toward relationships among African American youth. *Journal of Black Psychology, 34,* 356–380.

Conrad, K., Dixon, T., & Zhang, Y. (2007). *An examination of how rap and R & B music videos influence African American self identity.* Paper presented at the annual meeting of the National Communication Association, Chicago, IL.

Conrad, K., Dixon, T., & Zhang, Y. (2009). Controversial rap themes, gender portrayals and skin tone distortion: A content analysis of rap music videos. *Journal of Broadcasting & Electronic Media, 53,* 134–156.

Durham, M. G. (2008). *The Lolita effect: The media sexualization of young girls and what we can do about it.* Woodstock, NY: The Overlook Press.

Emerson, R. A. (2002). "Where my girls at?": Negotiating Black womanhood in music videos. *Gender & Society, 16,* 115–135.

Frisby, C. M., & Aubrey, J. S. (2012). Race and genre in the use of sexual objectification in female artists' music videos. *The Howard Journal of Communications, 23,* 66–87.

Gan, S. -L., Zillmann, D., & Mitrook, M. (1997). Stereotyping effect of Black women's sexual rap on White audiences. *Basic and Applied Social Psychology, 19,* 381–399.

Gordon, M. (2008). Media contributions to African American girls' focus on beauty and appearance: Exploring the consequences of sexual objectification. *Psychology of Women Quarterly, 32,* 245–256.

Gow, J. (1996). Reconsidering gender roles on MTV: Depictions in the most popular music videos of the early 1990s. *Communication Reports, 9*(2), 151–161.

Grabe, S., & Hyde, J. S. (2009). Body objectification, MTV, and psychological outcomes among female adolescents. *Journal of Applied Social Psychology, 39*, 2840–2858.

Hansen, C., & Hansen, R. (1988). How rock music videos can change what is seen when boy meets girl: Priming stereotypic appraisal of social interactions. *Sex Roles, 5/6*, 287–316.

Hansen, C. H., & Krygowski, W. (1994). Arousal-augmented priming effects: Rock music videos and sex object schemas. *Communication Research, 21*, 24–47.

Hust, S., & Lei, M. (2008). Sexual objectification, sports programming, and music television. *Media Report to Women, 36*, 16–23.

Jhally, S. (1995). *Dreamworlds II: Desire, sex, and power in music video*. Northampton, MA: Media Education Foundation.

Johnson, J. D., Adams, M. S., Ashburn, L., & Reed, W. (1995). Differential gender effects of exposure to rap music on African American adolescents' acceptance of teen dating violence. *Sex Roles, 33*, 597–605.

Jones, K. (1997). Are rap videos more violent? Style differences and the prevalence of sex and violence in the age of MTV. *Howard Journal of Communications, 8*, 343–356.

Kaestle, C., Halpern, C., & Brown, J. (2007). Music videos, pro wrestling, and acceptance of date rape among middle school males and females: An exploratory analysis. *Journal of Adolescent Health, 40*(2), 185–187.

Kalof, L. (1999). The effects of gender and music video imagery on sexual attitudes. *The Journal of Social Psychology, 139*, 378–385.

King, K., Laake, R., & Bernard, A. (2006). Do the depictions of sexual attire and sexual behavior in music videos differ based on video network and character gender? *American Journal of Health Education, 37*, 146–153.

Kistler, M., & Lee, M. J. (2010). Does exposure to sexual hip-hop music videos influence the sexual attitudes of college students? *Mass Communication and Society, 13*(1), 67–86.

Lin, C. (1998). The use of sex appeals in prime-time television commercials. *Sex Roles, 38*, 461–475.

Peterson, S., Wingood, G., DiClemente, R., Harrington, K., & Davies, S. (2007). Images of sexual stereotypes in rap videos and the health of African American female adolescents. *Journal of Women's Health, 16*(8), 1157–1164.

Roberts, D., Foehr, U., & Rideout, V. (2005, March). *Generation M: Media in the lives of 8–18 year olds*. Menlo Park, CA: Kaiser Family Foundation.

Seidman, S. A. (1992). An investigation of sex-role stereotyping in music videos. *Journal of Broadcasting & Electronic Media, 36*, 209–216.

Seidman, S. A. (1999). Revisiting sex-role stereotyping in MTV videos. *International Journal of Instructional Media, 26*, 11–22.

Signorielli, N. (2001). Television's gender role images and contribution to stereotyping: Past, present, and future. In D. Singer, & J. L. Singer (Eds.), *Handbook of children and the media* (pp. 341–358). Thousand Oaks, CA: Sage.

Sommers-Flanagan, R., Sommers-Flanagan, J., & Davis, B. (1993). What's happening on music television? A gender role content analysis. *Sex Roles, 28*, 745–753.

Squires, C., Kohn-Wood, L., Chavous, T., & Carter, P. (2006). Evaluating agency and responsibility in gendered violence: African American youth talk about violence and hip hop. *Sex Roles, 55*, 725–737.

Stephens, D., & Few, A. (2007). Hip hop honey or video ho: African American preadolescents' understanding of female sexual scripts in hip hop culture. *Sexuality & Culture, 11*, 48–69.

Stephens, D., & Phillips, L. (2003). Freaks, gold diggers, divas, and dykes: The socio-historical development of African American women's sexual scripts. *Sexuality & Culture, 7*, 3–49.

Strouse, J. S., Goodwin, M. P., & Roscoe, B. (1994). Correlates of attitudes toward sexual harassment among early adolescents. *Sex Roles, 31*, 559–577.

Tiggemann, M., & Pickering, A. S. (1996). Role of television in adolescent women's body dissatisfaction and drive for thinness. *International Journal of Eating Disorders, 20,* 199–203.

Tiggemann, M., & Slater, A. (2004). Thin ideals in music television: A source of social comparison and body dissatisfaction. *International Journal of Eating Disorders, 35,* 48–58.

Vincent, R. C. (1989). Clio's consciousness raised? Portrayal of women in rock videos, re-examined. *Journalism Quarterly, 66,* 155–160.

Vincent, R., Davis, D., & Boruszkowski, L. (1987). Sexism on MTV: The portrayal of women in rock videos. *Journalism Quarterly, 64,* 750–755, 941.

Wallis, C. (2011). Performing gender: A content analysis of gender display in music videos. *Sex Roles, 64,* 160–172.

Ward, L. M. (2002). Does television exposure affect emerging adults' attitudes and assumptions about sexual relationships? Correlational and experimental confirmation. *Journal of Youth and Adolescence, 31,* 1–15.

Ward, L. M., Hansbrough, E., & Walker, E. (2005). Contributions of music video exposure to Black adolescents' gender and sexual schemas. *Journal of Adolescent Research, 20,* 143–166.

West, C. M. (2009). Still on the auction block: The (s)exploitation of Black adolescent girls in rap(e) music and hip-hop culture. In S. Olfman (Ed.), *The sexualization of childhood* (pp. 89–102). Westport, CT: Praeger Publishers/Greenwood Publishing Group.

Zhang, Y., Dixon, T., & Conrad, K. (2009). Rap music videos and African American women's body image: The moderating role of ethnic identity. *Journal of Communication, 59,* 262–278.

Zhang, Y., Dixon, T., & Conrad, K. (2010). Female body image as a function of themes in rap music videos: A content analysis. *Sex Roles, 62,* 787–797.

Zhang, Y., Miller, L., & Harrison, K. (2008). The relationship between exposure to sexual music videos and young adults' sexual attitudes. *Journal of Broadcasting & Electronic Media, 52,* 368–386.

4

Athletics as Solution and Problem

Sport Participation for Girls and the Sexualization of Female Athletes

ELIZABETH A. DANIELS AND NICOLE M. LAVOI

> In my mind, this woman is dressed to look "beautiful" according to societies [sic] standards but these standards do not include the image of a basketball player (sweaty, ponytail, long shorts, fully covered upper torso, etc.)....I think that Lauren Jackson would be just as beautiful (if not more beautiful) if she were wearing her basketball jersey.
>
> *19-year-old college woman*

> This makes me feel somewhat inadequate, as I am not that tall, skinny, or tan. It saddens me slightly because she is more like an "ideal woman" to most men than I probably ever will be.
>
> *18-year-old college woman*

These are two responses from college women to a photograph of Lauren Jackson, a highly successful athlete in the Women's National Basketball Association (WNBA), posed in a bikini on the beach with her head tilted to the side, long blonde hair blowing in the wind and a big smile on her face. These quotations and dozens like them capture the feelings of many teenage girls and young women toward sexualized media images of female athletes (Daniels, 2012). Some view these images with a critical lens, whereas others uncritically accept them as yet another example of unattainable beauty portrayed in the media.

Many sociocultural influences in U.S. society prompt girls and women to feel dissatisfied with their bodies (see Chapters 1 and 3 of this volume). Objectification theory explains that Western societies routinely sexually objectify the female body (Fredrickson & Roberts, 1997; McKinley & Hyde, 1996). Women's bodies are scrutinized as objects for the pleasure and evaluation of others, specifically men (and boys). As a result, many girls and women self-objectify, focusing on how their bodies *appear* rather than what they can *do*.

Self-objectification has implications for girls' and women's mental health, including a heightened risk for disordered eating, negative body esteem, and negative effects on psychological well-being (Fredrickson, Roberts, Noll, Quinn, & Twenge, 1998; McKinley, 1999; Muehlenkamp, Swanson, & Brausch, 2005; Tiggemann & Lynch, 2001). In addition, individuals who experience severe dissatisfaction with their appearance are at risk for eating disorders, which can seriously negatively impact both psychological and physical health (Stice, 2002; Stice & Shaw, 2002).

As the opening quotations illustrate, media generally portray narrow and stereotypical representations of women and femininity that transmit unrealistic standards for physical appearance (Ward & Harrison, 2005), and girls and women judge themselves based on these idealized representations (Field et al., 1999; Grabe, Ward, & Hyde, 2008; Groesz, Levine, & Murnen, 2002; Levine, Smolak, & Hayden, 1994). Indeed, body dissatisfaction is a pervasive societal problem. Sports and physical activities are a potential avenue for the development of positive body concept, as well as for other positive self-perceptions, including higher levels of self-efficacy, confidence, self-esteem, physical competence and self-worth, character development, and more favorable body esteem (e.g., Biddle, Whitehead, O'Donovan, & Nevill 2005; Donaldson & Ronan, 2006; Richman & Shaffer, 2000). In addition, girls' sport involvement is associated with a functional body orientation (an appreciation of one's body for its athletic ability or what it can do, rather than for how it looks to others), which can contribute to more positive sexual health and sexual health behaviors among adolescent girls (Lehman & Koerner, 2004). Unfortunately, female athletes, like other women, are frequently sexualized in the media instead of portrayed as strong athletes— for example, tennis champion Maria Sharapova's multipage layout in *Sports Illustrated*'s 2006 Swimsuit Edition. Sexualized images depict an individual in provocative clothing or photograph an individual in such a way as to focus solely on sexual attributes; for example, centering attention on an athlete's breasts (Fink & Kensicki, 2002). Sexualized media images of female athletes, like other sexualized images of women, may negatively affect female viewers' body concept by increasing body dissatisfaction.

In this chapter, we will discuss the history of women's sport, which has contributed to the present day sexualization phenomenon, document the prevalence of this pattern, and assess its impact on viewers. Finally, in an effort to combat the negative, we will discuss sport involvement as a positive context for girls and young women. Before beginning, however, it is necessary to consider what constitutes a sexualized image of a female athlete. Some might question whether an athletic female body depicted in a bikini, or less, rather than in a sport uniform is necessarily sexualized (see Heywood & Dworkin, 2003, for an in-depth discussion). One argument is that elite female athletes have worked tremendously hard to reach the pinnacle of their sports and an ultra-fit, muscular, toned body often accompanies this level of training. Displaying such a body in its near-naked form is considered an act of empowerment, showing off the athlete's physical achievement. An opposing argument is that our society sexualizes and commodifies women's bodies as a dominant practice. Therefore, media images of female athletes posed in little clothing are, in effect, always objectified. Theoretical arguments aside, the compelling question is how do viewers read these images? Do teen girls and young women see them as empowering or objectifying? In truth, individuals' responses likely depend on a number of factors, including the viewer's gender, age, ethnicity, social class, and sexual orientation (Steele & Brown, 1995). Unfortunately, there is very little psychological research on viewers' experiences of media images of female athletes, sexualized or otherwise. The existing evidence, however, suggests that the objectification argument best represents teen girls' and college women's reactions to media images of female athletes depicted in bikinis or similar attire (Daniels, 2009, 2012).

History of Women's Sport

When thinking about the impact of the sexualization of female athletes on girls and women, it is relevant to consider why female athletes are sexualized in the media and why some female athletes contribute to the practice of sexualization. Concerns about femininity, heterosexuality, and lesbian stigma lie at the heart of the matter (see Cahn [1994], Lenskyj [1986], Griffin [1998], for comprehensive analyses of these issues). Historically, organized sport has been intimately tied to masculinity in the United States, and sport fields have been testing grounds for proving masculinity (Couturier & Chepko, 2001; Rader, 2004). Accordingly, girls and women have generally not been welcome in sporting arenas. When girls and women were afforded opportunities to play sports, their femininity was a primary concern among league owners and sport governing bodies (Cahn, 1994). For example, the All-American Girls Baseball League, which began during World War II as men went off to war, mandated that players wear pastel-skirted uniforms, makeup, long hair, and *not* wear shorts, pants, or jeans in public. In the early years of the league, spring training also included mandatory evening charm school. The concern was the players not appear "mannish," which referred to any so-called masculine behavior, including appearance and dress, or lesbian. Girls and women engaged in the "masculine" activity of sport had to demonstrate their femininity and heterosexuality.

Fast forward to 2008, when the WNBA included cosmetics lessons and fashion tips during rookie orientation, and one can see that the priority placed upon female athletes' femininity is alive and well in the twenty-first century.

Of these lessons, Renee Brown, the WNBA's vice president of player personnel said, "You're a woman first. You just happen to play sports" (Ryan, 2008). It is clear that demonstrating the womanhood and heterosexuality of their players is a main concern of the WNBA (see Banet-Weiser [1999] and McDonald [2002] for in-depth analyses of this practice). Indeed in May 2009, the WNBA's homepage featured a Mother's Day memories story and photographs of mothers in the WNBA, as well as video interviews with expectant mother, Candace Parker, and new mom, Lisa Leslie, which focused on motherhood rather than their many athletic accomplishments. This pattern is by no means unique to the sport of women's basketball. Similar practices exist in other women's sports, for example, in 1985, the Women's Tennis Association began publishing a calendar with its top players in evening gowns or bathing suits (Miller, 2001). In addition, numerous female athletes have personally opted to pose for magazines such as *Playboy, Maxim,* and *FHM (For Him Magazine).* Enough have posed in *Playboy* that AskMen.com devised a Top 10 list out of the pool of eligible candidates (Golokhov, 2008). In short, female athletes' femininity and heterosexuality are highly visible in media focused on them.

This emphasis on femininity and heterosexuality is meant to quiet fears that female athletes are lesbians. The association between women's sport and lesbianism can be traced to the 1930s, when Freudian beliefs stigmatizing same-sex relationships as "sex-role nonconformity" took root in the culture (Lenskyj, 1986). At the time, true fulfillment for women was defined by marrying a man, and all-female social contexts, such as sport teams, were viewed suspiciously. Sport, academic, or professional pursuits were not consistent with the "heterosexual goal" (marriage). Sport was thought to masculinize females in their physical appearance and deportment (Cahn, 1994; Griffin, 1998). By extension, sport was thought to also masculinize women's desire; that is, turn them into lesbians. To combat these accusations, some well-intentioned journalists wrote stories referencing athletes' interest in clothing, grooming, and hairstyles, as well as their "sweet and ladylike" behavior to demonstrate their femininity and, therefore, their heterosexuality (Griffin as cited in Lenskyj, 1986, p. 75). Thus began the pattern of focusing on female athletes' femininity and heterosexuality in the media. Nevertheless, "the mannish lesbian athlete" became a full-blown stereotype of females in sports by the late 1940s (Cahn, 1994; Griffin, 1998).

The threat of lesbian stigma has been a mechanism of social control in women's sports for decades. As Griffin (2001) described, "because lesbian stereotypes are severe (evil, sick, abnormal, predatory), many females do not want to be associated with them. Consequently, calling females in sport 'lesbians' is often an effective way to make females feel defensive or timid about expressing their athleticism" (p. 281). By associating females' sport involvement with homosexuality, the dominance of male sports is reinforced. Girls and women who would rather not have their femininity and sexual orientation critiqued avoid competitive sport. And, frequently, those who do play emphasize their femininity and heterosexuality, priorities that likely distract from their game. Currently, the manifestation of this focus on femininity and heterosexuality can be seen in media depicting female athletes in sexualized and objectified ways rather than as athletes. Female athletes who pose in sexualized ways for men's magazines may be doing so to highlight their own femininity and heterosexuality, thereby avoiding questions about their sexual orientation. Why specific individuals have made such a choice, however, is not well documented. Future research should investigate their motivations.

Prevalence of Sexualization of Female Athletes

In keeping with the broader cultural tendency to sexualize women in media, today's female athletes are often sexualized in print and visual media, as well as in color commentary (e.g., Christopherson, Janning, & McConnell, 2002; Schultz, 2005; Shugart, 2003). A clear illustration of this tendency can be seen in the popular GoDaddy.com commercial featuring seven-time Olympic medal winner, swimmer Amanda Beard, which debuted in 2007 during a college football game and is widely available on the Internet. Beard is depicted wearing a bathrobe while a male promoter urges her to "show them off," his hands cupping the air as if he is holding breasts. As Beard reluctantly agrees and throws open her robe to reveal her medals, Mark Spitz, a seven-time Olympic gold medalist, appears on the scene commenting that he has seven medals, too. The male promoter shakes his head and says, "yeah, I like hers better" as he turns away from Spitz and stares at Beard's chest. In addition to being a GoDaddy spokesperson, Beard has also graced the covers of *FHM*, *Maxim*, and *Playboy* magazines in a bikini, making her one of the most highly visible sexualized athletes today.

When considering the practice of sexualizing female athletes in media, it is important to consider the amount and type of media dedicated to women's sport. A large body of sport media research shows that female athletes are essentially "missing in action" despite the boom in female athletic participation since the passage of Title IX (e.g., Amateur Athletic Foundation of Los Angeles, 2001; Kane, 1996; Messner & Cooky, 2010; Messner, Duncan, & Cooky, 2003; Pedersen & Whisenant, 2003; Vincent, Imwold, Johnson, & Massey, 2003). Coverage of girls' and women's sports constitutes about 6–8% of all sport media (Kane & LaVoi, 2007). A recent study revealed that female sports constitutes as little as 1.4% of sport media on ESPN's *SportsCenter* and 1.6% of sport media on early evening and late night television sports news on three network affiliates in the Southern California market (Messner &

Cooky, 2010). In addition, coverage of female sports is often selective and ste-reotyped; for example, females participating in traditionally feminine sports, such as gymnastics, figure skating, and tennis, tend to receive more media cov-erage than do females in other sports (Kane, 1996). Further, media coverage of female sports tends to involve humorous stories of nonserious female sports and the sexual objectification of female athletes and audience members, such as commentary on tennis player Anna Kournikova's physical attractiveness (Messner, Duncan, & Cooky, 2003; Schultz, 2005). This pattern of objectify-ing female athletes mirrors that of focusing on girls' and women's sexual attrac-tiveness in media more generally (American Psychological Association, 2007; Ward & Harrison, 2005).

In an effort to establish the manner in which female athletes are typically depicted in sport media, Fink and Kensicki (2002) explored the coverage of female athletes in *Sports Illustrated* (*SI*) and the now-defunct *Sports Illustrated for Women* (*SIW*) from 1997 to 1999. The study was conducted following the highly publicized success of U.S. female athletes in the 1996 Atlanta Olympics. This study found that only 10% of the photographs in *SI* during this 3-year period were of female athletes, and 5% of these photographs were considered porno-graphic/sexually suggestive (compared to 0% of photographs of male athletes). The majority of the photographs were of female athletes in nonsport settings, such as at home with their families (55%) (compared to 23% of similar photographs of male athletes), and about a third depicted female athletes in action (34%) (com-pared to 66% of similar photographs of male athletes). *SIW* contained fewer por-nographic/sexually suggestive images of female athletes (2%) and more images of female athletes in action (56%), but 24% of images showed female athletes in nonsport settings. This study illustrates that, even in major sporting magazines, female athletes are depicted in nonsporting roles at a high rate, and a portion of these photographs present female athletes as sexual objects.

The existence of any sexually oriented images of female athletes in sport magazines is puzzling. Advertising for *SI* says that readers can expect "big bold photos that put you in the heart of the action" and content that "gives the reader a closer look at the biggest games, names and happenings from the world of sports" (www.amazon.com, 2009). The magazine lives up to neither promise in its portrayal of female sports. Indeed, SI.com, the magazine's website, featured a story in May 2009 entitled "The Real Greatest Spectacle in Racing" in which the author directs readers to a photo gallery of "56 Insanely Hot Indy Car Grid Girls," who "do everything from holding umbrellas for the racers to just stand-ing around looking sexy" (COEDmagazine.com, 2009; Traina, 2009). Clearly, *SI* prioritizes the sexual attractiveness of female athletes and women in sporting contexts over the actual athleticism of female athletes.

The sexualization of female athletes may be on the rise. So-called "lad mags," such as *Maxim* or *FHM*, have featured numerous bikini-clad female athletes, for example, race car driver Danica Patrick and golfer Natalie Gulbis in *FHM* and beach volleyball player Misty May and swimmer Dara Torres in *Maxim* (Popcrunch, 2008). Despite this anecdotal evidence, a systematic investigation of the prevalence of sexualized images of female athletes across various media sources has not been conducted to date. Instead, targeted investigations have explored treatment of female athletes during specific sporting events, such as the 1999 Women's World Cup (Christopherson et al., 2002; Shugart, 2003), or through a particular media publication, such as *Sports Illustrated*'s Swimsuit Edition (Davis, 1997). The absence of a comprehensive analysis documenting the extent to which female athletes are sexualized in media makes it difficult to lobby for more respectful coverage of female athletes and female sports. Individual examples of sexualization are more easily brushed off as insignificant or nonrepresentative, whereas a comprehensive analysis would be harder to ignore or rationalize.

In broadcast media, sexualized commentary about female athletes often centers on conformity to particular standards of beauty—white, hegemonic femininity, which emphasizes maintaining a thin body ideal and adhering to a rigid and narrow definition of beauty. Shugart's (2003) study on print and television coverage of the 1999 U.S. women's soccer team provides evidence of this pattern, as shown by the attention paid to particular members of the team, specifically Mia Hamm and Brandi Chastain, who fit these beauty standards. Shugart argued that media coverage of the team was sexualized in subtle ways, including through *passive objectification*, such as Mia Hamm's selection as one of *People Weekly*'s 50 Most Beautiful People and photographs that favor her face rather than her athletic performance. *Sexualizing women's athleticism* was another strategy. For example, when Brandi Chastain removed her jersey after scoring the winning goal of the World Cup, commentators called it a "striptease" and deemed her the owner of "the most talked-about breasts in the country" (pp. 12–13). Furthermore, the team was widely referred to as "booters with hooters" (p. 13) in several media sources. Shugart termed a third strategy of sexualization *"vigilant heterosexuality,"* in which the femininity of female athletes and their family lives are foregrounded in the press. For example, popular entertainer David Letterman raved about the soccer team regularly on his late night television show, calling the team "babe city" and its members "soccer mamas" (p. 20). On one show, he had several members of the team appear dressed in nothing but "Late Night" t-shirts. In short, the media coverage of the team was highly charged with a focus on femininity and heterosexuality.

Similarly, Schultz (2005) analyzed the decidedly sexualized media attention surrounding Serena Williams' outfit during the 2002 U.S. Open. Williams was described in the popular press, such as the *London Sunday Times*, as wearing "a body-clinging, faux leather, black cat-suit" (p. 338). The commentary surrounding the outfit widely critiqued the visibility of Williams' body in the outfit;

for example, one remark noted that only a thong came between Williams and her skin-tight apparel. In addition, commentators focused on Williams' sexuality because of the outfit, describing her as "pioneering the bondage look with her choice of garb" (Schultz, 2005, p. 350), and remarking that she looked like "a working girl of a different sort" (p. 350). Schultz (2005) noted the racist overtone of this commentary by contrasting it to similar commentary on Anna Kournikova, whose physical appearance was a frequent topic in the sport media during her career because it is consistent with traditional ideals of white femininity. Williams was said to have a "formidable" backside, whereas Kournikova was said to have a "sensational" one (p. 350). Moreover, although commentary on Kournikova was overtly sexualized, innuendo that she was a prostitute was not common. Female athletes of color, like women of color in general, continue to face racism and racial stereotypes in sport (see Corbett [2001], for an in-depth discussion). And, as Schultz's work demonstrates, in the case of African American female athletes, in particular, hypersexuality is a prominent component of this racism.

The most extreme example of the sexualization of women in sport on a large scale may be the Lingerie Bowl, which has been a pay-per-view alternative to the Super Bowl half-time show since 2004 (Daily News staff, 2008). A full-fledged lingerie league launched in the Fall of 2009 with 10 teams. In 2009, the league's website featured Erin Marie Garrett of the Dallas Desire promising viewers that the league "will feature some of America's most athletic and beautiful women" in 7-on-7 full contact football (www.lingeriebowl. com, 2009). Players, who are actresses and models—not athletes—wear "uniforms" of matching lace-trimmed bras, panties, and garters, and sexualized team names include the Los Angeles Temptation, the Dallas Desire, and the Atlanta Bliss. After the 2006 Lingerie Bowl, a columnist for ign.com, an entertainment website, summed up the experience of at least some, arguably most, male viewers as they watch lingerie football.

> What was really on our minds was whether or not we'd see something pop out! Then, just minutes into the second quarter our prayers were answered! Right where we were standing, on the 50 yard line, all we could hear from the guys was, "Oh $#1T!" Yup: it was quick, but still, it was some boob action. As the game continued we weren't paying any attention to the score; we were too busy watching super hot chicks beating up on each other. (Studio, 2006)

Clearly, lingerie football has very little to do with women playing the sport of football. In contrast to the Lingerie Football League, the Independent Women's Football League is a full-tackle women's football league with over 1,600 actual female athletes dressed in real football uniforms playing on

41 teams across North America. As scholars who pay close attention to media coverage of women's sports, we propose that the visibility in the media of this genuine women's football league and others like it pales in comparison to that of the Lingerie Bowl. Indeed, we suggest women's football does not register on the nation's consciousness at all. Future empirical research should be done to substantiate these perceptions.

In summary, the sexualization of female athletes, as well as females in sport settings, is a common practice. Some sexualization is overt, in which female athletes are depicted provocatively or nude. Other times, the sexualization is subtle and may seem innocuous; for example, a focus on female athletes' physical attractiveness. Taken together, however, current media coverage of female athletes emphasizes their physical appearance and heterosexual appeal while marginalizing their athleticism (Christopherson et al., 2002; Messner et al., 2003; Schultz, 2005; Shugart, 2003). Given that coverage of female sports constitutes less than 10% of sport media, there is little opportunity to view females as strong, skilled, and competitive athletes. Instead, the athleticism and athletic accomplishments of female athletes are obscured by the disproportionate attention paid to their femininity and sexual attractiveness.

Impact of Sexualization of Female Athletes on Viewers

Despite a robust research literature on media coverage of female sports by sport sociologists, there has been very little psychological research on the impact of media images, sexualized or otherwise, of female athletes on viewers' self-perceptions. There is reason to expect that sexualized images of female athletes negatively impact female viewers, given the large body of research documenting the problematic impact of other idealized and sexualized images of women on female viewers' body image (Grabe et al., 2008; Groesz et al., 2002; Holmstrom, 2004). Here, we review the limited body of psychological research on viewers' perceptions of athletes depicted in media, as well as research on viewers' own self-perceptions after exposure to media images of female athletes.

Viewers' Perceptions of Athletes

Knight and Giuliano (2001) examined male and female college students' perceptions of athletes portrayed in the print media that emphasized either physical attractiveness or athleticism. Both female and male participants perceived athletes (both male and female) whose attractiveness received more attention than their athleticism as less talented, less aggressive, and less heroic than athletes whose athleticism received more attention. Participants liked the article that focused on the athlete's attractiveness less than the article that focused on athleticism. Further, male and female participants who read the story emphasizing the female athlete's beauty rated her attractiveness higher than did participants who read the article focusing on her athleticism. A similar pattern was *not* found regarding the attractiveness of the male athlete. This study thus demonstrates that the type of coverage (attractiveness vs. athleticism focus), as well as the gender of the athlete, influenced people's perceptions of the athlete. Importantly, coverage of athletes that focuses on their athleticism is perceived more positively by the audience.

In a similar line of inquiry, Gurung and Chrouser (2007) investigated college women's perceptions of female athletes depicted in a sexually provocative manner as compared to sport attire. Female viewers rated the women in the sexualized images as significantly more attractive, more sexually experienced, more desirable, and more feminine, but less capable, less strong, less intelligent, less determined, and having less self-respect as compared to the sport attire images. In sum, athletes depicted provocatively were objectified by female viewers and considered less capable.

Finally, Parker and Fink (2008) examined female and male college viewers' attitudes toward female basketball players. They found that highly involved viewers, who reported being fans and following women's basketball, had more positive attitudes toward female athletes and their athletic abilities as compared to less involved viewers. In addition, college women had more positive attitudes toward female athletes and rated them as more athletic, aggressive, and respectable (i.e., good leaders, role models) as compared to college men. This work suggests the importance of considering gender as well as individual differences, such as level of interest and level of involvement, in investigating the impact of media on viewers.

To date, most of the research on people's perceptions of athletes has been conducted with men and women who are in late adolescence (college age) or older (exceptions include Daniels, 2009, 2012; Daniels & Wartena, 2011; Heywood & Dworkin, 2003). It is reasonable to expect that the perceptions of younger girls and boys will be similarly affected by the type of media coverage. Existing evidence suggests that performance-focused coverage leads to respect for female athletes' physical skills and abilities, whereas sexualized coverage leads to negative evaluations of athletic competence and a focus on female athletes' physical appearance. Further studies to test these predictions with children and teens are warranted.

Viewers' Self-Perceptions

The previous section reviewed studies on the effect of media coverage on people's perceptions of athletes. Perhaps even more important is the question of how such coverage can affect girls' perceptions of and beliefs about themselves. Thomsen, Bower, and Barnes (2004) examined adolescent girl athletes' reactions to photographs of women and well-known female athletes engaged in athletic activities in women's health, fitness, and sport magazines. In this study, images that explicitly emphasized aesthetic beauty rather than athleticism were used. Responses to images revealed that girls considered many of the women as role models. They compared themselves to these idealized images of adult female athletes and were left feeling "depressed" and "discouraged" because they felt they would never personally look like these women (p. 274). This study illustrates the potentially negative impact of images of female athletes that focus on their physical appearance rather than their athleticism. These images seem to promote self-objectification in teenage girls.

Newer research on media portrayals of female athletes (sexualized vs. performance) has examined both the impact of particular images on viewers' own self-perceptions and viewers' attitudes about female athletes. Daniels (2009) found that teenage girls and college women who viewed sexualized images of female athletes tended to make more self-descriptions about their own physical appearance as compared to girls and women shown images of female athletes performing a sport who, in contrast, were more likely to make self-descriptions about their own physical abilities. In addition, college men who viewed sexualized female athletes tended to make more self-descriptions about their own physical appearance as compared to college men shown images of female athletes performing a sport (Daniels & Wartena, 2009). Thus, sexualized images of female athletes prompted teenage girls, college women, and college men to self-objectify and focus on their own physical appearance.

In the same study, participants were asked to describe the female athletes (sexualized vs. performance) depicted in the photographs they viewed and discuss how the photographs made them feel (Daniels, 2012; Daniels & Wartena, 2011). Among girls' and women's responses to sexualized female athletes, 88% referenced the women's general physical appearance, body shape/ size, and/or weight; for example, her "perfect body." In contrast, responses to images of female athletes performing their sport referenced the women's general physical appearance, body shape or size, and/or weight at a far lesser rate (25%). Instead, performance athlete images elicited responses about the athletes' physical abilities; for example, "great athlete" (67%), and sport intensity; for example, "passion for the game" (72%). Sexualized athlete images evoked less commentary on the athletes' physicality (57%) and far less commentary on the athletes' sport intensity (less than 1%). Moreover, only 16% of the commentary on sexualized athletes' physicality was positive (e.g., "very skilled"), whereas the remainder was either neutral; for example, "sporty," (51%) or negative; for example, "sucks at tennis" (34%). A similar pattern was found among teenage boys' responses to the same photographs (Daniels & Wartena, 2011). In short, sexualized images of female athletes prompted viewers to focus on the athletes' physical appearance instead of their physical abilities, whereas the performance images evoked a focus on athleticism and physical skill. Similarly, participants of audience reception research indicate sexualized images of female athletes are rarely preferred over athletic images, and "sexy images" do not lead to increased interest in or support of women's sports (Kane & Maxwell, 2011).

In summary, studies on viewers' perceptions of athletes portrayed as attractive or sexually provocative in media demonstrate that these athletes are considered less capable and talented than athletes represented in a manner that focuses on their athleticism (Gurung & Chrouser, 2007; Kane & Maxwell, 2011; Knight & Giuliano, 2001). Sexualized images of female athletes seem to prompt a focus on the athlete's, and one's own, physical appearance, whereas performance images elicit a focus on the athlete's, and one's own, athleticism (Daniels, 2009, 2012; Daniels & Wartena, 2009, 2011).

Collectively, these studies demonstrate the negative effects of media images that focus primarily on female athletes' attractiveness, rather than their athleticism. Future research should address whether the sexualization of female athletes negatively affects positive results associated with girls' sport involvement, including increased self-esteem and more favorable body image (e.g., Donaldson & Ronan, 2006; Richman & Shaffer, 2000; Sabo & Veliz, 2008). Explicit interventions, like media literacy training, may be beneficial in sustaining a focus on physical abilities rather than physical appearance. In addition, social activism efforts aimed at increasing girls' sport and physical activity involvement should specifically critique sexualized media imagery of female athletes. The research described above has demonstrated the negative impact of these representations on female viewers. It is time to demand that female athletes be portrayed in media as athletes performing their sports.

More research should also investigate the impact of performance images of female athletes on girls in general, and particularly on girl athletes. In a recent study, female college athletes were asked to participate in a self-presentation photo essay project for younger athletes (Krane et al., 2010). The athletes reported preferences for depicting themselves in ways that displayed their athleticism (e.g., in an athletic pose) or conveyed their psychological strength (e.g., intensity, focus, and confidence). One athlete reported "I wanted to do this type of pose because it is something that you'll see a lot in an actual game" (p. 183). Another athlete stated her photograph conveys the message, "Have no fear. Be strong, determined, and ready to fight for what you want" (p. 186). More empirical research should be conducted to investigate whether performance media images, such as these, can bolster positive outcomes associated with girls' involvement in sport and physical activities.

Positive Impact of Sport Participation on Girls and Young Women

Although the media tends to trivialize female sports, physical activity can be a powerful counterweight to a cultural focus on female sexual attractiveness. Physical activities can be an important tool for teaching young girls to focus on—and honor—what their bodies can do versus what they can look like. Indeed, girls' involvement in sports and physical activities is related to increased physical self-perceptions (e.g., competence, self-worth), self-efficacy, internal locus of control, and instrumentality (i.e., being assertive and self-reliant) (Crocker, Eklund, Kowalski, 2000; Greenleaf, Boyer, & Petrie, 2009; Parsons & Betz, 2001). At the same time, there is some evidence that teen girls who participate in certain sports are at risk for self-objectification. Parsons and Betz (2001) found that college women who were highly involved in high school sports and physical activities and those who were involved in sports that tend to objectify the female body report increased body shame—that is, the potential to feel shame for not meeting cultural standards for the female body. They do not, however, report an increased tendency to monitor their bodies relative to nonathletes. Further research is clearly needed to investigate these patterns. Specifically, longitudinal research is necessary to determine whether participation in particular sports, for example lean sports, *causes* increased self-objectification.

In general, girls as well as boys have the potential to reap psychological, social, physiological, physical, and health benefits from participation in organized, structured, well-run sport programs (Wiese-Bjornstal & LaVoi, 2007). Scholars at the Tucker Center for Research on Girls & Women in Sports have developed an evidence-based model that specifies how to construct optimal sport and physical activity contexts for girls that increase the likelihood of positive youth development (Wiese-Bjornstal & LaVoi, 2007). An optimal sport context is characterized by simultaneously teaching sports skills along with life skills in a safe, fun, supportive, and challenging environment that involves caring relationships, well-trained adult leaders, facilitated and experiential learning, and moderate-to-vigorous physical activity (Perkins & Wechsler, 2009; Wiese-Bjornstal & LaVoi, 2007). In these contexts, positive outcomes for girls are more likely to accrue, but it should be noted that positive outcomes are not an automatic by-product of participation. Exploring all aspects of the optimal sport context model is beyond the scope of this chapter (see Kane & LaVoi, 2007).

In the following section, the psychological and environmental factors related to girls' involvement in sport and physical activities are discussed.

The Development of Girls' Psychological Assets in and through Sport

Involvement in structured physical activity is associated with positive psychological effects among various groups of girls and women. For middle school girls across socioeconomic groups (Barr-Anderson et al., 2007; Weiss, 2008), diverse urban adolescent girls (Pedersen & Seidman, 2004), Latina girls (Borden et al., 2006), and adolescent girls in general (Biddle et al., 2005; Donaldson & Ronan, 2006), participation in structured physical activities results in a host of positive outcomes, including higher levels of self-efficacy, confidence, self-esteem, physical competence and self-worth, character development, and more favorable body esteem. A recent national study found that girls in third to twelfth grade who participate in a team sport are more content with their lives, report a higher quality of life, and have higher self-esteem than do girls not on a sport team (Keane, 2004; Pedersen & Seidman, 2004; Sabo & Veliz, 2008). Further, when girls master physical skills and feel empowered in and through their bodies, positive body image can develop, which can translate into increased self-esteem (Gorely, Holroyd, & Kirk, 2003). Indeed, Richman and Shaffer (2000) found that girls' high school sport participation predicted global self-worth in college through increased self-perceived physical competence, positive body image, and gender-role flexibility.

A meta-analysis of 23 research studies shows that adolescent girls and college women who play sports report more satisfaction with their bodies than do nonathletes, and female high school athletes report fewer disordered eating problems than nonathlete girls (Smolak, Murnen, & Ruble, 2000). However, some female athletes are at risk for developing disordered eating problems, including dancers, girls and women who play "aesthetic sports" (in which bodies are judged as part of the competition, such as figure skating), "lean sports" (in which being slender is believed to be an advantage, such as distance running), and "elite athletes" (who play in professional leagues or compete at national or international events). Level of involvement in sports may also be an important factor in female athletes' body satisfaction. "Highly involved" girls, who report playing three or more sports a year, are more likely to report higher levels of body esteem as compared to girls who are moderately or not involved in sports (Sabo & Veliz, 2008).

Adolescent girls who are involved in sports also show a number of positive behaviors related to sexuality. Compared to adolescent girls who are not involved in sports, girl athletes start having sex later, engage in sex less often, have fewer sex partners, use condoms more often, and get pregnant less often (Erkut & Tracy, 2000; Lehman & Koerner, 2004; Miller, Sabo, Farrell, Barnes,

& Melnick, 1998). Overall, girl athletes engage in less risky sexual behavior and do more to protect their sexual health than do their nonathletic peers. Being involved in sports is related to higher levels of self-efficacy and a functional body orientation, which involves a greater focus on what one's body can do physically, rather than what it looks like (Lehman & Koerner, 2004). Evidence suggests that these factors could help girl athletes make positive decisions about their sexual behaviors and sexual health (Lehman & Koerner, 2004).

Existing research looking at the role of sport involvement in girls' choices about sexuality has not directly investigated *if* and *how* self-objectification is involved. A decreased tendency to self-objectify may partially explain why girl athletes make positive decisions about their sexuality. For example, it is possible that girl athletes are less likely to self-objectify and, thereby, more likely to make positive decisions about their sexual behaviors and sexual health. Future research should investigate this possibility.

Promoting Girls' Involvement in Sport and Physical Activities

Although many positives are associated with girls' involvement in sport and physical activities, girls continue to participate at lower rates than boys (Sabo & Veliz, 2008). Girls in all geographic areas—suburban, urban, and rural—lag behind their male peers' physical activity levels. Existing research suggests that participation is largely shaped by access and opportunities for sport. Underserved girls (i.e., girls of color, girls from low socioeconomic status families, urban and rural girls) face an array of complex and intertwined personal, social, structural, cultural, and societal barriers that make initiating and sustaining sport participation challenging (see LaVoi & Thul, 2009; Wiese-Bjornstal & LaVoi, 2007 for in-depth discussions). Girls of color are less active than their white female peers (Biddle et al., 2005; Crespo, 2005). A recent nationwide study found that whereas 1 in 4 white girls is not involved in organized sports, almost 1 in 2 Asian girls (47%) and more than 1 in 3 Latina and African American girls (36% for each group) are not involved in sports (Sabo & Veliz, 2008). Declines in African-American girls' physical activity from childhood to adolescence are also much greater than their white counterparts (Centers for Disease Control, 2008; Kim et al., 2002).

When girls have opportunities to participate in sports, social support and the creation of a "task-involving climate" created by parents, peers, and coaches are strong predictors of girls' physical activity participation and the accumulation of positive results for them (Neumark-Sztainer, Story, Hannan, & Rex, 2003; Wiese-Bjornstal, 2007). A task-involving climate is characterized by a focus on personal skill improvement, learning skills, positive reinforcement for effort and improvement, cooperation, supportive and warm relationships, perceptions of mistakes as part of the learning process, and an inherent belief in the value and unique role of each individual athlete. Coaches and parents can construct a task-involving climate by placing the primary focus on learning, skill development, enjoyment, and having fun, rather than on comparison to others and winning. This type of coach-created climate is superior in producing more enjoyment, greater satisfaction, prosocial sport behavior ("good sportspersonship"), intrinsically motivated behavior, sustained participation, positive relationships with others in the sport environment, positive self-perceptions and body image, and less anxiety, stress, burnout, and dropout (Galloway, 2004; Raedeke & Smith, 2004; Smith, Fry, Ethington, & Li, 2005; Wiese-Bjornstal, 2007).

Parents and peers occupy unique roles in the creation of a task-involving climate. For parents, encouragement, direct support and facilitation, positive expectations, valuing physical activity, a primary focus on learning and enjoyment (rather than winning), and active role modeling help facilitate sport participation for their daughters (Fredricks & Eccles, 2004; White, 1996). Dimensions of a positive task-involving peer climate include a focus on improvement, relatedness support, and effort rather than intrateam conflict and competition (Vazou, Ntoumanis, & Duda, 2006). Together, social agents—coaches, parents, and peers—in the lives of girls are salient in the psychological flourishing and positive youth development of girls.

Conclusion

In this chapter, we have demonstrated that female athletes and women in sport contexts are frequently sexualized in media (Christopherson et al., 2002; Messner et al., 2003; Schultz, 2005; Shugart, 2003), and this sexualization negatively affects viewers' attitudes toward female athletes (Daniels, 2012; Daniels & Wartena, 2011; Knight & Giuliano, 2001; Gurung & Chrouser, 2007) as well as their own self-perceptions (Daniels, 2009; Thomsen et al., 2004). We contend that the absence and erasure of women in sport, as well as their sexualization, are likely to affect children's and youth's beliefs about the role of women both in sport *and* more generally. Sport and physical activities have the potential to be contexts for girls' positive youth development (Wiese-Bjornstal & LaVoi, 2007). Parents, educators, and concerned citizens must work together to create optimal sport opportunities for girls. And the media need to depict female athletes as athletes, rather than as sex objects. Currently, girls and boys fail to regularly see healthy, active female role models in sport contexts. We need to change the message to girls and women that what their bodies can do is more important than how they look.

References

Amateur Athletic Foundation of Los Angeles, & ESPN. (2001). *Children and sport media.* Los Angeles, CA: Author.

American Psychological Association. (2007). *Report of the APA Task Force on the Sexualization of Girls.* Washington, DC: American Psychological Association. Retrieved from www.apa.org/pi/wpo/sexualization.html

Banet-Weiser, S. (1999). Hoop dream: Professional basketball and the politics of race and gender. *Journal of Sport and Social Issues, 23,* 403–420.

Barr-Anderson, D. J., Young, D. R., Sallis, J. F., Neumark-Sztainer, D. R., Gittelsohn, J., Webber, L., et al. (2007). Structured physical activity and psychosocial correlates in middle-school girls. *Preventive Medicine, 44,* 404–409.

Biddle, S. J. H., Whitehead, S. H., O'Donovan, T. M., & Nevill, M. E. (2005). Correlates of participation in physical activity for adolescent girls: A systematic review of recent literature. *Journal of Physical Activity and Health, 2,* 423–434.

Borden, L. M., Perkins, D. F., Villarruel, F. A., Carleton-Hug, A., Stone, M. R., & Keith, J. G. (2006). Challenges and opportunities to Latino youth development: Increasing meaningful participation in youth development programs. *Hispanic Journal of Behavioral Sciences, 28,* 187–208.

Cahn, S. K. (1994). *Coming on strong: Gender and sexuality in twentieth-century women's sport.* New York: The Free Press.

Centers for Disease Control and Prevention. (2008). *Physical activity and the health of young people.* Retrieved October 15, 2008, from http://www.cdc.gov/healthyyouth/physicalactivity/facts.htm

Christopherson, N., Janning, M., & McConnell, E. D. (2002). Two kicks forward, one kick back: A content analysis of media discourses on the 1999 Women's World Cup Soccer Championship. *Sociology of Sport Journal, 19,* 170–188.

COEDmagazine.com. (2009). *56 insanely hot Indy car grid girls.* (n.d.). Retrieved May 25, 2009, from http://coedmagazine.com/2009/05/21/56-insanely-hot-indy-car-grid-girls/

Corbett, D. R. (2001). Minority women of color: Unpacking racial ideology. In G. L. Cohen (Ed.), *Women in sport: Issues and controversies* (pp. 291–307). Reston, VA: National Association of Girls and Women.

Couturier, L., & Chepko, S. (2001). Separate world, separate lives, separate sporting models. In G. L. Cohen (Ed.), *Women in sport: Issues and controversies* (pp. 57–78). Reston, VA: National Association of Girls and Women.

Crespo, C. J. (2005). Physical activity in minority populations: Overcoming a public health challenge. *President's Council on Physical Fitness and Sports, 6,* 1–8. Retrieved November 7, 2007, from http://www.fitness.gov/Digest-June2005.pdf

Crocker, P. R. E., Eklund, R. C., & Kowalski, K. C. (2000). Children's physical activity and physical self-perceptions. *Journal of Sports Sciences, 18,* 383–394.

Daily News staff. (2008, October 8). *Putting the skin in pigskin, Lingerie Football League to debut in 2009.* Retrieved May 25, 2009, from http://www.nydailynews.com/sports/2008/10/08/2008-10-08_putting_the_skin_in_pigskin_lingerie_foo.html

Daniels, E. A. (2009). Sex objects, athletes, and sexy athletes: How media representations of women athletes can impact adolescent girls and young women. *Journal of Research on Adolescence, 24,* 399–422. doi: 10.1177/0743558409336748

Daniels, E. A. (2012). Sexy versus strong: What girls and women think of female athletes. *Journal of Applied Developmental Psychology, 33,* 79–90. doi:10.1016/j.appdev.2011.12.002

Daniels, E., & Wartena, H. A. (2009, April). *How do I look?: Men's reactions to media representations of women.* Poster presented at the Western Psychological Association Convention, Portland, OR.

Daniels, E.A. & Wartena, H. (2011). Athlete or sex symbol: What boys and men think of media representations of female athletes, *Sex Roles, 65,* 566–579. doi:10.1007/s11199-011-9959-7

Davis, L. R. (1997). *The swimsuit issue and sport: Hegemonic masculinity in Sports Illustrated.* Albany, NY: State University of New York Press.

Donaldson, S. J., & Ronan, K. R. (2006). The effects of sports participation on young adolescents' emotional well-being. *Adolescence, 41,* 369–389.

Erkut, S., & Tracy, A. J. (2000). *Protective effects of sports participation on girls' sexual behavior.* Wellesley, MA: Center for Research on Women.

Field, A. E., Cheung, L., Wolf, A. M., Herzog, D. B., Gortmaker, S. L., & Colditz, G. A. (1999). Exposure to mass media and weight concerns among girls. *Pediatrics, 103,* 54–60.

Fink, J. S., & Kensicki, L. J. (2002). An imperceptible difference: Visual and textual constructions of femininity in *Sports Illustrated* and *Sports Illustrated for Women. Mass Communication & Society, 5,* 317–339.

Fredricks, J. A., & Eccles, J. S. (2004). Parental influences on youth involvement in sports. In M. R. Weiss (Ed.), *Developmental sport and exercise psychology: A lifespan perspective* (pp. 145–164). Morgantown, WV: Fitness Information Technology.

Fredrickson, B. L., & Roberts, T. (1997). Objectification theory: Toward understanding women's lived experiences and mental health risks. *Psychology of Women Quarterly, 21,* 173–206.

Fredrickson, B. L., Roberts, T., Noll, S. M., Quinn, D. M., & Twenge, J. M. (1998). That swimsuit becomes you: Sex differences in self-objectification, restrained eating, and math performance. *Journal of Personality and Social Psychology, 75,* 269–284.

Galloway, M. K. (2004). In the classroom and on the playing field: Lessons from teachers and coaches for cultivating motivation in adolescence (Doctoral dissertation, Stanford University, 2004). *Dissertation Abstracts International, 64,* 3188.

Golokhòv, D. (2008, December 16). *Top 10: Athletes in Playboy.* Retrieved November 9, 2009, from http://www.askmen.com/top_10/celebrity/top-10-athletes-in-playboy.html

Gorely, T., Holroyd, R., & Kirk, D. (2003). Muscularity, the habitus and the social construction of gender: Towards a gender-relevant physical education. *British Journal of Sociology of Education, 24,* 429–448.

Grabe, S., Ward, L. M., & Hyde, J. S. (2008). The role of the media in body image concerns among women: A meta-analysis of experimental and correlational studies. *Psychological Bulletin, 134,* 460–476.

Greenleaf, C., Boyer, E. M., & Petrie, T. A. (2009). High school sport participation and subsequent psychological well-being and physical activity: The mediating influences of body image, physical competence, and instrumentality. *Sex Roles, 61,* 714–726.

Griffin, P. (1998). *Strong women, deep closets.* Champaign, IL: Human Kinetics.

Griffin, P. (2001). Heterosexism, homophobia, and lesbians in sport. In G. L. Cohen (Ed.), *Women in sport: Issues and controversies* (pp. 279–290). Reston, VA: National Association for Girls and Women in Sport.

Groesz, L. M., Levine, M. P., & Murnen, S. K. (2002). The effect of experimental presentation of thin media images on body satisfaction: A meta-analytic review. *International Journal of Eating Disorders, 31,* 1–16.

Gurung, R. A. R., & Chrouser, C. J. (2007). Predicting objectification: Do provocative clothing and observer characteristics matter? *Sex Roles, 57,* 91–99.

Heywood, L., & Dworkin, S. L. (2003). *Built to win: The female athlete as cultural icon.* Minneapolis, MN: University of Minneapolis Press.

Holmstrom, A. J. (2004).The effects of the media on body image: A meta-analysis. *Journal of Broadcasting & Electronic Media, 48,* 196–217.

Kane, M. J. (1996). Media coverage of the post Title IX Athlete: A feminist analysis of sport, gender, and power. *Duke Journal of Gender Law and Policy, 3,* 95–127. Retrieved July 31, 2004, from http://web/lexis-nexis.com/universe/printdoc

Kane, M. J., & LaVoi, N. M. (Eds.). (2007). *The 2007 Tucker Center Research Report, developing physically active girls: An evidence-based multidisciplinary approach.* Minneapolis, MN: Tucker Center for Research on Girls & Women in Sport, University of Minnesota.

Kane, M. J., & Maxwell, H. D. (2011). Expanding the boundaries of sport media research: Using critical theory to explore consumer responses to representations of women's sports. *Journal of Sport Management, 25,* 202–216.

Keane, S. H. (2004). Self-silencing behavior among female high school athletes and non-athletes (Doctoral dissertation, Walden University, 2004). *Dissertation Abstracts International, 64,* 6332.

Kim, Y. S., Glynn, N. W., Kriska, A. M., Barton, B. A., Kronsberg, S. S., Daniels, S. R., et al. (2002). Decline in physical activity in black girls and white girls during adolescence. *The New England Journal of Medicine, 347,* 709–715.

Knight, J. L., & Giuliano, T. A. (2001). He's a Laker; She's a "looker": The consequences of gender-stereotypical portrayals of male and female athletes by the print media. *Sex Roles, 45,* 217–229.

Krane, V., Ross, S. R., Miller, M., Rowse, J. L., Ganoe, K., Andrzejczyk, J. A., & Lucas, C. B. (2010). Power and focus: Self-representation of female college athletes. *Qualitative Research in Sport and Exercise, 2,* 175–195.

LaVoi, N. M., & Thul, C. M. (2009). The 2009 team-up for youth monograph series, *Sports-based youth development for underserved girls.* Oakland, CA: Team Up For Youth.

Lehman, S. J., & Koerner, S. S. (2004). Adolescent women's sport involvement and sexual behavior/health: A process-level investigation. *Journal of Youth and Adolescence, 33,* 443–455.

Lenskyj, H. (1986). *Out of bounds: Women, sport, and sexuality.* Toronto, Canada: Women's Press.

Levine, M. P., Smolak, L., & Hayden, H. (1994). The relation of sociocultural factors to eating attitudes and behaviors among middle school girls. *Journal of Early Adolescence, 14,* 471–490.

McDonald, M. G. (2002). Queering whiteness: The peculiar case of the Women's National Basketball Association. *Sociological Perspectives, 45,* 379–396.

McKinley, N. M. (1999). Women and objectified body consciousness: Mothers' and daughters' body experience in cultural, developmental, and familial context. *Developmental Psychology, 35,* 760–769.

McKinley, N. M., & Hyde, J. S. (1996). The Objectified Body Consciousness Scale: Development and validation. *Psychology of Women Quarterly, 20,* 181–215.

Messner, M. A., & Cooky, C. (2010). *Gender in televised sports: News and highlights shows, 1989–2009.* Los Angeles: Center for Feminist Research, University of Southern California.

Messner, M. A., Duncan, M. C., & Cooky, C. (2003). Silence, sports bras, and wrestling porn. *Journal of Sport & Social Issues, 27,* 38–51.

Miller, T. (2001). *Sportsex.* Philadelphia, PA: Temple University Press.

Miller, K. E., Sabo, D. F., Farrell, M. P., Barnes, G. M., & Melnick, M. J. (1998). Athletic participation and sexual behavior in adolescents: The different worlds of boys and girls. *Journal of Health and Social Behavior, 39,* 108–123.

Muehlenkamp, J. J., Swanson, J. D., & Brausch, A. M. (2005). Self-objectification, risk taking, and self-harm in college women. *Psychology of Women Quarterly, 29,* 24–32.

Neumark-Stzainer, D., Story, M., Hannan, P. J., & Rex, J. (2003). New moves: A school-based obesity prevention program for adolescent girls. *Preventive Medicine, 37,* 41–51.

Parker, H. M., & Fink, J. S. (2008). The effect of sport commentator framing on viewer attitudes. *Sex Roles, 58,* 116–126.

Parsons, E. M., & Betz, N. E. (2001). The relationship of participation in sports and physical activity to body objectification, instrumentality, and locus of control among young women. *Psychology of Women, 25,* 209–222.

Pedersen, S., & Seidman, E. (2004). Team sports achievement and self-esteem development among urban adolescent girls. *Psychology of Women Quarterly, 28,* 412–422.

Pedersen, P. M., & Whisenant, W. A. (2003). Examining stereotypical written and photographic reporting on the sports page: An analysis of newspaper coverage of interscholastic athletics. *Women in Sport and Physical Activity Journal, 12,* 67–86.

Perkins, D., & Wechsler, C. (2009). *Quality components of sports-based youth development programs.* Retrieved June 8, 2009, from http://www.up2us.org/uploads/reports/Up2Us%20 Research/Quality%20Components%20of%20SBYD.pdf

Popcrunch. (2008, February 6). *The 50 hottest women of sports.* Retrieved May 25, 2009, from http://www.popcrunch.com/the-50-hottest-women-of-sports-1-10/

Rader, B. G. (2004). *American sports: From the age of folk games to the age of televised sports* (5th ed.). Upper Saddle River, NJ: Prentice Hall.

Raedeke, T. D., & Smith, A. L. (2004). Coping resources and athlete burnout: An examination of stress mediated and moderation hypothesis. *Journal of Sport & Exercise Psychology, 26,* 525–541.

Richman, E. L., & Shaffer, D. R. (2000). "If you let me play sports:" How might sport participation influence the self-esteem of adolescent females? *Psychology of Women Quarterly, 24,* 189–1999.

Ryan, S. (2008, May 4). Banking on beauty: Trying to expand fan base by marketing its players, the WNBA for the first time offers rookies lessons in fashion and makeup. *Chicago Tribune.* Retrieved May 16, 2009, from http://archives.chicagotribune.com/2008/ may/04/sports/chi-04- wnbamay04

Sabo, D., & Veliz, P. (2008). *Go out and play: Youth sports in America executive summary.* East Meadow, NY: Women's Sport Foundation.

Schultz, J. (2005). Reading the catsuit: Serena Williams and the production of blackness at the 2002 U.S. Open. *Journal of Sport & Social Issues, 29,* 338–357.

Shugart, H. A. (2003). She shoots, she scores: Mediated constructions of contemporary female athletes in coverage of the 1999 U.S. Women's Soccer team. *Western Journal of Communication, 67,* 1–31.

Smith, S. L., Fry, M. D., Ethington, C. A., & Li, Y. (2005). The effect of female athletes' perceptions of their coaches' behaviors on their perceptions of motivational climate. *Journal of Applied Sport Psychology, 17,* 170–177.

Smolak, L., Murnen, S. K., & Ruble, A. E. (2000). Female athletes and eating problems: A meta-analysis. *International Journal of Eating Disorders, 27,* 371–380.

Sports Illustrated [product review]. (n.d.). Retrieved June 1, 2009, from http://www.amazon. com/Sports-Illustrated-1-year/dp/B00005R8BG/ref=sr_1_1?ie=UTF8&s=magazines& qid=1243018392&sr=1-1

Steele, J. R., & Brown, J. D. (1995). Adolescent room culture: Studying media in the context of everyday life. *Journal of Youth and Adolescence, 24,* 551–575.

Stice, E. (2002). Risk and maintenance factors for eating pathology: A meta-analytic review. *Psychological Bulletin, 128,* 825–848.

Stice, E., & Shaw, H. E. (2002). Role of body dissatisfaction in the onset and maintenance of eating pathology: A synthesis of research findings. *Journal of Psychosomatic Research, 53,* 985–993.

Studio, G. (2006, February 27). *Babes of Lingerie Bowl III: Ditchin' the Superbowl to watch scantily-clad models play full-tackle. Oh damn…*Retrieved May 25, 2009, from http:// stars.ign.com/articles/692/692215p1.html

Thomsen, S. R., Bower, D. W., & Barnes, M. D. (2004). Photographic images in women's health, fitness, and sports magazines and the physical self-concept of a group of adolescent female volleyball players. *Journal of Sport and Social Issues, 28,* 266–283.

Tiggemann, M., & Lynch, J. E. (2001). Body image across the lifespan in adult women: The role of self-objectification. *Developmental Psychology, 37,* 243–253.

Traina, J. (2009, May 22). *The real greatest spectacle in racing.* Retrieved May 22, 2009, from http://sportsillustrated.cnn.com/2009/extramustard/hotclicks/05/22/lucy-pinder-joha-cena-celebrities-at-lakers-game/index.html

Vazou, S., Ntoumanis, N., & Duda, J. L. (2006). Predicting young athletes' motivational indices as a function of the perceptions of the coach and peer created climate. *Psychology of Sport and Exercise, 7,* 215–233.

Vincent, J., Imwold, C., Johnson, J. T., & Massey, D. (2003). Newspaper coverage of female athletes competing in selected sports in the 1996 Centennial Olympic Games: The more things change the more they stay the same. *Women in Sport and Physical Activity Journal, 12,* 1–21.

Ward, L. M., & Harrison, K. (2005). The impact of media use on girls' beliefs about gender roles, their bodies, and sexual relationships: A research synthesis. In E. Cole, & J. H. Daniel (Eds.), *Featuring females: Feminist analyses of media* (pp. 3–23). Washington, DC: American Psychological Association.

Weiss, M. R. (2008). 2007 C. H. McCloy Lecture: "Field of dreams": Sport as a context for youth development. *Research Quarterly for Exercise and Sport, 79*(4), 434–449.

White, S. A. (1996). Goal orientation and perceptions of the motivational climate initiated by parents. *Pediatric Exercise Science, 8,* 122–129.

Wiese-Bjornstal, D. M. (2007). Psychological dimensions of girls' physical activity participation. In M. J. Kane, & N. M. LaVoi (Eds.), *The 2007 Tucker Center research report, Developing physically active girls: An evidence-based multidisciplinary approach* (pp. 7–27). Minneapolis, MN: Tucker Center for Research on Girls & Women in Sport, University of Minnesota.

Wiese-Bjornstal, D. M., & LaVoi, N. M. (2007). Girls' physical activity participation: Recommendations for best practices, programs, policies, and future research. In M. J. Kane, & N. M. LaVoi (Eds.), *The 2007 Tucker Center research report, Developing physically active girls: An evidence-based multidisciplinary approach* (pp. 63–90). Minneapolis, MN: Tucker Center for Research on Girls & Women in Sport, University of Minnesota.

5

It's Bad For Us Too

How the Sexualization of Girls Impacts the Sexuality of Boys, Men, and Women

DEBORAH L. TOLMAN

Emerging evidence suggests that the sexualization of girls has particular negative consequences on girls' development into healthy adult sexuality (see Lamb, 2013; Chapter 14, this volume; see also Hatch, 2011; Impett, Schooler, & Tolman, 2006; Tolman, 2000; Ward, 2002; Ward & Rivadeneyra, 1999; Wesley, 2009; Zurbriggen & Morgan, 2006). Although it creates problems for girls, it may be less obvious that the sexualization of girls impacts the sexuality of women, men, and boys. In this chapter, I present evidence for and theorize how the sexualization of girls is indeed bad for boys', men's, and women's sexuality as well. The sexual objectification of women itself has been reshaped by the saturation of society in sexualized images of girls. From a developmental perspective, imposing adult sexuality onto girls has a boomerang effect on men's and boys' expectations about what women and their sexuality is or should be like, and on women's conceptions of, beliefs about, and experiences of their own sexuality.

The chapter is separated into three sections. The first section is dedicated to the impact of the sexualization of girls on boys' sexuality development and men's sexuality.[1] The second section will cover the impact on adult women's sexuality. The third and final section addresses a striking recent phenomenon and the subject of vociferous debate in both popular culture and academia in response to the APA Task Force Report (2007): the question of whether the sexualization of girls may be a route to positive sexuality and sexual empowerment for young women (Else-Quest & Hyde, 2009; Lerum & Dworkin, 2009a,b; Liss, Erchull, & Ramsey, 2011; Vanwesenbeek, 2009).

Impact on Boys and Men

The sexualization of girls and women is endemic in the (hetero)sexual social-ization of boys and in the subsequent sexuality of men. One of the definitions of sexualization outlined in the Report is sexual objectification. The sexualiza-tion of girls has affected the ways in which women are sexually objectified, bootstrapping girlhood into the forms that women's sexual objectification now takes, what Gail Dines (2009) has called the "childification" of women in these portrayals. In still images, videos, and movies, the imposition of adult sexuality onto girls serves to normalize it, diminishing the sense of shock or concern that such images might have generated in the past. She also notes that such images are more pervasive with the technological development of computer-generated images of sexualized girls in pornography, a work-around to laws that prevent those under 18 from participating in its production. These technologies can produce images of "barely legal" models, all of which are disseminated as what "real women" are or should be like (see also Attwood, 2009). I will review the media research on how the sexualization of girls affects heterosexual male sexuality and its development, and then consider research informing our understanding of its impact on adult men's sexuality and intimate relationships.

Impact on Boys' and Men's Media: Sexualization of Girls in Old and New Technologies

The confluence of the sexualization of girls and its impact on the sexual objec-tification of women occurs in sexualized media aimed at boys and men, as both producing and providing contexts for the development of male sexuality and its expression. The pervasiveness and popularity of these sexually saturated genres continues to expand, in form and accessibility, in media comprised of print, network and cable television, movies, and new more interactive technolo-gies, including the Internet and video gaming. Dines (2009) analyzes how the sexualization of girls is part and parcel of the current landscape of pornography in multiple venues, including the Internet and magazines (in particular "lad mags" such as *Maxim*), but such images are no longer confined to the admit-tedly ineffectively regulated arena of official pornography. The constant objec-tification of girl celebrities as normative is enabled and fueled as a successful corporate strategy (Kim, 2011). Daniel and Wartena (2011) found that when adolescent boys were shown nonsexualized performance images of female ath-letes, they made instrumental evaluations. However, when shown sexualized images of female atheletes (and sexualized images of nonathletes), they focused on appearance and attractiveness; that is, objectified appraisals were induced.

What has been called the "pornification" of mainstream culture is a disturbing trend that not only increases sexualized images of girls and women geometrically (i.e., Hatton & Trautner, 2011) but also normalizes the sexualization of girls and generates unreal and unattainable notions of "normal" women (see also Coy & Horvath, 2011; Dines, 2009; Jensen, 2007; Paul, 2005). That is, the "spilling" of pornographic imagery out of formalized pornography into mainstream venues, such as music videos, cable television, and iPhone apps (Diaz, 2009), suggests the importance of considering media effects research on pornography as salient to everyday interactions with a broad array of media.

Video games are an especially problematic new arena in which the sexual objectification of women has been documented. Research has demonstrated that virtually the only way women are portrayed in these games is as sex objects, even in the rare instance that a woman is the heroine or star of the game (Burgess, Stermer, & Burgess, 2007). The interplay between sexualization and violence is particularly disturbing in this medium; because the user of the game is actually "doing" (virtually) the actions that are being portrayed, the interactive quality is cause for concern (Dill & Dill, 1998; Dill & Thill, 2007). Yao, Mahood, and Linz (2010), Dill and Dill (1998), and Dietz (1998) found that video games are powerful agents of socialization and that male participants who played a sexually explicit versus a nonsexual game were much more likely to view and treat women as sex objects. In particular, Dill and Dill (1998) found that a preponderance of games, especially those most popular with younger teenage males, emphasizes masculinity as tied to power, dominance, and aggression over women, coupled with images of femininity as tied to inferiority, sexual objectification, and enjoyment of or attraction to male sexual aggression. Although there is not yet an extensive empirical literature, this growing body of evidence regarding relatively mild or "soft" portrayals of female objectification, as in video games, constitutes cause for concern (Ezzell, 2009).

Although boys (and girls) are exposed to images of men "consuming" women's bodies as objects of their desire in G-rated movies (Martin & Kazyak, 2009), they are bombarded as never before with sexualized images of girls and women on the Internet (Bragg, Buckingham, Russell, & Willett, 2011). This pervasiveness has produced a new phenomenon: Boys (and girls) as young as 10 years old are inadvertently but regularly exposed to pornographic images and video (Davies, 2004; Greenfield, 2004). In addition, ubiquitous pornographic images on the Internet—both pretend and real— have yielded more intentional viewing (e.g., in 2006, 90% of boys and 70% of girls aged 13 and 14 had accessed sexually explicit media at least once in the previous year; cited in Ezzell [2009]). The phenomenon of tweens and young teens viewing these images is not limited to individuals seeking out this content by themselves. Young people's exposure is also on the rise due to the skyrocketing popularity of Internet-based social networking (such as

Facebook, Tumblr, Twitter, and MySpace), which has become a regular part of boys' and girls' everyday lives. The insidious effects of this daily dosage of sexualized images, constituting "business as usual," is that it both normalizes and numbs. In the context of such networks, young people construct components of this sexualized environments themselves (Greenfield, 2004), posting pictures of sexed-up girls and youthful-looking sexy women depicted as filled with desire for the young men who are looking at them. Constant interactive engagement with such portraits may be yielding an inadvertent and problematic sex education for boys (and girls).

There is no doubt that viewing pornography is part of the informal (and often only) sexuality education of the vast majority of boys, who have ever-easier access to these ever-younger sexually objectified females. Research demonstrates that some young men who watch pornography begin to derive sexual pleasure *only* from viewing pornography and from sexually objectifying women (Paul, 2005; see also Kimmel, 2008). Paul (2005) observed that the pervasiveness of more violent and humiliating pornography not only creates specific conditions for individual men to require an intensified level of sexual objectification but also infuses "enabling conditions" for male violence against girls and women (see also Attwood, 2005b; Garner, 2012). In what ways might adolescent boys' easier access to and likely increased use of such pornography to facilitate masturbation be shaping the sexuality development of boys and young men?

Research into this phenomenon has documented negative impacts with younger men, including unreal expectations of women's desires and behaviors, scripts to enable "breaking" women's resistance, intensification of sexual objectification of women, seeing sex with partners as boring, habituation and desensitization, dehumanization, and normalization of aggressive sexuality (Attwood, 2005b; Jensen, 2007; Paul, 2005; Purcell & Zurbriggen, 2013; Chapter 8, this volume; Vaes, Paladino, & Puvia, 2011). Linz, Donnerstein, and Penrod (1988) established the desensitization effects of sexually degrading explicit and nonexplicit films on beliefs about rape and the sexual objectification of women. The notion that "the more extreme, the more interesting the depiction is" is perpetuated by YouTube and the many vehicles outside of the official pornography industry that are unregulated and possibly unregulatable, in which such portrayals are pervasive.

Impact on Male Sexuality and Intimate Relationships

Objectifying another person is premised on the absence of empathy (Herman, 1992). A number of researchers have described how losing or not developing the capacity to empathize is problematic for, and undermining of, relationship building and maintenance (Kimmel, 2006; Kindlon & Thompson, 1999), which diminishes the humanity of boys and men themselves (Brooks, 1995). Studies of adult men's sexuality and difficulties with intimacy and in intimate relationships, and with younger men's interactions with and attitudes about young women as sexual and romantic partners, are beginning to suggest such patterns (Burn & Ward, 2005; England, Shafer, & Fogarty, 2007; Loftus, 2002; Weaver, Masland, & Zillmann, 1984), and research suggests these patterns may differ by race and class (i.e., Cox, 2009; Stephens & Phillips, 2003; Weekes, 2002). There is evidence that men who are exposed to soft core porn or mainstream sexualized images of girls are more likely to find their own partners less attractive and intimacy more difficult (Kenrick & Gutierrez, 1980; Schooler & Ward, 2006). Several experimental studies have shown that exposure to pornography leads men to indicate less satisfaction with their intimate partners' attractiveness, sexual performance, and level of affection and to express greater desire for sex without emotional involvement (Zillmann & Bryant, 1988). The infusing of the sexualization of girls into pornography is likely to intensify these reactions and expectations.

One of the central ways that boys and men establish and maintain masculinity is through the sexual objectification of women. The pressure to prove manhood begins in earnest in puberty (Pleck, Sonenstein, & Ku, 1993; Tolman, 2006; Tolman, Spencer, Rosen-Reynoso, & Porche, 2003), and the closest targets are the girls around them (Muhanguzi, Bennett, & Muhanguzi, 2011; Quinn, 2002). If boys are engaging with more and more mainstreamed and violent formal and informal pornography at younger ages through more interactive media, such sources may be how boys are learning sexual scripts and what is sexually exciting. Unreal portrayals of girls being sexually ravenous and ready at all times, who have bodies that are physically impossible to achieve or maintain in terms of the size and look of sexual parts, thinness, and looking perennially young, without comparable exposure to other images of girls and women, may be creating expectations and "sexual maps" that are not viable in real relationships. The growing phenomenon of boys and young men taping or web casting sexual assaults on women (i.e., Dobbin, 2008; see also Ezzell, 2009), reflecting the sense of normalization that is surrounding these behaviors, also raises the specter of spectatoring—are boys learning to watch rather than to experience their sexuality? Is their sexual experience about sexual feelings, or is it becoming intertwined with an increasing need to feel in control in a world that feels more and more out of control?

Kimmel (2008) observes how the sexual objectification of young women has been normalized for young men in what they do, as well as in what they see. In the guise of bonding, Kimmel found that young men are working hard to prove their masculinity and heterosexuality to themselves and one another. He recounts how young men sexualize and objectify young women as a group activity (see also Tolman et al., 2003), characterized by intensified expressions of aggression and violence that bode poorly for the development of intimacy, vulnerability, or mutuality with women as intimate and sexual partners into adulthood (Burn & Ward, 2005; Kimmel, 2008). Stombler (1994) recorded such behavior as fundamental to fraternity life. As Levy (2005) points out, women's collusion or participation in this process may yield more attributions of sexuality to women's behaviors than intended and render dating a context in which men may oversexualize women (Lindgren, Shoda & George, 2007; Rudman, & Borgida, 1995). The antithetical adherence to a strong sexual double standard by both men and women, even as women are incited by ostensibly "normal" circumstances to appear "slutty" or "pornified" (Coy & Garner 2010; Levy, 2005; Sweeney, 2008; Tolman, 2012; see below), may in fact make pathways to healthy adult sexuality ever more obscure, confusing, and littered with obstacles for young men (O'Sullivan & Majerovich, 2008).

There is some research indicating that young men report their wish for women to be the initiators in sexual and relational encounters, to share the "burden" of risk of rejection with women (Dworkin & O'Sullivan, 2007), rather than have women be only objects of their desire. However, at the same time, there is ample evidence that young women are also held accountable to a standard of femininity that reserves an ironically safer place for them as appealing only if they are not overly aggressive initiators of sexual interactions (McRobbie, 2009). The dual desire of young men to have more egalitarian scripts regarding initiation (and risk of rejection) with persistent pressure to treat young women as sexual objects may be confusing and undermine intimacy for both men and women (Bogle, 2008; Garner, 2012; Levy, 2005).

Impact on Adult Women

The sexualization of girls means that the impetus to be sexually attractive and desirable, to become a "good" sexual object, exerts a shaping force long before adult sexuality emerges. It also means that sexual objectification itself is looking younger. Women are not socialized to embrace their sexuality as part of themselves, but to be "good girls" (who grow up to be "good women"), who are not supposed to have strong sexual feelings, needs, or wishes of their own. In fact, these two dimensions of female sexual socialization are intertwined, as objects do not have feelings (Tolman & Debold, 1993). I will review two arenas of effects: the impact of the "youthification" of female sexual desirability on women, and the impact of being socialized as an increasingly "youthified" sexual object rather than as a mature sexual being on sexual functioning and on negotiating sexuality in heterosexual relationships. I will then illuminate how these impacts are exploited with the example of the fitness industry, creating and then relieving while further complicating the pressure to stay (and equate) young, "healthy," and attractive.

Youthification of Female Sexual Desirability

The sexualization of girls is problematic for girls on many fronts, as this book and the Report attest, including inappropriately imposing adult sexuality on them. The inappropriate sexuality in the case of adult women, however, is the "youthification" of female sexuality, the pervasiveness and cultural imposition of a youthful ideal of beauty (sexual appeal) and also the sexualization of young female bodies as a narrow ideal. In an era when young and younger is the new sexier and sexier, aging itself becomes a risk, not because of an increase in sexual dysfunction, but because of exclusion from the category of sexually attractive (Tasker & Negra, 2007). Youthification of sexual attractiveness poses unnatural and unattainable limits on available images and embodiments for women as they inevitably age. Women being fearful that getting older disqualifies them from being sexually appealing (to some men) may not be groundless. Studies demonstrate that exposure to pornography led to some men's diminished interest in their real-life partners and unrealistic expectations for their partners' appearance and sexual behavior (i.e., Kenrick & Gutierrez, 1980; see also Verhulst, 2010). The "youthification" of sexual objectification as an effect of the sexualization of girls (i.e., Graff, Murnen, & Smolak, 2012) intensifies and imparts another dimension to women's anxiety about aging and having a thin, youthful-looking body (Dittmar & Howard, 2004).

Middle-age and older women, whose naturally aging bodies contrast more and more with the omnipresence of young "sexy" bodies, have become vulnerable target consumer groups for many cosmetic surgeries designed to make their bodies look sexier by making them look younger, eliminating and undoing the aging process. Cosmetic surgeries, as a new option for achieving that forever-younger sexy body, have become normalized through reality makeover shows (Banet-Weiser & Portwood-Stacer, 2006), although in actual reality, such surgery is accessible only to a privileged few who can afford extraordinarily expensive procedures not covered by insurance. Data from the American Society of Plastic Surgeons show that common procedures designed to keep women's bodies looking young and sexually attractive have been steadily increasing. Between 2000 and 2005, annual rates of Botox injections rose from roughly three-quarters of a million to almost 4 million, amounting to a 388% increase. In the same 5-year period, there was also a 115% increase in tummy tucks annually and a 283% increase in buttock lifts (American Society of Plastic Surgeons, 2006b, cited in the Report). Evidence that these procedures reflect adult women's attempts and leveraged financial ability to retain a sexy young body is apparent in the age differentials for these procedures: The rates for women 35–50 years of age who receive breast lifts, buttock lifts, tummy tucks, and liposuction are approximately double those of women 19–34 years of age (American Society of Plastic Surgeons, 2006a, cited in the Report). These surgeries are not medically indicated, can have negative medical side effects, and can even be fatal (Chalker, 2009). Some of these procedures actually reduce sexual sensations and the ability to express emotions (i.e., breast and Botox procedures) (Braun, 2010).

The notion of a young and sexy female body has spread to the genitals themselves, as in the recent emergence of "vaginal rejuvenation" and a new industry of other female cosmetic genital surgeries, such as labiaplasty (the cutting back of what are deemed "overly large" labia), which are solely for aesthetics and that promise more beautiful, tighter, and "more appealing" genitals (Braun, 2005, 2010; Tiefer, 2008). Women who have received cosmetic labiaplasty range in age from early teens (requests as young as 10) through to 50s or 60s, with those in their 20s and 30s predominating (cited in Braun, 2010). These surgeries have no established medical indications or regulations and can produce (an underreported) lack of sensation and pain. Risks are also underreported, and outcome reports have been problematized as scientifically unsound and conducted more as consumer satisfaction than clinical outcome surveys (Liao et al., 2007, cited in Braun, 2010).

Aging female bodies are not the only ones left out of the category of "sexually attractive/desirable woman," which has become more exclusionary, marginalizing, and obfuscating, pushing and leaving out large numbers of other women who do not look young, supple, girlish, or white and heterosexual (i.e., elderly [Loe, 2004], fat [Levy, 2005], disabled [Gill, 2008; Rousso, 1994], lesbian [Hill & Fischer, 2008], women of color [Gill, 2008; Ward, 2004]). A very particular type of young, thin, and highly sexualized celebrity African American and Latina woman peppers the cultural visual landscape (Stephens & Phillips, 2003; Ward, Hansbrough & Walker, 2005). However, these primarily young, thin, and light-skinned women's bodies do not represent the bodies of most African American and Latina women (Ward & Rivadeneyra, 2002). Several analyses have suggested that being excluded from the category of "object of male sexual desire" in society, including being older, larger, darker, disabled, or not fitting into bodily conventions of sexy or attractive, could be a "protective" factor for those women (Gill, 2009; McRobbie, 2009; Tolman, 2002), but the denial of this aspect of one's humanity, including for those who derive esteem or pleasure from being admired, could have other negative consequences.

Impact on Women's Sexual Relationships and Sexual Functioning

Sexualization can induce negative feelings in girls about their bodies in adolescence, which ultimately may lead to sexual problems in adulthood

(Graham, Saunders, Milhausen, & McBride, 2004; Wiederman, 2000). Some studies indicate that women with high body dissatisfaction engage in less sexual activity and are especially apprehensive about sexual situations in which their bodies can be seen; conversely, women who feel more positively about and comfortable with their bodies are more comfortable with their own sexual feelings (Ackard, Kearney-Cooke, & Peterson, 2000; Trapnell, Meston, & Gorzalka, 1997; Wiederman, 2000). Women who report more body dissatisfaction report a later onset of masturbation (Wiederman & Pryor, 1997) and are less likely to receive (but not to perform) oral sex (Wiederman & Hurst, 1998). Schooler, Ward, Merriwether, and Caruthers (2005) found that greater levels of body discomfort and body self-consciousness each predicted lower levels of sexual assertiveness, sexual experience, and condom use self-efficacy, as well as higher levels of sexual risk-taking. When self-objectification was experimentally induced in one study, women reported decreased interest in the physical aspects of sex (Roberts & Gettman, 2004). Cosmetic surgeries for "vaginal rejuvenation" may be contributing to physiological sexual problems (Braun, 2010; Tiefer, 2008).

Such findings demonstrate that the interplay between being sexualized as girls and socialized into sexual objects may inhibit women's ability to advocate for, or even acknowledge, their own sexual feelings or pleasure in adulthood. A woman who has been socialized to separate from her experiences of sexual arousal and desire may find it difficult to be aware of her desires, assert her desires, or feel entitled to satisfaction in sexual situations (Brotto, Heiman, & Tolman, 2009). Such sociocultural ideas of women's sexual attractiveness predict their intentions regarding and acceptance of sexualizing behavior, resulting in a lack of subjective experience of their own sexuality (Nowatzki & Morry, 2009). Empirical evidence that young women do opt to let events unfold based on their (male) partner's wants and interests supports these concerns (Cotton, Mills, Succop, Biro, & Rosenthal, 2004; Morgan & Zurbriggen, 2007). The historical hypersexualization of African American girls and women (Collins, 2000; hooks, 1992), recently intensified in the media (Ward et al., 2005), results in African American young women's not feeling entitled to protection from sexually transmitted infections and pregnancy or to sexual pleasure (Burson, 1998; Belgrave, Van Oss Marin, & Chambers, 2000).

There is recent evidence that sexual objectification has negative impacts on women's sexual functioning. Sanchez and Kiefer (2007) found that body shame in women was more strongly linked to greater sexual problems than in men, including lower sexual arousability, lower ability to reach orgasm, and having less pleasure from physical intimacy, which was mediated by sexual self-consciousness, regardless of relationship status or age. Donaghue (2009) found negative implications of body dissatisfaction for women's sexual self-schemas. Yamamiya, Cash, and Thompson (2006) found that women feeling bad about their bodies during sex with a partner was associated with lower sexual self-efficacy, more ambivalence in sexual decision making, and more emotional disengagement. Another study found that self-objectification was related to self-consciousness during sexual activity and decreased sexual functioning via body shame and appearance anxiety for women, with women in an exclusive relationship reporting relatively less self-consciousness during sexual activity (Steer & Tiggemann, 2008; see also Aubrey, 2006; Sanchez & Broccoli, 2008). Focusing attention during sexual encounters on how one looks rather than on how one feels can also lead to diminished sexual pleasure (Wiederman, 2000, 2001).

"Moving Targets": Exploitation of the Impact on Women's Sexuality

The sexualization of girls and the ensuing "youthified" sexual objectification of women has worked its way into the multibillion-dollar fitness industry for women by subtly co-opting sexualizing activities, preying on women's latest anxieties about being sexually attractive or "good enough" sexual objects, and on women's disconnection from their bodies as a way to sell. By using the language of "empowerment" while obfuscating yet exploiting its sexualizing associations, this fitness fad is exemplified by the promotion of strip tease as exercise, performing fitness activities in stiletto heels, and the immense popularity of pole dancing as a route to fitness (i.e., Pilates "on the pole," Dunn-Camp [2007]; Donoghue & Kurz [2011]).

In an interview study in which Whitehead and Kurz (2009) identified ways that young women make sense of pole dancing, they found that embracing it as a "fun" fitness activity was predicated on distancing the activity from its associations with unwanted or "dirty" sexual objectification and from women who pole dance to make money as sexual objects for male customers. However, their participation in a practice of sexual objectification, divorced from women's sexual feelings or pleasure, is premised on their explicit denial of the origins of the practice in sex work. If women must distance themselves from the "dirty" associations they describe about "real" pole dancing, then why pole dance for fitness rather than engage in other bodily practices as a source of personal power? The women said that they felt what their instructors promised, empowered, "amazing," and youthful but only by desexualizing and not experiencing this practice as sexual. The elephant in the room is the pole itself.

Pole dancing as a physical fitness activity underscores and reifies how *looking* youthfully sexy trumps *feeling* sexy or even sexual, while ironically taking advantage of the disconnection that so many women experience from their bodies in the wake of their sexual socialization and the sexualization of girls. If pole dancing were a route to sexual empowerment for women themselves, shouldn't there be directions for how to use the pole for women's own sexual pleasure?

Impact on Young Women: Sexual Objectification as Sexual Empowerment?

One current public discussion that has been linked to the sexualization of girls is that it could be a positive reflection of a new acceptance of young women's sexuality: that young women and society have transcended the sexual double standard that denies active female sexuality (Lerum & Dworkin, 2009a, 2009b). Indeed, in recent and frequent depictions of young women, their sexuality is everywhere. In advertisements, in movies, on television (network as well as cable and especially in the guise of "reality" TV), they appear to flaunt their bodies by choice to show off their unabashed sexuality; coy flirtation has given way to in-your-face sexy. Young women voluntarily shaking booty and flashing waxed privates, laughing along with the admiring male crowds captured on reality programs (such as the wildly successful franchise *Girls Gone Wild*) could be interpreted as a new day dawning for young women's sexuality. It has been asserted that women's sexual agency—sexual assertiveness, taking the initiative, shedding a demure seductive look for portrayals of sexual voraciousness more reminiscent of their male counterparts than their female foremothers, say and know what they want as much as the next guy—is the new expected norm for young women and that it is synonymous with sexual empowerment (Gill, 2008; Lerum & Dworkin, 2009a, 2009b; Peterson, 2010). In this final section, I will review the relevant literature and provide a critical lens for approaching this issue.

Recent Research: Complicating Pictures of Empowerment with the Objectification of Women's Sexual Agency

The most recent research suggests that young women continue to be negatively affected by sexualized portrayals of young, lithe women, in particular leading them not to feelings of sexual empowerment but to more constrained and stereotypical notions about gender roles and sexual roles—that is, that women are sexual objects (Smolak & Murnen, 2012; Ward, 2002; Zurbriggen & Morgan, 2006). Ward and Averitt (2005) reported that heavier reading of popular men's magazines and stronger identification with popular male TV characters was associated with undergraduate (male and female) virgins' expectation that their first experience with sexual intercourse would be more negative. Among undergraduate women, more frequent viewing of reality dating television programs was correlated with greater acceptance of a sexual double standard and the belief that dating is a game and that men and women are adversaries (Zurbriggen & Morgan, 2006; see also Ward, 2002). Roberts and Gettman (2004) found that after exposure to objectifying words found on magazine covers, young women expressed reduced interest in sexual relationships. Young women have been found to have ambivalent and contradictory responses to viewing pornography, for instance disliking it but finding it sexually arousing (Ciclitira, 2004).

Even given this evidence that the sexual double standard still "operates" to organize young women's sexuality, the power and ubiquity of a sense that young women are now unabashed and unadulterated in their sexual aggression requires attention. I suggest that it has become more difficult than ever to analyze these questions, *as young women's sexual agency itself has been objectified* (Tolman, 2012). That is, rather than sexual agency being anchored in women knowing what they feel and acting on it, it is now the latest command performance: to appear to have sexual agency. This phenomenon has occurred at the same time in images of sexy and sexual young women and in young women's engagement with their own sexuality. This perspective is supported by the work of communications researchers, who have identified how new images of women's sexual agency are used in advertising (Gill, 2008; McRobbie, 2009). Although such research does not investigate the impact of media, it does provide avenues for reading "between the lines" of the proliferation of images of sexy, assertive young women.

These researchers observe how fashion, consumerism, bodily pleasure, and sexuality are talked about and portrayed in order to crystallize women into a new market by proffering "new" female sexualities (which are, in fact, a commodification of old sexualities) (Attwood, 2005a, 2006; Harris, 2004; see also McRobbie, 2009). Farvid and Braun (2006), in a content analysis of portrayals of male and female sexuality in *Cosmopolitan* (U.S.) and *Cleo* (U.K.) magazines, observed pervasive contradictory messages directed toward young women (be sexually confident but don't speak your mind directly, be "subtle" about sexual communication to get him to pleasure you without bruising his ego), yielding what they call "pseudo liberation and sexual empowerment" (p. 306). Gill (2008) has noted that the "girl" version of sexual empowerment includes being "hot," constituted by a narrow set of bodily and comportment characteristics, and is not accompanied by young women's (or television producers,) demands that men bare it all for women to enjoy. These researchers ask whether these portrayals and how young people are making sense of them constitute a parody of female sexual power rather than its expression.

McRobbie (2009) notes that what she calls the performance of being a sexy and assertive young women must be tempered with a kind of soft femininity that precludes masculine sexual aggression in order for it to be of interest.

Alternatively, Gill (2009) suggests that white, heterosexual women have shifted from sexual objectification to "sexual subjectification"; that is, rather than being shown as passive objects of desire, these young women (and only these young women) are portrayed as being active "subjects" of their own sexuality. However, rather than being "liberating," such portraits may constitute a new set of limiting mandates about how young women should express or appear to express their sexuality that is anchored in the "midriff bearing," actively desiring young woman, requiring a toned but not too strong body that looks youthful but should not be too physically capable. To support this analysis, she shows how another new image of female sexuality evident in advertising, the "hot lesbian," is completely disconnected from lesbian sexuality itself and being used to sell products not to lesbians but to men. These media analysts argue that these new depictions of gender relations visually posit that the solution to male bad behavior is for women to be badder; portrayals of the desirable, desiring young woman to always be "up for it" reflect how advertisers have recuperated and commodified a kind of feminist consciousness and offered it back to women sanitized of its political critique of gender relations, male sexual violence against women, and heteronormativity (Gill, 2008, 2009; Harris, 2004; McRobbie, 2009).

Young Women's Sexual Empowerment?: Choice, Contradiction, and the Absence of Embodied Sexual Desire

Although images are one significant arena in which ideas about young women's sexuality circulate, the contested question on the table is whether or how young women have taken up being sexual objects as an "ironic" new form of sexual agency. Given that in the not-too-distant past, being sexually assertive and being positioned as a sexual object were to be avoided at all costs, it seems remarkable that such a profound 180-degree turnaround of female sexuality has occurred. However, new media cycles and the speed with which new images, forms, and performances sweep through social networks may make such quick transformations possible in ways that are unprecedented. Are women being acknowledged and not suffering consequences for being sexual on their own terms, agents of their own sexuality, if you will, empowered to be sexually assertive or to pursue their own sexual feelings on their own behalf?

One simple assertion is that it is what it seems—young women voluntarily stripping for crowds and the camera, even masturbating on camera, having fun like and with the guys by being sexual free agents—is unequivocal evidence of sexual empowerment: the power to choose to engage in any sexual action (Lamb & Peterson, 2012; Peterson, 2010). Another simple analysis is that young women have been sold and bought a bill of goods: that what they want is to be as raunchy as guys, that the "girl version" is to make the choice to be fantastic (literally, to bring heterosexual male sexual fantasies to life), and that they are being duped into believing they have achieved sexual freedom. A third way to evaluate this conundrum is anchored in a set of psychological questions about young women's experience of this ostensible sexual empowerment (Tolman, 2012). These psychological questions are about the place of dissociation and embodied desire—sexual and emotional—in sexual empowerment. By *dissociation*, I mean a literal disconnection from one's feelings, both emotional and physical. Embodied sexual desire is the experience of sexual feelings, passions, desire, and arousal in one's own body; that is, desire not only as what one wants at an intellectual or cognitive level but as bodily experience.

Although there is virtually no peer-reviewed research to date that enables an evaluation of these interpretations, there is one very rich and thorough source that enables the investigation of these three interpretations. Ariel Levy has named the infusion of highly sexualized media into the mainstream "raunch culture" (Levy, 2005), an outcome of the pornification of culture that has already been discussed. Her journalistic investigations provide an account of how this culture gained ascendance, who produces it, what roles young women are playing in it, and what young women say about their experiences of participating in it. She offers some pointed analyses that go beneath the surface of portrayals and actual performances of young women's sexuality to reveal the only sexual agency we know—male sexual agency. In trying to make sense of "raunch culture," Levy discovered a kind of double-speak in the uncritical embrace of sexual object turned sexual actor status by these young women. She and others (Gill, 2009; Harris, 2004; McRobbie, 2009) observe that being a "great sexual object" who also acts like a porn star is a performance rather than the embodiment of a new form of female sexuality, one that, in the past, has been desired but condemned but that now accrues attention, popularity, and new versions of old experiences of power—the power to turn men on, the power to tease men who are bursting at the seams at the sight of their sexual fantasies come to life, and the power to accept or reject them.

Specifically, Levy noted a widespread absence of any discussion of female sexual pleasure (save for the pleasure of feeling power over a "vulnerable" other), a consistent lack of or explicit denial of feeling sexual (rather, only enjoyment of being perceived as sexy), the pervasiveness of alcohol in all of the settings she observed (including the production of "reality" TV), and the still-present and even eroticized threat and reality of male sexual violence that makes it all more exciting—unless it happens. Young women did not describe their wanting or demanding what felt good or right to them sexually, as the new sexual empowerment is about doing—performing—rather than feeling, adopting a girl version of sexuality as conquest that, when queried, seems less about sexual agency and more to do with other rewards—being admired as fantastic sexual objects to the point of embodying the pornographic, which Levy found was ultimately embarrassing, humiliating, or the undesired end-point of sexual experiences. This seemingly limited and disembodied sexuality is complemented and intensified by how young men are (more than ever) sexually socialized to be disconnected consumers of these very young women.

Levy identifies the paucity of choice and missing multiplicity of ideas about what sexuality and sexual expression are or might be—for women and even for men if unencumbered by persistent gender inequality—and how the current landscape obscures that limit while at the same time holding it in place. It is difficult to evaluate claims of acting on or acting out sexual choices when, as Farvid and Braun (2006) note, these sexual choices are invisibly limited. That is, women are partaking at *a very sparse buffet* without a sense of what is not on the menu or their right or wish to want those choices. As Braun (2010) observes, "if social control is enacted through advertising and media, which creates the guise of free choice... free choice becomes culturally circum-scribed" (see also Harris, 2004). That is, more than ever, "free choice" is lim-ited to what's on sale, but the ways in which these choices are a subset of the range of choices women have as sexual beings are in fact regulatory—and that circumstance is not visible to the naked or untrained eye. Corsianos (2007) contends that the production of what looks like choice in the content of main-stream pornography contributes to the constraint on sexual choice itself. Coy and Garner (2010) suggest that empowerment through self-sexualization to form sexual agency is problematic.

Levy concludes "we are afraid of real female power...to figure out what we internally want from sex instead of mimicking whatever popular culture holds up to us as sexy" (pp. 199–200). In the wide range of anecdotal accounts she collected, the theme of young women going for sexy looks and acting sexy while at the same time expressing discomfort or lack of interest in being sex-ual (thinking about the way they are experienced rather than what they are experiencing) reflects the strong hold that sexual objectification has over what might constitute one's sexuality. In her interviews, young women narrated their embrace of "the male sexual gaze" as the only apparent option for sexual agency, conveying "if you can't beat them, join them" mentality (see Thompson, 2013; Chapter 7, this volume, for supportive and contradictory views).

This line of thinking suggests the need *to distinguish between embodied sexuality and performances of sexuality that are now portrayed as sexual freedom.* The spectre of disembodiment that echoes in available accounts by young women and analyses of portrayals in advertising and the media raise a red flag about the role of sexual objectification in sexual empowerment. Even orgasm—the one form of women's sexual pleasure that is acknowledged, albeit itself objectified—appears to be more about doing a good performance than one's own pleasure, evidenced by one young woman Levy observed after she did a masturbation scene for *Girls Gone Wild*, who was concerned that she had not done it right, because she had taken too long to produce her orgasm.

Teasing apart the complex, contradictory, and commercial dimensions of the "new sexual empowerment" and raising challenges about what is missing from it—women's embodied sexual pleasure as an anchor to sexual subjectivity, real choices that flesh out rather than laminate female sexual agency—within or perhaps missing from the lived experiences of real young women is a vital next step for public discourse, education, and research. Additionally, interrogating cultural conditions that yield analysis and discussion of women's sexual empowerment primarily at the individual level, enabling a kind of "intimate injustice" (McClelland, 2010) that is systematic or difficult to discern, may prove the very concept to be too compromised to be useful (Gavey, 2012). With the exception of Levy's account, research and analysis addressing the question of young women's sexual empowerment reflects dissections of images rather than real young women's experiences. The question of how they are to make sense of "sexual empowerment" remains up for grabs: Is it authentic, or what does it mean to have to be (or appear to be) sexual in a new kind of way that forefronts appearance but makes irrelevant whether or not a woman's desire is real or embodied? Investigating younger and older women's negotiations of embodiment and pressures to disembody may provide a way of navigating questions about and analyses of sexual empowerment that appear to defy, diffuse, defuse, or obfuscate young women's sexuality under the newest "youthified" regime of pervasive sexual objectification.

Conclusion

In this chapter, I have reviewed what we know about the consequences of the sexualization of girls and the current youthified forms of sexual objectification of women for boys', and men's and women's sexuality. In some ways, this is a literature that awaits development, and the leads that we have currently underscore the urgency for such a research agenda. What may be most problematic and challenging is the way that these representations and, increasingly, enactments of sexual objectification seem more and more to be "normal" in general and what real people's sexuality is supposed to be like. Media literacy campaigns that reveal the commercial interests embedded in the depiction and simultaneous cooptation and commercialization of female sexual agency as the latest product to consume, crave, create, and maintain are needed, as is "choice education." Young people deserve the tools to discern and challenge the limited choices put forth as a sparse menu for sexuality. These choices barely offer any sense of sexuality as part of our humanity, and young people must demand more and better options for how they are represented and how they can be.

For women, boys, and men, sexual objectification as sexuality is continuous with education that fails to teach children and teenagers to differentiate their sexual desires from their desire for attention, to differentiate being sexual from being sexy, and to distinguish sex as consumption from sex as experience. Gill (2009) argues that being for or against sexualization is less useful than is breaking it out as a multifaceted—not homogeneous—process. Sexual rights for girls and women, including rights to pleasure, knowledge, and the freedom to enact what one does and does not desire (Tolman & Costa, 2010) are predicated on an understanding of and refusal to embrace the divisions left standing among women and girls predicated on their sexual behavior regardless of what is motivating it.

In all of this stew of sexual objectification and inappropriate sexualization, however, it is important to keep in mind that boys, men, women, and girls themselves are not empty vessels into which images and constructions of girls and women as (only) sexual objects and sexualized body parts are deposited. Media, feminist, and psychological theories posit individuals as at least potentially "active agents" in determining how they will make sense of and "consume" what these various cultural contexts provide, thus underscoring avenues for critique, resistance, and change, both individual and social. Not all boys are trolling the Internet for porn and playing video games with interactive options for sexualized violence, nor are all men disengaged from their emotional lives; not all young women are baring it all for cameras (or want to), and not all women buy into (literally and figuratively) the impossible portrayals that define sexy or deny feeling sexual.

Acknowledgements

The author wishes to thank Rachel Liebert for assistance in research, Christin Bowman and Amy Baker for assistance in preparing the manuscript, and the editors and anonymous reviewer for their feedback and guidance.

Note

1. Although there is evidence that the sexual objectification and self-objectification of boys' and men's bodies is on the rise, this line of argument is not included in this chapter because it falls outside of its scope. Although boys' and men's focus on their appearance may be a subject of increased concern, it is also neither a socially mandated absolute nor a pervasive part of their self-identity on a broad scale (boys and men are, without question, more than their bodies, albeit male adolescent anxieties can certainly be about their physical development), as is the case with girls and women.

References

Ackard, D. M., Kearney-Cooke, A., & Peterson, C. B. (2000). Effect of body image and self-image on women's sexual behaviors. *International Journal of Eating Disorders, 28*(4), 422–429.

Attwood, F. (2005a). Fashion and passion: Marketing sex to women. *Sexualities, 8*(4), 392–406.

Attwood, F. (2005b). What do people do with porn?: Qualitative research into the consumption, use and experience of pornography and other sexually explicit media. *Sexuality & Culture, 9*(2), 65–86.

Attwood, F. (2006). Sexed up: Theorizing the sexualization of culture. *Sexualities, 79*(1), 77–94.

Aubrey, J. S. (2006). Effects of sexually objectifying media on self-objectification and body surveillance in undergraduates: Results of a 2-year panel study. *Journal of Communication, 56*(2), 366–386.

Banet-Weiser, S., & Portwood-Stacer, L. (2006). "I just want to be me again!": Beauty pageants, reality television and post-feminism. *Feminist Theory, 7*(2), 255–272.

Belgrave, F. Z., Van, O. M., & Chambers, D. B. (2000). Culture, contextual, and intrapersonal predictors of risky sexual attitudes among urban African American girls in early adolescence. *Cultural Diversity and Ethnic Minority Psychology, 6*(3), 309–322.

Bogle, K. A. (2008). *Hooking up: Sex, dating and relationships on campus.* New York: New York University Press.

Bragg, S., Buckingham, D., Russell, R., & Willett, R. (2011). Too much, too soon? Children, 'sexualization' and consumer culture. *Sex Education: Sexuality, Society and Learning, 11*(3), 279–292.

Braun, V. (2005). In search of (better) sexual pleasure: Female genital "cosmetic" surgery. *Sexualities, 8*(4), 407–424.

Braun, V. (2010). Female genital cosmetic surgery: A critical review of current knowledge and contemporary debates. *Journal of Women's Health, 19*(7), 1393–1407.

Brooks, G. R. (1995). *The centerfold syndrome: How men can overcome objectification and achieve intimacy with women.* San Francisco: Jossey-Bass.

Brotto, L. A., Heiman, J. R., & Tolman, D. L. (2009). Narratives of desire in mid-age women with and without arousal difficulties. *Journal of Sex Research, 46*(5), 387–398.

Burgess, M. C. R., Stermer, S. P., & Burgess, S. R. (2007). Sex, lies, and video games: The portrayal of male and female characters on video game covers. *Sex Roles, 57*(5–6), 419–433.

Burn, S. M., & Ward, A. Z. (2005). Men's conformity to traditional masculinity and relationship satisfaction. *Psychology of Men and Masculinities, 6*, 254–263.

Burson, J. A. (1998). AIDS, sexuality and African-American adolescent females. *Child and Adolescent Social Work Journal, 15*(5), 357–365.

Chalker, R. (2009). *The "perfect" porn vulva: More women demanding cosmetic genital surgery.* Retrieved February 20, 2010, from http://www.alternet.org/sex/141479/the_%5C%27perfect%5C%27_porn_vulva:_more_women_demanding_cosmetic_genital_surgery/

Ciclitira, K. (2004). Pornography, women and feminism: Between pleasure and politics. *Sexualities, 7*(3), 281–301.

Collins, P. H. (2000). *Black feminist thought.* New York: Routledge.

Corsianos, M. (2007). Mainstream pornography and "women": Questioning sexual agency. *Critical Sociology, 33*(5–6), 863–885.

Cotton, S., Mills, L., Succop, P. A., Biro, F. M., & Rosenthal, S. L. (2004). Adolescent girls' perceptions of the timing of their sexual initiation: "Too young" or "just right"? *Journal of Adolescent Health, 34*(5), 453–458.

Coy, M. (2009). Milkshakes, lady lumps and growing up to want boobies: How the sexualization of popular culture limits girls' horizons. *Child Abuse Review, 18*(6), 372–383.

Coy, M., & Garner, M. (2010). Glamour modelling and the marketing of self-sexualization. *International Journal Of Cultural Studies, 13*(6), 657–675.

Coy, M., & Horvath, M. H. (2011). Lads' mags, young men's attitudes towards women and acceptance of myths about sexual aggression. *Feminism & Psychology, 21*(1), 144–150.

Daniels, E. A., & Wartena, H. (2011). Athlete or sex symbol: What boys think of media representations of female athletes. *Sex Roles, 65*(7–8), 566–579.

Davies, G. (2004). Over half of children see net porn. *Times Educational Supplement* (4595), 9. Retrieved February 25, 2010 from Education Research Complete database

Diaz, J. (2009). *First Apple-approved iPhone porn app.* Retrieved February 25, 2010 from http://gizmodo.com/5302365/first-apple+approved-iphone-porn-app/gallery/

Dietz, T. L. (1998). An examination of violence and gender role portrayals in video games: Implications for gender socialization and aggressive behavior. *Sex Roles, 38*(5–6), 425–442.

Dill, K. E., & Dill, J. C. (1998). Video game violence: A review of the empirical literature. *Aggression and Violent Behavior, 3*(4), 407–428.

Dill, K. E., & Thill, K. P. (2007). Video game characters and the socialization of gender roles: Young people's perceptions mirror sexist media depictions. *Sex Roles, 57*(11–12), 851–864.

Dines, G. (2009). Childified women: How the mainstream porn industry sells child pornography to men. In S. Olfman (Ed.), *The sexualization of childhood.* (pp. 121–142). Westport, CT: Praeger Publishers/Greenwood Publishing Group.

Dittmar, H., & Howard, S. (2004). Thin-ideal internalization and social comparison tendency as moderators of media models' impact on women's body-focused anxiety. *Journal of Social and Clinical Psychology, 23,* 768–791.

Dobbin, M. (2008). *Victim slams YouTube over rape footage.* Retrieved January 22, 2010, from http://www.theage.com.au/news/technology/rape-victim-slams-youtube-for-fo otage/ 2008/03/05/1204402501579.html

Donaghue, N. (2009). Body satisfaction, sexual self-schemas and subjective well-being in women. *Body Image, 6*(1), 37.

Donaghue, N., Whitehead, K., & Kurz, T. (2011). Spinning the pole: A discursive analysis of the websites of recreational pole dancing studios. *Feminism & Psychology, 21*(4), 443–457.

Dunn-Camp, S. (2007). Pole-ates? Teaser takes on new meaning in this sexy new twist on the method. *Pilates Style Magazine,* May/June, 21.

Dworkin, S. L., & O'Sullivan, L. (2007). "It's less work for us and it shows us she has good taste": Masculinity, sexual initiation, and contemporary sexual scripts. In M. Kimmel (Ed.), *The sexual self: The construction of sexual scripts* (pp. 105–121). Nashville, TN: Vanderbilt University Press.

Else-Quest, N., & Hyde, J. (2009). The missing discourse of development: Commentary on Lerum and Dworkin. *Journal of Sex Research, 46*(4), 264–267.

England, P., Schafer, E. F., & Fogarty, A. (2007). Hooking up and forming romantic relationships on today's college campuses. In M. Kimmel, & A. Aronson (Eds.), *The gendered society reader* (pp. 531–547). New York: Oxford University Press.

Ezzell, M. (2009). Pornography, lad mags, video games, and boys: Reviving the canary in the cultural coal mine. In S. Olfman (Ed.), *The sexualization of childhood.* (pp. 7–32). Westport, CT: Praeger/Greenwood.

Farvid, P., & Braun, V. (2006). "Most of us guys are raring to go anytime, anyplace, anywhere": Male and female sexuality in *Cleo* and *Cosmo. Sex Roles, 55*(5–6), 295–310.

Garner, M. (2012). The missing link: The sexualisation of culture and men. *Gender & Education, 24*(3), 325–331.

Gavey, N. (2012). Beyond "empowerment"? Sexuality in a sexist world. *Sex Roles, 66*(11–12), 718–724.

Gill, R. (2008). Empowerment/sexism: Figuring female sexual agency in contemporary advertising. *Feminism & Psychology, 18*(1), 35–60.

Gill, R. (2009). Beyond the "sexualization of culture" thesis: An intersectional analysis of "sixpacks," "midriffs" and "hot lesbians" in advertising. *Sexualities, 12,* 137.

Gill, R. (2012). Media, empowerment and the 'sexualization of culture' debates. *Sex Roles, 66*(11–12), 736–745.

Greenfield, P. M. (2004). Inadvertent exposure to pornography on the internet: Implications of peer-to-peer file-sharing networks for child development and families. *Journal of Applied Developmental Psychology, 25*(6), 741–750.

Graff, K., Murnen, S. K., & Smolak, L. (2012). Too sexualized to be taken seriously? Perceptions of a girl in childlike vs. sexualizing clothing. *Sex Roles, 66*(11–12), 764–775.

Graham, C. A., Sanders, S. A., Milhausen, R. R., & McBride, K. R. (2004). Turning on and turning off: A focus group study of the factors that affect women's sexual arousal. *Archives of Sexual Behavior, 33*(6), 527–538.

Harris, A. (Ed.). (2004). *All about the girl: Culture, power, and identity.* New York: Routledge.

Herman, J. L. (1992). *Trauma and recovery: The aftermath of violence—from domestic abuse to political terror.* New York: Basic Books.

Hill, M. S., & Fischer, A. R. (2008). Examining objectification theory: Lesbian and heterosexual women's experiences with sexual- and self-objectification. *The Counseling Psychologist, 36,* 745–776.

Hatton, E., & Trautner, M. (2011). Equal opportunity objectification? The sexualization of men and women on the cover of *Rolling Stone. Sexuality & Culture: An Interdisciplinary Quarterly, 15*(3), 256–278.

hooks, b. (1992). *Black looks: Race and representation.* Cambridge, MA: South End Press.

Impett, E. A., Schooler, D., & Tolman, D. L. (2006). To be seen and not heard: Femininity ideology and adolescent girls' sexual health. *Archives of Sexual Behavior, 35*(6), 129–142.

Jensen, R. (2007). *Getting off: Pornography and the end of masculinity.* Cambridge, MA: South End Press.

Kenrick, D. T., & Guttierez, S. E. (1980). Contrast effects and judgments of physical attractiveness: When beauty becomes a social problem. *Journal of Personality and Social Psychology, 38,* 131–140.

Kim, Y. (2011). Idol republic: The global emergence of girl industries and the commercialization of girl bodies. *Journal of Gender Studies, 20*(4), 333–345.

Kimmel, M. (2008). *Guyland: The perilous world where boys become men.* New York: Harper.

Kindlon, D., & Thompson, M. (1999). *Raising Cain: Protecting the emotional life of boys.* New York: Ballantine Books.

Lamb, S. (2013). Toward a healthy sexuality for girls and young women: A critique of desire. In E. L. Zurbriggen & T.- A. Roberts (Eds.), *The sexualization of girls and girlhood: Causes, consequences, and resistance* (Chapter 14). New York: Oxford University Press.

Lamb, S., & Peterson, Z. D. (2012). Adolescent girls' sexual empowerment: Two feminists explore the concept. *Sex Roles, 66*(11–12), 703–712.

Lerum, K., & Dworkin, S. L. (2009a). "Bad girls rule": An interdisciplinary feminist commentary on the report of the task force on the sexualization of girls. *Journal of Sex Research, 46*(3), 1–14.

Lerum, K., & Dworkin, S. L. (2009b). Toward the interdisciplinary dialogue on youth, sexualization, and health. *Journal of Sex Research, 46*(4), 271–273.

Levy, A. (2005). *Female chauvinist pigs: Women and the rise of raunch culture.* New York: Free Press.

Lindgren, K. P., Shoda, Y., & George, W. H. (2007). Sexual or friendly? Associations about women, men and self. *Psychology of Women Quarterly, 31*(2), 190–201.

Linz, D. G., Donnerstein, E., & Penrod, S. (1988). Effects of long-term exposure to violent and sexually degrading depictions of women. *Journal of Personality and Social Psychology, 55*(5), 758–768.

Loe, M. (2004). Sex and the senior woman: Pleasure and danger in the Viagra era. *Sexualities, 7,* 303–326.

Loftus, D. (2002). *Watching sex: How men really respond to pornography.* New York: Thunder's Mouth.

Martin, K. A., & Kazyak, E. (2009). Hetero-romantic love and heterosexiness in children's G-rated films. *Gender & Society, 23*(3), 315–336.

McClelland, S. I. (2010). Intimate justice: A critical analysis of sexual satisfaction. *Social and Personality Psychology Compass, 4,* 663–680.

McRobbie, A. (2009). *The aftermath of feminism: Gender, culture, and social change.* London: Sage Publications.

Morgan, E. M., & Zurbriggen, E. L. (2007). Wanting sex and wanting to wait: Young adults' accounts of sexual messages from first significant dating partners. *Feminism & Psychology, 17*(4), 515–541.

Muhanguzi, F., Bennett, J., & Muhanguzi, H. D. (2011). The construction and mediation of sexuality and gender relations: Experiences of girls and boys in secondary schools in Uganda. *Feminist Formations, 23*(3), 135–152.

Nowatzki, J., & Morry, M. M. (2009). Women's intentions regarding, and acceptance of, self-sexualizing behavior. *Psychology of Women Quarterly, 33*(1), 95–107.

O'Sullivan, L. F., & Majerovich, J. (2008). Difficulties with sexual functioning in a sample of male and female late adolescent and young adult university students. *Canadian Journal of Human Sexuality, 17*(3), 109–121.

Paul, P. (2005). *Pornified: How pornography is damaging our lives, our relationships, and our families.* New York: Holt.

Pleck, J., Sonenstein, F., & Ku, L. (1993). Masculinity ideology: Its impact on adolescent males' heterosexual relationships. *Journal of Social Issues, 49*(3), 11–29.

Purcell, N. J., & Zurbriggen, E. L. (2013). The sexualization of girls and gendered violence: Mapping the connections. In E. L. Zurbriggen & T.- A. Roberts (Eds.), *The sexualization of girls and girlhood: Causes, consequences, and resistance* (Chapter 8). New York: Oxford University Press.

Quinn, B. A. (2002). Sexual harassment and masculinity: The power and meaning of "girl watching." *Gender Society, 16,* 386–402.

Roberts, T., & Gettman, J. Y. (2004). Mere exposure: Gender differences in the negative effects of priming a state of self-objectification. *Sex Roles, 51*(1–2), 17–27.

Rousso, H. (1994). Daughters with disabilities: Defective women or minority women. In J. Irvine (Ed.), *Sexual cultures and the construction of adolescent identities* (pp. 139–171). Philadelphia, PA: Temple University Press.

Rudman, L. A., & Borgida, E. (1995). The afterglow of construct accessibility: The behavioral consequences of priming men to view women as sexual objects. *Journal of Experimental Social Psychology, 31*(6), 493–517.

Sanchez, D. T., & Broccoli, T. L. (2008). The romance of self-objectification: Does priming romantic relationships induce states of self-objectification among women? *Sex Roles, 59*(7–8), 545–554.

Sanchez, D. T., & Kiefer, A. K. (2007). Body concerns in and out of the bedroom: Implications for sexual pleasure and problems. *Archives of Sexual Behavior, 36*(6), 808.

Schooler, D., & Ward, L. M. (2006). Average Joes: Men's relationships with media, real bodies and sexuality. *Psychology of Men and Masculinity, 7,* 27–41.

Schooler, D., Ward, L. M., Merriwether, A., & Caruthers, A. S. (2005). Cycles of shame: Menstrual shame, body shame, and sexual decision-making. *Journal of Sex Research, 42*(4), 324–334.

Steer, A., & Tiggemann, M. (2008). The role of self-objectification in women's sexual functioning. *Journal of Social & Clinical Psychology, 27*(3), 205–225.

Stephens, D. P., & Phillips, L. D. (2003). Freaks, gold diggers, divas, and dykes: The socio-historical development of adolescent African American women's sexual script. *Sexuality & Culture: An Interdisciplinary Quarterly, 7*(1), 3–49.

Stombler, M. (1994). "Buddies" or "slutties": The collective sexual reputation of fraternity little sisters. *Gender & Society. Special Issue: Sexual identities/Sexual Communities, 8*(3), 297–323.

Sweeney, B. N. (2008). Dangerous and out of control: College men, masculinity, and subjective experiences of sexuality. *Dissertation Abstracts International: Section A: Humanities and Social Sciences, 68*(9-A), 4094.

Tasker, Y., & Negra, D. (Eds.). (2007). *Interrogating postfeminism: Gender and the politics of popular culture.* Durham, NC: Duke University Press.

Thompson, E. M. (2013). "If you're hot, I'm bi": Implications of sexualization for sexual minority girls. In E. L. Zurbriggen & T.- A. Roberts (Eds.), *The sexualization of girls and girlhood: Causes, consequences, and resistance* (Chapter 7). New York: Oxford University Press.

Tiefer, L. (2008). Female genital cosmetic surgery: Freakish or inevitable? Analysis from medical marketing, bioethics, and feminist theory. *Feminism & Psychology, 18*(4), 466–479.

Tolman, D. (2000). Object lessons: Romance, violation, and female adolescent sexual desire. *Journal of Sex Education & Therapy, 25*(1), 70.

Tolman, D. L. (2002). *Dilemmas of desire: Teenage girls talk about sexuality.* Cambridge, MA: Harvard University Press.

Tolman, D. L. (2006). In a different position: Conceptualizing female adolescent sexuality within compulsory heterosexuality. *New Directions for Child and Adolescent Development, 2006*(112), 71–89.

Tolman, D. L. (2012). Female adolescents, sexual empowerment and desire: A missing discourse of gender inequity. *Sex Roles, 66*(11–12), 746–757.

Tolman, D. L., & Costa, S. H. (2010). Sexual rights for young women: Lessons from developing countries. In. P. Aggleton, & R. Parker (Eds.). *Routledge Handbook of Sexuality, Health and Human Rights* (pp. 389–398). New York: Routledge.

Tolman, D. L., & Debold, E. (1993). Conflicts of body and image: Female adolescents, desire, and the no-body body. In P. Fallon, M. Katzman, & S. Wooley (Eds.), *Feminist perspectives on eating disorders* (pp. 301–317). New York: Guilford Press.

Tolman, D. L., Spencer, R., Rosen-Reynoso, M., & Porche, M. V. (2003). Sowing the seeds of violence in heterosexual relationships: Early adolescents narrate compulsory heterosexuality. *Journal of Social Issues, 59*(1), 159–178.

Trapnell, P. D., Meston, C. M., & Gorzalka, B. B. (1997). Spectatoring and the relationship between body image and sexual experience: Self-focus or self-valence? *Journal of Sex Research, 34*(3), 267–278.

Vaes, J., Paladino, P., & Puvia, E. (2011). Are sexualized women complete human beings? Why men and women dehumanize sexually objectified women. *European Journal of Social Psychology, 41*(6), 774–785.

Vanwesenbeeck, I. (2009). The risks and rights of sexualization: An appreciative commentary on Lerum and Dworkin's "Bad girls rule." *Journal of Sex Research, 46*(4), 268–270.

Verhulst, J. (2010). Review of 'Male sexuality: Why women don't understand it—and men don't either.' *Journal of Sex & Marital Therapy, 36*(3), 298–300.

Ward, L. M. (2002). Does television exposure affect emerging adults' attitudes and assumptions about sexual relationships? Correlational and experimental confirmation. *Journal of Youth & Adolescence, 31*, 1–15.

Ward, L. M. (2004). Wading through the stereotypes: Positive and negative associations between media use and black adolescents' conceptions of self. *Developmental Psychology*, 40, 284–294.

Ward, L. M., & Averitt, L. (2005). *Associations between media use and young adults' perceptions of first intercourse.* Paper presented at the annual meeting of the National Communication Association, Boston.

Ward, L. M., Hansbrough, E., & Walker, E. (2005). Contributions of music video exposure to black adolescents' gender and sexual schemas. *Journal of Adolescent Research*, 20(2), 143–166.

Ward, L. M., & Rivadeneyra, R. (1999). Contributions of entertainment television to adolescents' sexual attitudes and expectations: The role of viewing amount versus viewer involvement. *Journal of Sex Research*, 36(3), 237–249.

Ward, L. M., & Rivandeneyra, R. (2002, August). *Dancing, strutting and bouncing in cars: The women of music videos.* Paper presented at the annual meeting of the American Psychological Association, Chicago.

Weaver, J., Masland, J. L., & Zillmann, D. (1984). Effect of erotica on young men's aesthetic perception of their female sexual partners. *Perceptual and Motor Skills*, 58, 929–930.

Weekes, D. (2002). Get your freak on: How black girls sexualise identity. *Sex Education*, 2(3), 251–262.

Wesely, J. K. (2009). "Mom said we had a money maker": Sexualization and survival contexts among homeless women. *Symbolic Interaction*, 32(2), 91–105.

Whitehead, K., & Kurz, T. (2009). "Empowerment" and the pole: A discursive investigation of the reinvention of pole dancing as a recreational activity. *Feminism & Psychology*, 19(2), 224–244.

Wiederman, M. W. (2000). Women's body image self-consciousness during physical intimacy with a partner. *Journal of Sex Research*, 37(1), 60–68.

Wiederman, M. W. (2001). "Don't look now": The role of self-focus in sexual dysfunction. *The Family Journal: Counseling and Therapy for Couples and Families*, 9, 210–214.

Wiederman, M. W., & Hurst, S. R. (1998). Body size, physical attractiveness, and body image among young adult women: Relationships to sexual experience and sexual esteem. *Journal of Sex Research*, 35(3), 272–281.

Wiederman, M., & Pryor, T. (1997). Body dissatisfaction and sexuality among women with bulimia nervosa. *International Journal of Eating Disorders*, 21, 361–365.

Yamamiya, Y., Cash, T. F., & Thompson, J. K. (2006). Sexual experiences among college women: The differential effects of general versus contextual body images on sexuality. *Sex Roles*, 55(5–6), 421–427.

Yao, M., Mahood, C., & Linz, D. (2010). Sexual priming, gender stereotyping, and likelihood to sexually harass: Examining the cognitive effects of playing a sexually-explicit video game. *Sex Roles*, 62(1/2), 77–88.

Zillmann, D., & Bryant, J. (1988). Pornography's impact on sexual satisfaction. *Journal of Applied Social Psychology*, 18, 438–453.

Zurbriggen, E. L., & Morgan, E. M. (2006).Who wants to marry a millionaire? Reality dating television programs, attitudes toward sex, and sexual behaviors. *Sex Roles*, 54, 1–17.

PART THREE

INTERPERSONAL CONTRIBUTIONS AND CONSEQUENCES

6

Sexual Harassment by Peers

JENNIFER L. PETERSEN AND JANET SHIBLEY HYDE

A common approach to understanding the sexualization of girls involves a focus on impersonal, large-scale cultural forces such as the media. Yet, some sexualization occurs at a very individual, personal level. Sexual harassment is one of these very personal factors. Although much theorizing and research has focused on sexual harassment by older, more powerful individuals, such as teachers, in fact, what is most common in the lives of girls is sexual harassment by peers (American Association of University Women [AAUW], 2001; Timmerman, 2003). Here, we review what is known about peer sexual harassment, what factors predict who is victimized and who is the perpetrator, and what some of the consequences may be. We focus especially on peer sexual harassment in the schools, but also include research on some of the new electronic forms of sexual harassment.

Scope of the Problem

The American Psychological Association Task Force on the Sexualization of Girls (TFSG) says that sexualization occurs when "sexuality is inappropriately imposed upon a person" (Zurbriggen et al., 2007). This definition closely mimics the definition of peer sexual harassment victimization. The American Association of University Women (AAUW) defined peer sexual harassment victimization as any "unwanted or unwelcome sexual behavior that interferes with one's life" (AAUW, 2001). They identified 14 different behaviors that constitute peer sexual harassment victimization, including both physical and verbal sexual behaviors such as being called gay or lesbian and having clothes pulled off or down. According to this definition, as many as 81% of students between grades 8 and 11 have experienced some form of peer sexual harassment in their school lives (AAUW, 2001). Table 6.1 lists all 14 sexually harassing behaviors identified by the AAUW and their incidence rates. The most common sexually harassing behavior is being the victim of sexual comments, jokes, gestures, or looks (AAUW, 2001; Petersen & Hyde, 2009). The least common behavior was being spied on while dressing or showering (AAUW, 2001). As evidenced in Table 6.1, verbal forms of sexual harassment (e.g., hearing a sexual joke) are more prevalent than physical sexual harassment (e.g., having clothes pulled off or down).

Research on peer sexual harassment in adolescence indicates no gender difference in overall victimization incidence (see Table 6.1, AAUW, 2001). However, girls are more commonly victims of frequent and severe sexual harassment than are boys (Hand & Sanchez, 2000). Gender differences also emerge when a distinction is made between same-gender and cross-gender harassment (Craig, Pepler, Connolly, & Henderson 2001; McMasters, Connolly, Pepler, & Craig, 2002; Petersen & Hyde, 2009). Studies indicate that there is no gender difference in victimization incidence for cross-gender harassment; that is, girls are just as likely to harass boys as boys are to harass girls. However, boys are more likely to harass other boys than girls are to harass other girls (Craig et al. 2001; McMasters et al., 2002; Pelligrini, 2002; Petersen & Hyde, 2009). This finding indicates that same-gender and cross-gender sexual harassment victimization are distinct from one another and should be studied as separate phenomena.

Although boys and girls are equally likely to report peer sexual harassment, girls are more likely to be upset by harassment (AAUW, 2001). Forty-eight percent of students of both genders report feeling upset by harassment, but when this statistic is broken down by gender, 70% of girls, but only 24% of boys, report being upset by peer sexual harassment victimization (AAUW, 2001). A meta-analytic review of research on gender differences in perceptions of sexual harassment indicated that girls and women considered a larger range of sexual behaviors to be upsetting than did boys and men ($d = 0.30$, Rotundo, Nguyen, & Sackett, 2001). This gender differences was even larger when the perpetrator was the victim's peer ($d = 0.43$). Sexual harassment perpetrated by peers is often more ambiguous than harassment perpetrated by someone with more power, such as in workplace harassment or harassment by teachers, because interactions are more casual and may include discussions about sexuality that are not harassing. When harassment is ambiguous, such as peer sexual harassment victimization, girls were more likely than boys to interpret the behavior as harassing (Rotundo et al., 2001).

Issues of strength and power likely contribute to gender differences in perceptions of sexual harassment. Late adolescent boys are, on average, physically stronger and larger than girls (Marshall & Tanner, 1969, 1970), and, regardless of their size, boys typically report more interpersonal power than girls do (Sheets & Braver, 1999). Therefore, girls are likely to be more fearful of harassment because boys are stronger and more powerful. For example, boys are likely

Table 6.1 **Types of Sexual Harassment Experienced in School**

Behavior	Girls	Boys	Total
Sexual comments, jokes, gestures, or looks	76%	56%	61%
Touched, grabbed, or pinched in a sexual way	60%	41%	53%
Intentionally brushed up against in a sexual way	57%	36%	46%
Flashed or mooned	48%	41%	45%
Had sexual rumors spread about them	42%	34%	37%
Had clothing pulled at in a sexual way	37%	37%	33%
Shown, gave, or left sexual pictures, messages, or notes	32%	34%	32%
Had their way blocked in a sexual way	37%	16%	27%
Sexual graffiti written about them on the bathroom walls, locker room, etc.	20%	17%	19%
Forced to kiss someone	23%	13%	18%
Called gay or lesbian	10%	23%	16%
Had clothes pulled off or down	16%	16%	16%
Forced to do something sexual other than kissing	12%	9%	11%
Spied on while dressing or showering	6%	8%	7%

to feel flattered by sexually harassing behaviors, particularly when perpetrated by girls (AAUW, 2001; Duffy, Wareham & Walsh, 2004). However, girls are likely to be fearful or feel dirty as a consequence of peer sexual harassment (AAUW, 2001; Duffy et al., 2004). In fact, one study found that sexual harassment perpetrated by boys was more upsetting than sexual harassment perpetrated by girls, regardless of the gender of the victim (McMasters et al., 2002). In addition, girls are more commonly victims of rape and sexual assault than are boys (Anderson, 2007). Therefore, it is not surprising that the sexualization of girls in the form of peer sexual harassment is particularly upsetting for girls.

Developmental Patterns

Students report sexual harassment victimization at a very early age, with 38% of high school students reporting that they were sexually harassed before sixth grade (AAUW, 2001). Alarmingly, victimization increases throughout middle school and into high school, then drops off again in college (Craig et al., 2001; Goldstein, Malanchuk, Davis-Kean, & Eccles, 2007; McMasters et al., 2002; Petersen & Hyde, 2009).

As adolescents begin to experience the changes of pubertal development, they have an increased interest in sexuality. Because youth have little experience expressing sexual attraction, they may do so in inappropriate ways (Petersen & Hyde, 2009). Sexual teasing in the form of peer sexual harassment may allow youth to express their romantic attraction without the risk of being rejected. Therefore, sexual harassment, particularly cross-gender harassment, may increase through early adolescence as youth experiment with ways of expressing attraction. As they become more experienced, most teens develop more mature ways of expressing attraction that do not include sexual harassment (Petersen & Hyde, 2009).

This increase in victimization across adolescence may also be a product of changes in peer relationships during the transition from grade school to middle school and from middle school to high school. Changes in peer social structure often accompany these transitions as youth establish power hierarchies among unfamiliar peers in their new schools (Pelligrini, 2001). Friendship hierarchies become increasingly important from early to middle adolescence, and youth may use peer victimization to establish dominance (Pelligrini & Long, 2002). Peer sexual harassment may increase as adolescents express dominance over their peers in an attempt to develop a hierarchy in their social relationships.

Which Girls Are Likely to Be Victims?

As with all victimization research, researchers must be careful not to blame the victim when they look for predictors of sexual harassment. No one is ever responsible for being the victim of unwanted sexual harassment, and it is important for researchers to stress that sexual harassment is never the victim's fault. That being said, it is important to identify girls who are often targets of sexual harassment so that these victims may be protected from future harassment. Therefore, much research has focused on the predictors of sexual harassment victimization. Research and theory suggest that pubertal status, perceived power, school climate, and peer groups are predictors of peer sexual harassment victimization.

Pubertal Status

Youth with more advanced pubertal status are more likely than their less advanced peers to be victims of peer sexual harassment (Craig et al., 2001; Goldstein et al., 2007; McMasters et al., 2002; Petersen & Hyde, 2009). As girls enter pubertal development and develop secondary sex characteristics, such as larger breasts and wider hips, their peers may respond with sexual interest. These secondary sex characteristics might signal to teens that these girls are sexually ready. For example, in one qualitative interview, a girl reported "I have large breasts and they [boys] pay me out for it. They all know my bra size and they tease me about it" (Shute, Owens, & Slee, 2008). Although multiple studies document a correlation between pubertal status and peer sexual harassment victimization (Craig et al., 2001; Nadeem & Graham, 2005; McMasters et al., 2002; Petersen & Hyde, 2009), it is not clear whether the association applies across gender and harassment type. For example, some studies have found that girls, but not boys, with advanced pubertal status were more likely to be victims of sexual harassment than their less advanced peers (Goldstein et al., 2007; Stattin & Magnusson, 1990), whereas others found the correlation for both genders (Craig et al., 2001; McMasters et al., 2002). The results of studies that distinguished between same-gender and cross-gender harassment have not been consistent. One study found that youth with advanced pubertal status were more likely to be victims of cross-gender harassment, but not same-gender harassment (McMasters et al., 2002), whereas another found the correlation for both same- and cross-gender harassment (Craig et al., 2001).

We conducted a longitudinal study to better understand the relationship between sexual harassment and pubertal development (Petersen & Hyde, 2009). In this study, 242 adolescents reported their stage of pubertal development (as assessed from Tanner stages, Marshall & Tanner, 1969, 1970) and frequency of peer sexual harassment victimization after they completed fifth, seventh, and ninth grades. In all three grades, youth with advanced pubertal status were more often victims of overall sexual harassment in comparison to youth who were less advanced. However, analysis of harassment type revealed that only youth with advanced development during seventh grade were more likely to be harassed by cross-gender peers in ninth grade, whereas advanced pubertal status in all grades predicted ninth-grade same-gender harassment.

There are multiple possible explanations for why adolescents may target physically advanced peers of their same gender for sexual harassment. First, Craig and colleagues (2001) proposed that youth with advanced pubertal status are more conspicuous than their less advanced peers, and, therefore, they may receive more attention from their peers through sexual harassment. Second, youth who are advanced in development may surround themselves with an older or more deviant peer group who may find more situations to be sexual and express their sexuality by harassing their younger associates (Magnusson, Stattin, & Allen, 1985; Goldstein et al., 2007). Third, youth with advanced pubertal status are more commonly perpetrators of peer harassment (Schreck, Burek, Stewart, & Mitchell, 2007). Adolescents who are perpetrators may be more likely to be victims of harassment than their peers (AAUW, 2001; Fineran & Bennett, 1999; McMasters et al., 2002).

Power

Bullying and other forms of victimization often target low-power youth. The perpetrator is motivated to gain social status and express dominance over the victim (Cillessen & Rose, 2005; Pelligrini & Long, 2002). For example, children who are low in power are more likely to be bullied than are their high-power peers (Coleman & Byrd, 2003). Our longitudinal study predicted a similar relationship for peer sexual harassment, in which low-power youth would be likely victims of sexual harassment (Petersen & Hyde, 2009). However, in contrast to this hypothesis, youth with high perceived power were more likely to be victims of harassment than youth with low power. In fact, youth with high perceived power at all grades were more likely to be victims of ninth-grade cross-gender harassment than their peers (Petersen & Hyde, 2009). Powerful adolescents have increased influence among their peers and thus are likely objects of romantic interest. Adolescents might use sexually harassing behaviors to gain the attention of their powerful, cross-gender peers. For example, powerful youth may be told a sexual joke or left sexual messages intended to attract romantic attention rather than cause emotional distress. An interaction of power and gender in ninth grade indicated that girls in particular may be more likely to harass their powerful male peers than less powerful boys. Girls are attracted to powerful boys who gain status through aggression and dominance (Bukowski, Sippola, & Newcomb, 2000; Pelligrini & Bartini, 2001). Therefore, cross-gender harassment may be bidirectional. Boys who sexually harass girls may be harassed in return by girls who find this dominance attractive. Other research, which indicates that perpetrators are often also victims, supports this bidirectional effect (AAUW, 2001; Fineran & Bennett, 1999; McMasters et al., 2002).

School Climate

Teacher reports indicate that both male and female teachers hold intolerant attitudes toward peer sexual harassment (Stone & Couch, 2004). Teachers report that they almost always notice peer sexual harassment, intervene as soon as they are able, and punish perpetrators (Stone & Couch, 2004). However, other research suggests that these teacher reports may be false or at least misguided (Hand & Sanchez, 2000). The majority of students report that teachers do not intervene to stop peer sexual harassment, even though the majority of harassment occurs in public places such as school hallways and in classrooms (AAUW, 2001).

Only 7% of students report peer sexual harassment to their teachers (AAUW, 2001). Girls, in particular, may be unlikely to report sexual harassment because they fear that teachers will not believe them, or may even blame and punish them (Ormerod, Collinsworth, & Perry, 2008). This type of passive tolerance toward sexual harassment leads to more sexual harassment in the schools (Ormerod et al., 2008). In fact, girls who report that their schools have a tolerant attitude toward sexual harassment, where perpetrators are rarely punished and sexual harassment goes largely unnoticed, are not only more likely to experience sexual harassment, but are also more likely to report negative consequences as a result (Ormerod, et al., 2008).

Peer Group

Peers become increasingly important to youth as they enter adolescence. Although adolescents benefit from a strong group of friends, peer groups may lead to aggressive behavior, such as sexual harassment. Teens are more likely to be harassed by their peers than by a stranger or dating partner (Fineran & Bennett, 1999). Therefore, adolescents who spend time with aggressive friends or older friends are more likely to be harassed than their peers (Magnusson et al., 1985; Goldstein et al., 2007). These peer groups may use sexual harassment to form a dominance hierarchy, or they may just consider sexual harassment a part of teen culture.

In contrast, other research indicates that a positive peer group may buffer the effects of peer sexual harassment. For example, sexual minorities who are victims of peer sexual harassment are less likely to report depression and externalizing symptoms if they have supportive friends (Williams, Connolly, Pepler, & Craig, 2005).

Who Are the Perpetrators?

Unfortunately, the majority of research on peer sexual harassment has focused on the victims, and very little research has been done to identify the perpetrators of peer sexual harassment. This pattern is not surprising, given that youth would be reluctant to admit perpetrating peer sexual harassment. Some research suggests that perpetrators, particularly early adolescents, may not even be aware that their behavior is unwanted (AAUW, 2001). Nevertheless, the majority of boys (66%) and girls (57%) admitted that they had sexually harassed someone in their school at least once (AAUW, 2001).

The majority of female victims of peer sexual harassment report that boys are the perpetrators (AAUW, 2001; McMasters et al., 2002; Petersen & Hyde, 2009). Eighty-six percent of girl victims report that sexual harassment was perpetrated by a boy acting alone, and 57% report that they were victimized by a group of boys (AAUW, 2001). Girls are much less likely to report that girls are the perpetrators. Only 10% of girls report harassment perpetrated by a single girl, and 3% report harassment from a group of girls (AAUW, 2001).

Some research suggests that perpetrators of sexual harassment may not know that their actions are inappropriate. According to one study, 25% of perpetrators thought the victim would like the behavior, and an additional 20% of youth said they did it to get a date with the victim (AAUW, 2001). Social skills training may help these perpetrators to identify appropriate ways of flirting and showing romantic interest in a way that is not offensive or unwanted.

Interestingly, perpetrators of peer sexual harassment are also likely to be victims of harassment. Of the teens who admitted sexual harassment in the AAUW study (2001), 94% said that they had also been victims of sexual harassment. Perhaps adolescents use sexual harassment as a defense against further sexual harassment, or perhaps the dynamics of some peer groups are such that sexual harassment is so prevalent that teens are both perpetrators and victims.

Since very little research has been done to identify the perpetrators of peer harassment, we may look to research on workplace sexual harassment in adulthood to determine variables that may be associated with perpetrator frequency. Research on workplace harassment suggests that endorsement of traditional gender-role values is related to the likelihood to sexually harass (Pryor, 1987). Perhaps boys who hold traditional gender-role beliefs in high school are more likely than their egalitarian peers to sexually harass girls (Fineran & Bennett, 1999). Cultural messages that sexualize girls may increase these traditional gender-role beliefs, thus increasing sexualization in the form of peer sexual harassment.

Some researchers suggest that the media is at fault for peer sexual harassment perpetration (e.g., Brown & L'Engle, 2009; Montemurro, 2003). A recent content analysis of television programs reported that sex scenes on television nearly doubled from 1998 to 2003 (Kunkel et al., 2003). Many of these programs portray sexually harassing behaviors in a positive light, trivializing it with humor (Montemurro, 2003). Some research suggests that exposure to sexualized media in men increases masculine identity that is associated with negative views about women (Ward, Merriwhether, Caruthers, 2006). These negative views may be expressed in the form of peer sexual harassment. For example, one study indicated that exposure to pornographic media increased peer sexual harassment perpetration for boys, but not for girls (Brown & L'Engle, 2009). Another study found that boys, but not girls, who reported watching three or more hours of television per day had more accepting attitudes toward sexual harassment than did boys who watched fewer than three hours of television each day (Strouse, Goodwin, & Roscoe, 1994). These studies indicate that the sexualization of girls in the media may lead to more sexualization in the form of peer sexual harassment.

Electronic Harassment

The news media have recently reported many stories about a relatively new phenomenon termed "sexting." The media use this term to refer to the act of sending or receiving sexually explicit messages or pictures or spreading sexual rumors electronically. Popular ways of sending these electronic messages include e-mail, text messaging, online instant messaging, blogging, and social networking sites. Sexting may be a form of sexual harassment itself, if the pictures or messages are unwanted. Alternatively, sexting may lead to sexual harassment if unintended recipients receive these pictures and messages and use them to spread sexual rumors or direct offensive comments toward the person who sent them. Sexual harassment on the Internet, including blogs and social networking sites, may be particularly harmful for teens because these messages and images may be viewed by anyone with Internet access. Although it is important for teens to be cautious about whom they send sexual messages and pictures to and how they transmit these messages, it is important to remember that no one, no matter how sexually explicit their messages may be, should be blamed for being the victim of sexual harassment. Instead, youth should be taught to be respectful and courteous toward their peers and express their sexual interest in appropriate ways that do not involve harassment.

Very little empirical research has been done to investigate the prevalence of "sexting." The National Campaign to Prevent Teen and Unplanned Pregnancy (2008) conducted a preliminary study to investigate this issue. In this study, 653 teens (aged 13–19) and 627 young adults (aged 20–26) from across the United States answered an online questionnaire about their experiences with "sexting." Results indicate that 20% of teens and 33% of young adults reported sending nude or semi-nude pictures to someone electronically, and an astounding 39% of teens and 59% of young adults sent sexual messages. Although the majority (70% of teens and 80% of young adults) sent messages to their boyfriend or girlfriend, many of them (46%) said that it is common for sexually explicit messages to be shared with someone other than the intended recipient. When asked about the reasons that they sent sexually explicit messages or images, 51% of girls, but only 18% of boys, said they were pressured by their boyfriend or girlfriend.

This survey reveals striking results about the prevalence of sending sexually explicit messages, yet some limitations of the research suggest that these numbers might be inflated when compared with the general population. Specifically, results may be biased because this research was conducted online. Teens who have access to the Internet and are willing to take an online survey are likely proficient with technology and may be more likely to use technology to send sexually explicit messages than are teens who are less tech savvy. More research must be conducted on this topic to get more conclusive evidence about the prevalence of using technology to send sexually explicit images and messages to others.

Another form of electronic sexual harassment is unwanted online sexual solicitation. This has been defined as "the act of encouraging someone to talk about sex, to do something sexual, or to share personal sexual information on the Internet when the person doesn't want to" (Ybarra, Espelage, & Mitchell, 2007). Research indicates that the majority of youth have no experience as either the victims or perpetrators of online sexual solicitation (Ybarra et al., 2007). However, youth who are victims of online sexual solicitation are also likely to be perpetrators of online sexual solicitation and are likely to be victims and perpetrators of sexual harassment offline as well (Ybarra et al., 2007).

What Are the Consequences?

Negative consequences of peer sexual harassment are particularly severe when sexual harassment occurs repeatedly or is intense (Duffy et al., 2004). Girls are more likely than boys to experiences negative consequences of peer harassment, partially because girls are more likely than boys to be victims of frequent and severe harassment and more likely to be upset by peer sexual harassment (AAUW, 2001, Duffy et al., 2004; Hand & Sanchez, 2000). Research indicates that female victims of sexual harassment report negative educational and psychological consequences.

Educational Consequences

Girls who are victims of frequent or intense sexual harassment are often unwilling to face their harasser at school. They are more likely than girls who are not harassed to report not wanting to go to school, cutting class, and think about changing schools (AAUW, 2001). Persistent and intense sexual harassment also affects girls' ability to concentrate at school, likely because victims are worried about their next encounter with their harasser. Girls who are sexually harassed report not talking as much in class, making lower grades on school assignments, finding it hard to study, and even doubting whether they will be able to graduate (AAUW, 2001; Duffy et al., 2004). In particular, being the victim of sexual rumors, sexual jokes, comments, gestures, and looks, or sexual pictures, messages, or notes increases negative educational consequences (Duffy et al., 2004). Reducing the rates of sexual harassment, particularly for girls, may increase students' academic performance, in addition to increasing psychological well-being.

Psychological Consequence

A broad range of psychological consequences are correlated with sexual harassment victimization. For girls, these consequences typically include internalizing behaviors such as depression, body shame, anxiety, and low self-esteem.

Depression

A gender difference in depression begins to emerge in adolescents, with girls twice as likely to report symptoms of depression as are boys (Hyde, Mezulis, & Abramson, 2008; Kaltiala-Heino, Kosunun, & Rimpela, 2003). This gender difference emerges at the same time that peer sexual harassment becomes more prevalent in the schools, suggesting a link between the two. Research suggests that girls who are victims of sexual harassment are more likely than their nonharassed peers to report depressed mood, such as reduced appetite, loss of interest and pleasure, and sleep disturbances (Nadeem & Graham, 2005).

Body Shame and Disordered Eating

Sexualization in the form of peer sexual harassment focuses negative attention on the victim's body, which may decrease body esteem. Girls who report peer sexual harassment victimization have higher levels of body surveillance, or increased attention to having an ideal body type, than do their peers. Body surveillance is, in turn, associated with feelings of shame about one's body (Lindberg, Grabe, & Hyde, 2007; Petersen & Hyde, in press). Even elementary school girls who have been sexually harassed report lower body esteem than do their nonharassed peers (Murnen & Smolak, 2000).

As girls develop a decreased sense of body esteem, they are likely to try to alter their body shape by engaging in disordered eating behaviors, such a bulimia and anorexia nervosa. Sexual harassment has been associated with disordered eating among women in the workplace, particularly when the sexual harassment is severe and distressing (Harned, 2000; Harned & Fitzgerald, 2002). In a qualitative interview, a teacher described the association between sexual harassment and anorexia for one of her students: "one of the boys made a comment about her being fat and put it on the computer screen in the computing room. Um, and so she, you know, that triggered her off, was a trigger, not the total reason I think, for her anorexia" (Shute, Owens, & Slee, 2008).

There are many possible reasons for the association of distressing harassment to disordered eating. First, girls may cope with the distress associated with peer sexual harassment victimization by controlling their eating behaviors. Girls might feel that their sexual image is causing unwanted sexual attention, so they might control their eating in order to reduce body fat and return to a skinny, nonsexual body (Harned & Fitzgerald, 2002). Second, girls may resort to extreme dieting or anorexic behaviors in order to physically reduce their size and presence among their peers, in the hopes that this will make them less conspicuous and decrease unwanted attention. Third, they may feel that peer sexual harassment is out of their control and may wish to compensate for this lack of control by controlling other aspects of their life, including their weight (Surgenor, Horn, Plumridge, & Hudson, 2002). Finally, both peer sexual harassment and disordered eating may be caused by a third variable—namely, sexualization of girls in the media. The media increasingly depict young girls as sexual beings (Kunkel et al., 2003). This is likely to increase sexual objectification in the form of sexual harassment and self-objectification, which may reduce body esteem and increase disordered eating behaviors in order to obtain an ideal body (Petersen & Hyde, in press).

The association between peer victimization and body shame may partially explain why peer victimization is associated with adverse outcomes such as depression (Grabe, Hyde & Lindberg, 2007; Lindberg et al., 2007). Girls who are commonly victims of peer sexual harassment are at risk of body objectification, which in turn increases depressive symptoms (Grabe et al., 2007). Acknowledging these processes provides hope for reducing the connection between peer victimization and depression by increasing body esteem for girls.

Anxiety

Sexual harassment, at least in the workplace, may be so severe that it may cause posttraumatic stress disorder (Murdoch, Polusny, Hodges, & Cowper, 2006). Women who report posttraumatic stress symptoms as a result of sexual harassment tend to reexperience the event and purposefully avoid situations and people who remind them of it (Murdoch et al., 2006). Although these severe anxiety symptoms have not been researched as consequences of peer sexual harassment in adolescents, symptoms such as avoiding certain people, changing seats in a classroom, feeling self-conscious or embarrassed, and feeling afraid are common documented consequences of adolescent peer sexual harassment for girls (Duffy et al., 2004).

Peer sexual harassment not only increases anxiety for the victim, but also increases anxiety for witnesses (Nishina & Juvonen, 2005). Eighty percent of middle school boys and girls report witnessing sexual harassment (Nishina & Juvonen, 2005). Students who witness harassment may view harassment as a frequent occurrence and may fear that they will be the victims of sexual harassment the next time it occurs. Alternatively, witnesses of sexual harassment may have increased anxiety because they are torn between wanting to help the victim and fearing the consequences of doing so.

Self-Esteem

Common consequences of peer sexual harassment include feeling less sure of oneself, less confident, and more self-conscious (Duffy et al., 2004). Girls who are victims of peer sexual harassment also report a lower sense of global self worth than do girls who are not victimized (Nadeem & Graham). Girls as young as third, fourth, and fifth grade who reported being victims of sexual harassment also reported lower levels of self-esteem than their nonharassed peers (Murnen & Smolak, 2000).

A gender difference in self-esteem develops during the adolescent years, with girls reporting somewhat lower levels of self-esteem than boys (Kling, Hyde, Showers, & Busswell, 1999; Polce-Lynch, Myers, Kliewer, & Kilmartin, 2001). Girls' self-esteem may decrease in adolescence more than boys' because they are more commonly victims of frequent and severe sexual harassment (Duffy et al., 2004). Reducing the rates of peer sexual harassment, particularly for female victims, may help to reduce the gender difference in self-esteem that emerges in adolescence.

Intervention Programs

Intervention programs for peer sexual harassment in the schools are only beginning to be used, and data on long-term results are not yet available. However, intervention programs for peer sexual harassment may benefit from knowledge about successful interventions to reduce other forms of victimization, specifically bullying. Intervention programs for bullying have had mixed results. Although some programs have been very successful in reducing bullying (Olweus, 1993), others have not been successful, and may have actually increased the rates of bullying (Roland, 2000). A meta-analysis of 16 intervention programs concluded that the majority of intervention program had no effect (Merrell, Gueldner, Ross, & Isava, 2008). The key to a successful program seems to be a "whole-school" approach (Olweus, 1993). This approach includes educational materials and interventions with teachers, school principals, bullies, victims, and parents to teach social skills and warn against the consequences of bullying. The whole-school approach involves follow-up sessions and assessment of procedures throughout the intervention. Interventions that pass out materials to teachers or school principals and do not follow-up with them are not likely to significantly reduce bullying (Roland, 2000).

Expect Respect was an intervention program designed to reduce the rates of bullying and sexual harassment among fifth graders in six elementary schools (Meraviglia, Becker, Rosenbluth, Sanchez, & Robertson, 2003). This program used the whole-school approach and included education for students, teachers, school administrators, and parents to recognize bullying and sexual harassment, minimize its occurrence, and help the victims cope. When compared with control schools, schools in the intervention program were better able to recognize sexual harassment after the intervention, but were not better at recognizing bullying. This indicates that intervention programs for sexual harassment might be even more effective than bullying interventions. Future research should examine whether interventions such as these can reduce the prevalence of sexual harassment in the schools.

Prevention of sexual harassment may be more effective than intervention programs for victims. Students should be taught to recognize and avoid sexual harassment before it becomes a problem. They should be taught appropriate ways of expressing sexual attraction and cautioned that sexual harassment may occur both within and across genders. Teachers should also be taught to recognize sexual harassment, to avoid blaming the victim, and to implement consequences for inappropriate behaviors.

An organization called Equal Rights Advocates discusses sexual harassment in the schools and lists several things that girls can do if they have been sexually harassed (http://www.equalrights.org/publications/kyr/shschool.asp). First, girls should not blame themselves. Regardless of the situation, the victim is never the one at fault for being sexually harassed; the perpetrator has done something wrong and should be the one who is blamed. Parents and teachers can support the victim by helping them realize that they are not at fault. Second, the target should be clear that the harassment is unwanted by saying "No!" or by telling the harasser explicitly that the behavior is offensive. The perpetrator may not know that his or her behavior is unwanted or may not be aware of how uncomfortable it makes the victim feels. If the perpetrator does not stop, the victim should report the behavior to a school official, such as a teacher, guidance counselor, or principal. The victim may also want to consult the school's sexual harassment policy. All schools should have a Title IX grievance policy, which should list the behaviors that the school considers to be sexual harassment. Each school or district should also have a Title IX officer who can explain these policies and how to file a complaint about sexual harassment with the school. Finally, if the school does not act, a complaint may be filed with the U.S. Department of Education's Office of Civil Rights or a law suit may be filed.

Future Directions

Research in this area has a number of limitations. First, most samples have been primarily White and middle class. Only a few studies have examined the role of ethnicity in peer sexual harassment victimization, and they have indeed found that patterns of sexual harassment victimization differ as a function of ethnicity (AAUW, 2001; Goldstein et al., 2007; Nadeem & Graham, 2005). For example, African American boys are more likely to be sexually harassed than are White or Hispanic boys, but there were no ethno-racial differences for victimization among girls (AAUW, 2001). In one study, African American women reported difficulty in separating harassment based on race versus gender, thus creating a type of racialized sexual harassment (Buchanan & Ormerod, 2002). This suggests that the specific behaviors that constitute peer sexual harassment victimization and the meaning of these behaviors may be different for ethnic minorities and those with low socioeconomic status. Additionally, sexual harassment may be different when it is perpetrated within or across races. For example, in one study, African American women reported being more upset by harassment from White men than from African American men (Woods, Buchanan, & Settles, 2009). Future research should include participants from all ethno-racial groups in order to determine the predictors and consequences of peer sexual harassment for all people and include forms of racialized sexual harassment in sexual harassment measures.

Research on sexual harassment among sexual minorities is also scarce. Sexual minorities are at particular risk of experiencing sexual harassment victimization. One study reports that sexual harassment victimization is more commonly reported by sexual minority high school students than by heterosexual students, regardless of gender (Williams et al., 2005). This victimization also mediated the relationship between sexual minority status and externalizing symptoms and depression. Future research on peer sexual harassment should include sexual minorities and seek to identify which types of sexual harassment are targeted toward them. Reducing sexual harassment victimization targeted toward sexual minorities may help reduce depression and externalizing behaviors in this population.

Is measurement a problem in this research area? On the one hand, all studies reviewed here have used youth self-reports of behaviors, and self-reports can be biased. We know of no study that has attempted direct observations of these behaviors or used others' reports of peer sexual harassment victimization. Research on other forms of peer victimization, such as bullying, often relies on peer and teacher nomination to identify students who are frequent victims of harassment. Although students are likely the best reporters of their own experiences, they may be unwilling to admit that they were victimized. We believe that including peer nominations in peer sexual harassment research, in combination with self-reports, would strengthen this field of study. We also believe that some of these behaviors could be observed, but many, if not most, remain concealed from adults. Therefore, an observational study would represent a major advance, yet, at the same time, might miss many of the incidents that can be tapped using self-report.

Peer sexual harassment researchers have consistently followed the excellent measurement principles established in the path-breaking research of Mary Koss and her colleagues (1987) in the study of rape. Rather than asking women, "Have you ever been raped?" which leads to substantial underreporting for a variety of reasons, Koss instead asked about whether specific behaviors had occurred. Our research and that of others have used this same model. We do not ask teens, "have you ever been sexually harassed by a peer?" because responses might be distorted by the respondent's lack of knowledge of the definition of sexual harassment, unwillingness to acknowledge it to the self, and so on. Instead, we ask whether specific behaviors have occurred, such as "has anyone ever made sexual comments, jokes, gestures, or looks toward you?" and "has anyone ever called you gay or lesbian?" (AAUW, 2001). This should lead to optimal accuracy of self-reports.

The majority of sexual harassment research to date has focused on predictors and consequences of harassment victimization. Future research should identify the perpetrators of sexual harassment. Models used by research in workplace harassment (Pryor, 1987), bullying, and other forms of victimization (Olweus, 1993) may provide insight about the characteristics of peer sexual harassment perpetrators to be applied to research on peer sexual harassment.

Researchers should also attempt to identify protective factors. Current research indicates that a supportive peer group may buffer against the negative effects of peer harassment (Pelligrini, 2001). What other victim characteristics might reduce the effects of peer victimization? Researchers may wish to examine victim characteristics, such as emotion regulation, a supportive family environment, or a supportive school environment. These factors, among others, may help buffer teens from the harmful effects of peer victimization. Identifying and strengthening protective factors may help reduce the negative consequences of peer harassment.

Finally, additional research must be done on intervention programs for peer sexual harassment. Research indicates that this problem is pervasive and may have severe negative consequences. Intervention programs should be a priority to help prevent and reduce the incidence of harassment, support the victims, and increase observational skills and victim sensitivity for teachers and parents.

Conclusion

Peer sexual harassment is a thorny problem for adolescents and for the adults responsible for guiding them. From the research reviewed here, it is clear that there is more than one kind of peer sexual harassment in adolescence. A spectacular diversity exists in the behaviors that fall into the category of peer sexual harassment. Moreover, the meaning of the behavior to the victim and to the perpetrator may differ considerably, and the meaning of a behavior may vary from one victim to the next. A behavior that flatters one teen may frighten another.

We believe that, in some cases, early adolescents engage in sexually harassing behaviors as a way of making sense of their developing sexualities. In particular, cross-gender sexual harassment may be a typical part of sexual development in which adolescents experiment with expressing romantic attraction toward their peers. The transition into associating with other-gender peers allows youth to determine appropriate ways of expressing romantic attraction by testing the boundaries of sexual teasing. Sexual attention in the form of low levels of harassment (e.g., telling sexual jokes) may not always be harmful, but rather may be a typical part of development in which adolescents experiment with expressing romantic attraction toward their peers. In one study, 39% of students reported that sexual harassment was "just a part of school life" or "no big deal," and over half of students (52%) reported not being upset by harassment (AAUW, 2001). For some peer sexual harassment, the perpetrator may have the intent of hurting the victim, so the activity represents bullying. In other cases, the perpetrator may intend to attract romantic or sexual attention, but due to inexperience, may engage in inept flirtation in the form of sexual harassment. For example, in one qualitative study, boys indicated that girls sometimes hit or slapped them, but said "Its not serious hitting, just flirtation" (Shute et al., 2008). In this way, sexual harassment is distinct from other forms of peer victimization in which the uniform intent is to physically or emotionally harm the victim.

Although some forms of sexual harassment may be innocuous, instances of sexual aggression should not be ignored. Eleven percent of perpetrators report that they harass to express power over the victim (AAUW, 2001). Sexual harassment intended to express dominance may have far-reaching consequences for its victims and is important to eliminate. Moreover, even when the perpetrator's intentions are harmless, the target of the harassment may be distressed by this unwanted attention, and this may cause negative psychological and educational consequences for the victim. Regardless of the perpetrator's intentions, negative perceptions of harassment by the victim are associated with a variety of negative outcomes ranging from embarrassment to a severe drop in self-esteem or even depression (AAUW, 2001; Nadeem & Graham, 2005). The alarming increase in sexual harassment during early adolescence requires more research to expand on existing knowledge and identify additional predictors and sequelae of this complex form of sexualization among peers.

References

American Association of University Women (AAUW). (2001). *Hostile hallways: Bullying, teasing, and sexual harassment in school.* New York: Harris/Scholastic Research.

Anderson, I. (2007). What is a typical rape: Effects of victim and participant gender in female and male rape perceptions. *British Journal of Social Psychology, 46,* 225–245.

Brown, J. D., & L'Engle, K. L. (2009). X-rated: Sexual attitudes and behaviors associated with U.S. early adolescents exposure to sexually ecplicit material., *Communication Research, 36,* 129–151.

Buchanan, N. T., & Ormerod, A. (2002). Racialized sexual harassment in the lives of African American women. *Women and Therapy, 25,* 107–124.

Bukowski, W. M., Sippola, L. K., & Newcomb, A. F. (2000). Variations in patterns of attraction to same- and other-sex peers during early adolescence. *Developmental Psychology, 36,* 147–154.

Cillessen, A. H. N., & Rose, A. J. (2005). Understanding popularity in the peer system. *Current Directions in Psychological Science, 14,* 102–105.

Coleman, P. K., & Byrd, C. P. (2003). Interpersonal correlates of peer victimization among young adolescence. *Journal of Youth and Adolescence, 32,* 301–314.

Craig, W., Pepler, D., Connolly, J., & Henderson, K. (2001). Developmental context of peer harassment in early adolescence. In J. Juvonen, & S. Graham (eds.), *Peer harassment in school: The plight of the vulnerable and victimized* (pp. 242–261). New York: Guilford.

Duffy, J., Wareham, S., & Walsh, M. (2004). Psychological consequences for high school students of having been sexually harassed. *Sex Roles, 50,* 811–821.

Fineran, S., & Bennett, L. (1999). Gender and power issues of peer sexual harassment among teenagers. *Journal of Interpersonal Violence, 14,* 626–641.

Goldstein, S. E., Malanchuk, O., Davis-Kean, P. E., & Eccles, J. S. (2007). Risk factors of sexual harassment by peers: A longitudinal investigation of African American and European American adolescents. *Journal of Research on Adolescence, 17,* 285–300.

Grabe, S., Hyde, J. S., & Lindberg, S. (2007). Body objectification and depression in adolescents: The role of gender, shame, and rumination. *Psychology of Women Quarterly, 31,* 164–175.

Hand, J. Z., & Sachez, L. (2000). Badgering or bantering? Gender differences in experience of, and reaction to, sexual harassment among U.S. high school students. *Gender and Society, 14,* 718–746.

Harned, M. S. (2000). Harassed bodies: An examination of the relationships among women's experiences of sexual harassment, body image, and eating disorders. *Psychology of Women Quarterly, 24,* 336–348.

Harned, M. S., & Fitzgerald, L. F. (2002). Understanding a link between sexual harassment and eating disorder symptoms: A meditational analysis. *Journal of Counseling and Clinical Psychology, 70,* 1170–1181.

Hyde, J. S., Mezulis, A. H., & Abramson, L. Y. (2008). The ABCs of depression: Integrating affective, biological, and cognitive models to explain the emergence of the gender difference in depression. *Psychological Review, 115,* 291–313.

Kaltiala-Heino, R., Kosunen, E., & Rimpela, M. (2003). Pubertal timing, sexual behavior and self reported depression among middle adolescence. *Journal of Adolescence, 26,* 531–545.

Kling, K. C. Hyde, J. S., Showers, C., & Buswell, B. (1999). Gender differences in self-esteem: A meta-analysis. *Psychological Bulletin, 125,* 470–500.

Koss, M. P., Gidycz, C. A., & Wisniewski, N. (1987). The scope of rape: Incidence and prevalence in a national sample of higher education students. *Journal of Consulting and Clinical Psychology, 55,* 162–170.

Kunkel, D., Biely, E., Eyal K., Cope-Farrar, K., Donnerstein, E., & Fandrich, R. (2003). *Sex on TV III: A biennial report to the Kaiser Family Foundation.* Menlo Park, CA: Kaiser Family Foundation.

Lindberg, S. M., Grabe, S., & Hyde, J. S. (2007). Gender, pubertal development, and peer sexual harassment predict objectified body consciousness in early adolescence. *Journal of Research on Adolescence, 17,* 723–742.

Magnusson, D., Stattin, H., & Allen, V. (1985). Biological maturation and social development: A longitudinal study of some adjustment processes from mid-adolescence to adulthood. *Journal of Youth and Adolescence, 14,* 267–283.

Marshall, W. A., & Tanner, N. M. (1969). Variations in the pattern of pubertal changes in girls. *Archives of Diseases in Childhood, 44,* 291–303.

Marshall, W. A., & Tanner, N. M. (1970). Variations in the pattern of pubertal changes in boys. *Archives of Diseases in Childhood, 45*, 15–23.

McMasters, L., Connolly, J., Pepler, D., & Craig, W. (2002). Peer to peer sexual harassment in early adolescence: A developmental perspective. *Development and Psychopathology, 14*, 91–105.

Meraviglia, M. G., Becker, H., Rosenbluth, B., Sanchez, E., & Robertson, T. (2003). The expect respect project: Creating a positive elementary school climate. *Journal of Interpersonal Violence, 18*, 1347–1360.

Merrell, K. W., Gueldner, B. A., Ross, S. W., & Isava, D. M. (2008). How effective are school bullying intervention programs? A meta-analysis of intervention research. *School Psychology Quarterly, 23*, 26–42.

Montemurro, B. (2003). Not a laughing matter: Sexual harassment as "material" on workplace-based situation comedies. *Sex Roles, 48*, 433–445.

Murdoch, M., Polusny, M. A., Hodges, J., & Cowper, D. (2006). The association between in-service sexual harassment and post-traumatic stress disorder among department of veterans' affairs disability applicants. *Military Medicine, 171*, 166–173.

Murnen, S. K., & Smolak, L. (2000). The experience of sexual harassment among grade-school students: Early socialization of female subordination? *Sex Roles, 43*, 1–17.

Nadeem, E., & Graham, S. (2005). Early puberty, peer victimization, and internalizing symptoms in ethnic minority adolescents. *Journal of Early Adolescence, 25*, 197–222.

The National Campaign to Prevent Teen and Unplanned Pregnancy. (2008). *Sex and technology*. Washington, DC: Author.

Nishina, A., & Juvonen, J. (2005). Daily reports of witnessing and experiencing peer harassment in middle school. *Child Development, 76*, 435–451.

Olweus, D. (1993). *Bullying at school: What we know and what we can do*. Oxford, UK: Blackwell.

Ormerod, A. J., Collingsworth, L. L., & Perry L. A. (2008). Critical climate: Relations among sexual harassment, climate, and outcomes for high school girls and boys. *Psychology of Women Quarterly, 32*, 113–125.

Pelligrini, A. D. (2001). A longitudinal study of heterosexual relationships, aggression, and sexual harassment during the transition from primary school through middle school. *Applied Developmental Psychology, 22*, 119–133.

Pelligrini, A. D. (2002). Bullying, victimization, and sexual harassment during the transition to middle school. *Educational Psychologist, 37*, 151–163.

Pelligrini, A. D., & Bartini, M. (2001). Dominance in early adolescent boys: Affiliative and aggressive dimensions and possible functions. *Merrill-Palmer Quarterly, 47*, 142–163.

Pelligrini, A. D., & Long, J. D. (2002). A longitudinal study of bullying, dominance, and victimization during the transition from primary school through secondary school. *British Journal of Developmental Psychology, 20*, 259–280.

Petersen, J. L., & Hyde, J. S. (2009). A longitudinal investigation of peer sexual harassment victimization in adolescence. *Journal of Adolescence, 32*, 1173–1188.

Petersen, J. L., & Hyde, J. S. (in press). Peer sexual harassment and disordered eating in early adolescence. *Developmental Psychology*.

Polce-Lynch, M., Myers, B. J., Kliewer, W., & Kilmartin, C. (2001). Adolescent self-esteem and gender: Exploring relations to sexual harassment, body image, media influence, and emotional expression. *Journal of Youth and Adolescence, 30*, 225–244.

Pryor, J. B. (1987). Sexual harassment proclivities in men. *Sex Roles, 17*, 269–290.

Roland, E. (2000). Bullying in schools: Three national innovations in Norwegian schools in 15 years. *Aggressive Behavior, 26*, 135–143.

Rotundo, M., Nguyen, D., & Sackett, P. R. (2001). A meta-analytic review of gender differences in perceptions of sexual harassment. *Journal of Applied Psychology, 86*, 914–922.

Schreck, C. J., Burek, M. W., Stewart, E. A., & Mitchell, J. M. (2007). Distress and violent victimization among young adolescence. Early puberty and the social interactionist explanation. *Journal of Research in Crime and Delinquency, 44,* 381–405.

Sheets, V. L., & Braver, S. L. (1999). Organization status and perceived sexual harassment: Detecting the mediators of a null effects. *Personality and Social Psychology Bulletin, 25,* 1159–1171.

Shute, R., Owens, L., & Slee, P. (2008). Everyday victimization of adolescent girls by boys: Sexual harassment, bullying, or aggression? *Sex Roles, 58,* 477–489.

Stattin, H., & Magnusson, D. (1990). *Pubertal maturation in female development.* Hillsdale, NJ: Lawrence Erlbaum Associates.

Stone, M., & Couch, S. (2004). Peer sexual harassment among high school students: Teachers' attitudes, perceptions, and response. *The High School Journal, 88*(1), 1–13.

Strouse, J. S., Goodwin, M. P., & Roscoe, B. (1994). Correlates of attitudes toward sexual harassment among early adolescents. *Sex Roles, 31,* 559–577.

Surgenor, L. J., Horn, J., Plumridge, E. W., & Hudson, S. (2002). Anorexia nervosa and psychological control: A reexamination of selected theoretical accounts. *European Eating Disorder Review, 10,* 85–101.

Timmerman, G. (2003). Sexual harassment of adolescents perpetrated by teachers and by peers: An exploration of the dynamics of power, culture, and gender in secondary schools. *Sex Roles, 48,* 231–306.

Ward, L. M., Merriwether, A., & Caruthers, A. (2006). Media, masculinity ideologies, and men's beliefs about women's bodies. *Sex Roles, 55,* 703–714.

Williams, T., Connolly, J., Pepler, D., & Crais, W. (2005). Peer victimization, social support, and psychosocial adjustment of sexual minority adolescents. *Journal of Youth and Adolescence, 34,* 471–482.

Woods, K. C., Buchanan, N. T., & Settles, I. H. (2009). Sexual harassment across the color line. Experiences and outcomes of cross- versus intraracial sexual harassment among Black women. *Cultural Diversity and Ethnic Minority Psychology, 15,* 67–76.

Ybarra, M. L., Espelage, D. L., & Mitchell, K. J. (2007). The co-occurrence of internet harassment and unwanted sexual solicitation victimization and perpetration: Associations with psychosocial indicators. *Journal of Adolescent Health, 41,* 31–41.

Zurbriggen, E. L., Collins, R. L., Lamb, S., Roberts, T., Tolman, D. L., Ward, L. M., & Blake, J. *Sexualization of girls: Executive Summary.* Washington, DC: American Psychological Association.

7

"If You're Hot, I'm Bi"

Implications of Sexualization for Sexual Minority Girls

ELISABETH MORGAN THOMPSON

As I was leaving the gym several months ago, I saw a young woman wearing a t-shirt that took me by surprise—not because of what it said, but because I had never seen it before. I had seen the t-shirts that sexualized and objectified women ("Who needs brains when you have these [breasts]?" or "Tell your boyfriend to call me"), but they were always focused on specific body parts or presumptions of heterosexuality—the typical sexualization of women's bodies. What made this shirt different was its blatant sexualization of sexual minority women; it read, "If You're Hot, I'm Bi," suggesting that this woman's sexual interest does not see gender but rather "hotness." Through a simple t-shirt, she was not only sexualizing herself and encouraging others to sexualize her (as this shirt in many ways reduced her to her sexuality), but she was also engaging in the sexualization of other women, particularly bisexual women.

In 2007, the American Psychological Association's (APA) Task Force on the Sexualization of Girls (TFSG) reviewed the evidence for and effects of sexualization on girls' health and well-being. The report recommendations encouraged researchers to explore differences in content and effects of sexualized images on sexual minority girls in particular. To date, very little research has systematically studied or described if and how sexual minority women are sexualized and are affected by that sexualization. In most cases, researchers can only speculate on the effects of sexualization on sexual minority girls based on what is known about the sexualization of girls and women in general, because this population has not been prioritized in research. The few studies conducted with this population have provided evidence consistent with that described in the TFSG report; that is, sexual minority women experience sexualization, and this sexualization is detrimental to their psyches, bodies, sexuality, and identity development. The purpose of this chapter is to provide evidence of the sexualization of sexual minority women in sociocultural and interpersonal contexts. A second purpose is to review the limited research with this population and describe some of the already determined consequences and projected implications of sexualization for sexual minority girls. Finally, I provide suggestions for future research with this un(der)examined population.

(How) Are Sexual Minority Women Sexualized?

To establish the sexualization of sexual minority women as an issue to be addressed, we must first know whether sexual minority women are sexualized, and if so, how? In this section, I will use the TFSG's (American Psychological Association [APA], 2007) description of sexualization in answering this question. The TFSG defined sexualization broadly as it pertains to women in general, and their definition included emphasis and value placed on one's attractiveness/sexiness/sex appeal; and/or experiences of sexual objectification, exploitation, or victimization. Sexualization can occur in several domains: culturally (e.g., by the media or other social institutions), interpersonally (e.g., by partners, peers, family members, or strangers), and internally (i.e., self-sexualization). The following review provides evidence that the definition of sexualization provided by the TFSG is relevant to sexual minority women's experiences.

Sexualization in the Media

The sexualization of sexual minority women and same-sex experiences between women is probably most evident in media and popular culture outlets; this sexualization has been noted by theorists (Diamond, 2005c; Gill, 2003, 2008; Jackson & Gilbertson, 2009; Levy, 2005; Thompson, 2006; Wilkinson, 1996) and journalists alike (Forcella, 2008; Lo, 2005; Warn, 2003a, 2003b, 2003c, 2005). Images and storylines sexualizing same-sex sexual behavior between women or "lesbian sex" that were at one time primarily relegated to pornography (Jensen, 1995; Leitenberg & Henning, 1995) have now surfaced in mainstream genre-crossing outlets, such as television, magazines, music, movies, and advertising (for examples, see Diamond, 2005c, and Thompson, 2006).

The last decade boasted a number of sexualized images of young women's same-sex sexuality, the most notable of which have occurred between women who did/do not identify as sexual minorities (e.g., the Britney Spears-Madonna-Christina Aguilera kiss at the *MTV Video Music Awards* in 2003). In the Summer of 2008, a new pop artist, Katy Perry, released her first single *I Kissed a Girl* from her album entitled *One of the Boys*, which has since topped the "Billboard Hot 100" and become an international chart-topping hit in more than 20 countries (Amos, 2008; billboard.com, 2009). In this highly popular song (e.g., 2009 Kids Choice Awards Favorite Song nominee; nick. com, 2009), Katy sings about enjoying her first kiss with a girl who wears cherry lip balm. Katy sexualizes this girl by saying that she just "wants to try [her] on," and "I don't even know [her] name; it doesn't matter; [she's] my experimental game."

Iconic girl-on-girl kissing scenes from movies like *Cruel Intentions* (received "Best Kiss" at the 2000 MTV Movie Awards; Benson-Allot, 2005) and *American Pie 2* are frequently referenced and replicated in other media forms. For example, the music video for Pittsburgh Slim's (2007) *Girls Kiss Girls*, a song whose lyrics are dedicated to sexualizing same-sex behavior among women, reenacts a webcam version of a combination of scenes from the original *American Pie* movie and its aptly named sequel, *American Pie 2* (Pittsburgh Slim begins the video by telling his girlfriend "you should get your 'American Pie' on"). In this video, two girls kiss and touch each other while he (Pittsburgh Slim) voyeuristically watches and even directs their behavior from the other side of the camera. Same-sex sexualized images (primarily kissing) and references to "girl-on-girl action" can be found on most network and cable channels (e.g., Fox, ABC, MTV, E!) during prime-time hours (e.g., *Grey's Anatomy, Nip Tuck*) and in shows intentionally directed at young audiences (e.g., *The OC, One Tree Hill, The Real World, The Hills*). The CW's *Gossip Girl*, a racy teen drama popular with girls and young women aged 12–34, provides a recent example of this kind of sexualization, when the camera focused on two leading female characters kissing during an implied threesome with a male character on the show (Season 3, Episode 9; Lasher & McLean, 2009).

In addition to same-sex sexual behavior, sexual minority identities (e.g., "bisexual" or "curious") are also sexualized in the media and popular culture, especially when those identities imply attractions to, or histories with, both men and women. Identifying as "bi" is a recent Hollywood trend (Warn, 2003a), and several female celebrities' popularity can be attributed in part to the sexualization of their current/past public same-sex relationships. In September 2008, Megan Fox participated in an interview for *GQ* magazine (i.e., a men's fashion and lifestyle magazine) in which she disclosed her same-sex sexual history. Most of the interview was focused on other topics, such as her childhood obsession with comic books, her relationship with her boyfriend, her adolescent rebellion, and her career aspirations. However, senior editor and author Mark Kirby (2008) contributed to the sexualization of her same-sex sexual history by returning repeatedly to her passing mention of a brief relationship with a female stripper at age 18, and he entitled the article based on this interview, "Megan Fox was a Teenage Lesbian!" Since this interview, Megan has "come out" as bisexual, and this has been the topic of many Internet and entertainment stories (just googling "Megan Fox, bisexual" solicits 2,010,000 hits). Other popularizations of "sexy" sexual minority women in the media include Tila Tequila, an Internet model on MySpace, who became a household name when she was cast on *MTV* as the bachelorette on the first-ever bisexual reality dating television show, *A Shot at Love with Tila Tequila*. The viewership for the finale in its first season was nearly 6 million in the 12–34 age bracket, the highest on MTV since 2005 (Weprin, 2008). As a result of the popularity of this show as MTV's highest rated new series, MTV subsequently telecast a second season with Tila, and produced a spin-off—*A Double Shot at Love* with bisexual twins who were also commercial models and have appeared on several daytime talk shows to discuss their bisexuality.

Although the increase in sexual minority representation in the media may seem like a social progression, these same-sex images are only possible because they are highly sexualized, often fleeting or unserious, and have commercial appeal (Diamond, 2005c; Wilkinson, 1996). Acceptable images of same-sex sexuality between women are very specific images of attractive, hyperfeminine, "hot" women intended to cater to the heterosexual male fantasy (Diamond, 2005c; Gill, 2008; Jackson & Gilbertson, 2009). The power of this fantasy results in images of same-sex desire between women that are meant to be less threatening because they are presented as purely "experimental" and dictated by male rather than female desire (Diamond, 2005c; Wilkinson, 1996), and, in fact, adolescent viewers tend to read these images in this way (Jackson & Gilbertson, 2009).

Interpersonal and Peer Sexualization (Sexualization of/by Others)

These movies, music, and images are primarily directed toward those growing up in the MTV generation (Benson-Allot, 2005), bombarded by a reality television, "viral," and *Girls Gone Wild*, porno-chic culture (Hall & Bishop, 2007; Levy, 2005), in which young people are exposed to a set of sexual norms that differs markedly from previous cohorts (Wells & Twenge, 2005). These images have arguably influenced young people's behavior, such that Malernee (2003), Forcella (2008), and Jackson and Gilbertson's (2009) data suggest it is not unusual to attend a high school party and see adolescent girls making out with other girls in the presence of boys. Hence, not only is the sexualization of sexual minority women and same-sex behavior evident in the media, it is experienced interpersonally as well.

Research has shown that sexual minority women report experiencing various forms of interpersonal sexualization, including childhood sexual abuse and adult sexual assault (Balsam, Rothblum, & Beauchaine, 2005), appearance pressure from peers (Beren, Hayden, Wilfley, & Striegel-Moore, 1997), and sexual objectification by others, both men (Engeln-Maddox, Miller, & Doyle, 2009; Hill, 2002; Hill & Fischer, 2008; Kozee & Tylka, 2006) and women (Hill, 2002; Hill & Fischer, 2008). My dissertation (2009) was one of the first empirical examinations of the role of peers in the sexualization of same-sex behavior and sexual minority women. In this study, I interviewed 111 female undergraduates (aged 18–25) of varied ethnicities and sexualities (i.e., exclusively/mostly straight or lesbian, bisexual, curious, questioning, queer, unlabeled) about their own same-sex experiences or a time when they witnessed other women's same-sex experiences (mostly "kissing") with men present. There had been much theoretical discussion of this "popular phenomenon" in peer culture but no systematic examination of the ways it manifests on the ground—the primary purpose of my study (i.e., Who are the major players? At what age and in what contexts is this occurring? What are the primary motivations behind these occurrences?). The feminist critiques of this phenomenon have posed it as objectifying to women and sexual minorities, in that the "(heterosexual) male gaze" is presumed responsible for much of this behavior (Diamond, 2005c; Levy, 2005). As a result, a secondary purpose of this study was to explore whether young women saw this as a site of the sexualization (or objectification) of their bodies and/or a space to explore their sexual agency and identity. Results from this study relevant to the sexualization of sexual minority women in peer culture will be discussed at various points throughout this chapter.

Many of the stories these young women told fit the expected profile of the sexualization of same-sex behavior among women in peer culture. A subset of my sample reported intentionally kissing other women in order to be seen as "sexy" by, or to gain the attention of, men. That is, some of these young women were "experimenting" with each other, under the guise of boys thinking it is "hot." Other women participated in the phenomenon because men encouraged or cheered them on. Whereas most of these young women identified as heterosexual and were actively participating in the sexualization of themselves and their peers, the sexual minority women in this study were not exempt from this behavior. In fact, many of their experiences dated back to high school, and some to as early as middle school, often prior to their identification as sexual minorities. The early onset of this sexualization of themselves and others in peer culture has direct implications for the sexualization of (sexual minority) girls.

All of the young women in my study were aware of the "heterosexual male fantasy" surrounding same-sex behavior, and several blamed society as a source of ideas for and promotion of this phenomenon. For example, "Christine" (pseudonyms were provided by all participants), a white, bisexual young woman, articulated the role of mainstream media, "You can't turn on the TV without seeing two girls making out." Others echoed Christine by referencing society in general and mainstream media in particular, "Society tells you to do this...you see all these movies like you know girls 'Jell-O wrestling' and so you think like 'oh that's what happens in college' and then you get there and you try to make that happen" (Jasmine, white, sexually open), and "It's just kind of like a given with all the *Girls Gone Wild* material…I just feel like our culture is really interested in two hot girls making out…and I feel [women] see that too and perpetuate this cultural construction more" (Ness, white, curious).

Even though discussions of this phenomenon have presumed the male gaze as dictating much of this behavior, it is important to note that the young women in my study (several of whom were sexual minorities) also perpetuated the sexualization of (sexual minority) women through their language and behavior. Several of the young women themselves used objectifying terms when describing the women they were kissing, and others discussed their sexual exploits as meaningless or a competition/game. Women's sexualization of other women has been evident in both peer culture and the media as well (Levy, 2005), through young women wearing t-shirts like "If You're Hot, I'm Bi," *Girls Gone Wild* videos of young women kissing and touching each other while flashing the camera, and reality shows (e.g., the *Real World*) with young women making out in drunken stupors, screaming "You're Hot!" These experience-based phenomena in peer culture provide the basis for the interpersonal sexualization of sexual minority women.

In reviewing these examples, the definition of sexualization provided by the TFSG (APA, 2007) can clearly characterize the experiences of sexual minority women in American culture. In summary, sexual minority women have reported high levels of peer sexualization, sexual objectification, childhood sexual abuse, and sexual victimization as adults, providing evidence for the interpersonal sexualization of sexual minority women in our culture (Balsam et al., 2005; Beren et al., 1997; Hill, 2002; Hill & Fischer, 2008; Kozee & Tylka, 2006). When sexual minority women are sexualized in the media, there is an overrepresentation of feminine, "hot," sexy women who meet rigid societal standards of attractiveness, intended to cater to the heterosexual male gaze. These women's value is located in their sexual appeal to men, not unlike images of sexualized heterosexual women. What differs for sexual minority women is the presence of multiple minority stressors, where they are sexualized at least twice, as both women and sexual minorities. These images and experiences are different in that sexual minority women do not meet the standards of hegemonic femininity—which Tolman (2006) describes as "expectations of how women and girls should and should not feel, behave, and think regarding themselves, their own bodies, their roles in relationships" (p. 76), all of which presupposes and requires heterosexuality.

Because hegemonic femininity assumes and requires heterosexuality (Rich, 1980; Tolman, 2006), sexual minorities are defined primarily by their sexual "deviance." This deviance is almost exclusive to their same-sex sexual behavior, and there is little emphasis placed on the way their sexuality fits into their whole person. This reductionism is in line with the TFSG definition of sexualization and is evident in the sexualized images and experiences of sexual minority women, in which the focus is almost exclusively on their same-sex sexual behavior. It is not hard to see how the sexualization of same-sex behavior and sexual minority women has the potential to psychologically and physically impact girls in general and sexual minority girls in particular. As this is a relatively unexplored area, little research has discussed the implications of this sexualization—the focus of the next section of the chapter.

What Are the Implications of Sexualization of/for Sexual Minority Girls?

The TFSG (APA, 2007) dedicated a section of its report to providing examples and evidence of the ways in which women in general are sexualized, both culturally and interpersonally. The authors also reviewed the research on the effects of sexualization of women in general; however, they acknowledged the research was limited in its understanding of diverse populations, especially sexual minority women. In the previous section, I provided examples and evidence of the sexualization of same-sex behavior and/or sexual minority women. The following sections will address what we know about how sexual minority women are affected by the sexualization of women in general, and the ways in which all girls could be affected by the sexualization of same-sex experiences and sexual minority identities.

Are Sexual Minorities Protected?

Several schools of thought have driven the research on sexual identity and sexualization. Because sexual minority women are raised in the same sexist and objectifying contexts as heterosexual women, some researchers have expected them to have the same experiences and consequences of objectification as heterosexual women (Dworkin, 1988). In contrast, others believe that sexual minority women are shielded or "protected" from the negative effects of objectification because of the less stringent beauty norms within the lesbian community (Brown, 1987) and a lack of use of the "male gaze" as a measuring stick (Siever, 1994). However, there has been little support for the "protection" hypothesis. That is, sexual minority women are not exempt from sexualization or appearance standards; in fact, they are socialized in the same sociocultural and objectifying contexts as heterosexual women, and are subject to both mainstream and "lesbian" subcultural standards. These identities/ subcultural communities may provide a different set of appearance standards against which they measure themselves, but only in some instances (Beren et al., 1997; Bergeron & Senn, 1998; Rothblum, 1994). In addition, I argue that these "protective" community appearance standards are not particularly far-reaching, particularly because of their timing and (lack of) applicability to all sexual minority women.

In regards to timing, sexual minority women are not raised within a social vacuum, but instead have many of the same socialization experiences as their heterosexual peers. Because most young women do not begin to identify as a sexual minority until the age of 17 (and even later for bisexuals) (Rust, 1993; Savin-Williams & Diamond, 2000), they experience similar socialization to their heterosexual counterparts during the majority of their childhood and adolescent years. These young women's access to a sexual minority community that may foster less rigid beauty norms comes well after being exposed to the powerful messages of what it means to be a girl in this society, not the least of which includes excessive value placed on appearance and (hetero)sexual appeal (APA, 2007). Thus, it is important to note that these girls' gender socialization is both salient and relevant to understanding the implications of sexualization for them.

Another problem with the "protection" hypothesis is applicability—"sexual minority" is not a monolithic category and does not only mean "lesbian." Rather, a variety of identities and subtypes comprise sexual minority women, including many with a combination of both same-sex and other-sex attractions, behaviors, and desires (Diamond, 2005a; Savin-Williams, 2005; Thompson & Morgan, 2008). Even lesbians have reported sexual experiences with and attraction toward men both currently (Diamond, 2005a) and in the past (Kitzinger & Wilkinson, 1995), and evidence suggests that women's sexual identity trajectories are fluid and nonexclusive toward one sex (Diamond, 2008). The belief that sexual minority women are not interested in men as partners or in seeking the "male gaze" (Siever, 1994), again, only applies to a subset of sexual minority women. Hence, not all sexual minority women are automatically protected from mainstream appearance norms, and not all sexual minority women have access to a community that fosters their own norms (Berenson, 2002; Bradford, 2004). For instance, the most visible and viable community for sexual minority women historically has been the lesbian community, which has been unwelcoming to those who are sexual/partnered with men or do not fit the "look" (Bradford, 2004; Bower, Gurevich, & Mathieson, 2002; Clarke & Turner, 2007; Drechsler, 2003). Protection within the lesbian community is predicated on more separatist or politicized versions of lesbianism, which younger generations of sexual minority women are less likely to endorse or identity with (Golden, 1996, 2006; Savin-Williams, 2005). Rather, younger sexual minority women are trending toward individualistic notions, placing more emphasis on appearance and seemingly identifying as post-feminist and even post-gay (Golden, 2006; Levy, 2005; Savin-Williams). Ultimately, this recent shift in the "lesbian community" has implications for sexual minority women's (lack of) exemption and protection from sexualization.

Consequences of the Sexualization of Women in General (for Sexual Minority Girls)

Much of the research on sexualization has focused narrowly on the "objectification" of women's bodies as its working definition (APA, 2007), and most of the unhealthy consequences of sexualization have been examined using objectification theory as a guiding framework (Fredrickson & Roberts, 1997; McKinley & Hyde, 1996). Few studies have examined experiences of objectification and its consequences for sexual minority populations in particular, but the few that exist have mostly compared heterosexuals and lesbians on the typically examined outcomes of objectification (e.g., self-esteem, body dissatisfaction, body shame, eating disorder symptomatology).

Psychological and Bodily Consequences

Overall, research has shown the physical and mental health consequences of objectification to be similar for heterosexual and lesbian women, ultimately suggesting that the sexualization of women is equally damaging regardless of one's sexual identity. One of the consequences of being sexualized by the media and/or interpersonally is the internalization of that sexualization. To have a constant "gaze" on one's body results in the internalization of that gaze (i.e., self-sexualization or self-objectification). With few exceptions (Brand, Rothblum, & Solomon, 1992; Siever, 1994), studies have shown that gender trumps sexual identity in that bisexual and lesbian women are as likely as heterosexual women to self-objectify, value thinness, and perceive themselves as overweight (Beren et al., 1997; Downs, James, & Cowan, 2006; Kozee & Tylka, 2006). These similarities in self-sexualization make sense in that lesbians and heterosexual women report similar recent and lifetime experiences with objectification, and these experiences are associated with higher levels of self-objectification (Hill, 2002; Kozee & Tylka).

Similarly, the more that women internalize the sexualization of their bodies, the more detrimental the effects of that self-sexualization, regardless of sexual identity. Higher internalization is associated with more negative attitudes and shame toward one's body (Bergeron & Senn, 1998; Engeln-Maddox et al., 2009; Haines et al., 2008) and disordered eating (Haines et al., 2008;

Kozee & Tylka, 2006) for both lesbian and heterosexual women. Lesbians tend to have similar levels of body dissatisfaction (Beren, Hayden, Wilfley, & Grilo, 1996; Brand et al., 1992; Siever, 1994; Striegel-Moore, Tucker, & Hsu, 1990), body shame (Engeln-Maddox et al., 2009), and eating disorder symptomatology (Striegel-Moore et al., 1990) as heterosexual women (for exceptions, see Bergeron & Senn, 1998; Siever, 1994). That there are few reliable differences between heterosexual and lesbian women's experiences of sexualization, self-sexualization, and the consequences of sexualization supports some research that has shown affiliation with the lesbian community is unrelated to negative body outcomes in lesbians (Beren et al., 1996). Thus, the "protective factors" (if they exist) that come with identifying as a lesbian are not enough to counteract already internalized beliefs and values (Striegel-Moore et al., 1990).

It is important to note that sexist appearance norms are not the only rigid sociocultural standards that sexual minority women internalize. Rather, in a heterosexist culture, sexual minorities also have to contend with compulsory heterosexuality (Rich, 1980), which can lead to additional feelings of inadequacy and internalized heterosexism (Szymanski, Kashubeck-West, & Meyer, 2008). The internalization of heterosexism has been shown to have physical and mental health consequences for sexual minority women. In an interview study by Beren et al. (1997), many of the lesbian participants explained negative stereotypes about lesbians as "ugly" and "masculine," and feelings that they were not fulfilling their proper "feminine" social role affected the way they viewed their bodies and influenced their feelings about their appearance. Here, these lesbians were aware that they were not meeting the rigid standards of hegemonic femininity that worked together to require them to be both "sexy" and "heterosexual." Lesbians' disordered eating and depression (Haines et al., 2008), as well as their lowered self-esteem, greater interpersonal distrust, and increased difficulties in identifying their own emotions (Striegel-Moore et al., 1990), may have as much to do with "living in a homophobic society and all [tha]t entails" (p. 498) as it does with living in a sexist society that sexualizes and objectifies women.

Implications of the Sexualization of Sexual Minority Women (for Girls)

The increased sexualization and mainstream representation of sexual minority women and same-sex behavior among women in our culture will likely lead to even greater internalization of cultural beauty norms—the current construct that theoretically "protects" sexual minority women from the negative effects of self-objectification (e.g., Bergeron & Senn, 1998). As we have seen from the research on the effects of sexualization of women in general, we can expect

these emergent and specific images and experiences to magnify the internalization of sexism and heterosexism in sexual minority women. This, then, can
result in similar (if not more intense) psychological and body image concerns
as have already been found, along with other potential consequences not yet
addressed in research.

Sexual Identity Concerns

One area that has been especially overlooked in the literature pertains to
the implications of sexualization for sexual identity development concerns in
girls. Patriarchy both relies on and perpetuates compulsory heterosexuality
(Pharr, 1988; Rich, 1980; Tolman, 2006), such that young women are socialized to think that they need men's protection and provision and that their
feelings for or relationships with women are not "natural" or sufficient. The
internalization of a heterosexual imperative might result in identity issues for
sexual minority women.

The general sexualization of all women's bodies in our culture can result
in sexual minority women feeling uncertain about their same-sex attractions,
delaying the identification of their same-sex feelings as erotic (Diamond, 2002;
Diamond, 2005b; Morgan & Thompson, 2006). That is, sexual minority
women find themselves in the unique position of wondering whether they are
really attracted to and desire women or if they are merely attracted to a cultural aesthetic ideal. Several of the participants in my study (Thompson, 2009)
explained their identity uncertainty as the result of the sexualization of women
in general and sexual minority women in particular. For example, Davis, a
newly queer-identified, biracial (black/German) young woman offered this
perspective when she was encircled and cheered by men as she was kissing a
girl she was interested in at a party:

> I went on like a huge feminist rant just about how it's really disre-
> spectful to objectify us for your own entertainment. Where we're just
> like an object of your fantasy. It's just really...dehumanizing.... We
> definitely were like way more gay after this. I think *at the same time it's
> all really convoluted and complicated....* It's *hard for me to understand my
> sexuality because I view it through the lens that a man has created*...view-
> ing myself through the eyes of men, and identifying in that like false
> ideal of like what a woman's sexuality should be. It's like women's
> sexuality is for men, by men.... I think that's why...*my sexuality is so
> confusing.* (emphasis added)

This identity uncertainty is often resolved later into a more stable sexual
minority identity (which for Davis is "queer"); however, the delay that can

occur as a result of this sexualization has implications for less than authentic earlier sexual and relational experiences (which Davis alludes to later in her narrative, as she continued a relationship with a boyfriend in high school for some time despite no longer being interested in him).

Another implication of the sexualization of sexual minority women is a depoliticization or invalidation of one's identity. If the predominant representation of same-sex sexuality is to appease the "male gaze," then sexual minority women's same-sex desires and experiences are less likely to be viewed as legitimate (Diamond, 2005c). The implications of a lack of validation for one's identity can extend to viewing one's own experiences and identity as illegitimate or inauthentic. This internalization of negativity toward a sexual minority identity can result in various mental and physical health risks, including increased sexual shame and psychosocial difficulties (e.g., psychological distress, depression, lower self-esteem; Szymanski et al., 2008). Internalized heterosexism can also result in delays in sexual identity development. For example, many of the women in my dissertation study (Thompson, 2009) dismissed or denied a bisexual identity, primarily as a result of the specific sexualization of a bisexual identity in our culture. That is, young women whose experiences and desires may otherwise fit a bisexual identity strategically avoided this label because of its association with trendiness, attention-seeking behavior, and promiscuity (see also Thompson, 2008)—evaluations that are all tied to heterosexist construals of sexual minorities' expressions of desire. These findings suggest that the sexualization of sexual minority women has implications for the application of an appropriate label to one's experiences and identity.

Sexual Risk

The sexualization of sexual minority women (especially in peer culture) also has implications for sexually unhealthy behavior in girls, regardless of sexual identity. In my study (Thompson, 2009), the combination of alcohol impairment and desire to gain attention from young men by engaging in same-sex behavior had the potential to lead to sexual compromises and other more serious and risky sexual behaviors. For example, several of the young women in my study shared a story of how they kissed another woman to gain explicit sexual attention from men—that is, to "hook-up" with a guy they were interested in. Engaging in same-sex behavior (which is "out of character" for some women) leads to assumptions about who these young women are and what they are willing to do sexually (perhaps making it difficult to convincingly request condoms to protect oneself against sexually transmitted infections). Several of the participants in my study suggested that others, especially young men, view those who participate in the phenomenon as "one-night stand type of girls" or "up for anything." Because this behavior has the potential to affect young women's reputations as "easy" or promiscuous, it then also has implications for young men's expectations in subsequent sexual situations with these young women.

Women's Objectification of Women

The internalization of both sexism and heterosexism as a product of the sexualization of sexual minority women also has implications for women's objectification of other women. The male gaze shifts to an internalized "self-policing gaze" (Bartky, 1990; Fredrickson & Roberts, 1997; Gill, 2003, 2008), which then translates into an "other-critical gaze." In a compulsory heterosexist society, young sexual minority women learn how to sexually and relationally engage with other women on men's terms (Levy, 2005). The primary language available to them is one of games, adversarial competitions, and power struggles. For example, Taryn, a sexually unlabeled, biracial (black/white) woman from my study (Thompson, 2009), equated male objectification and female objectification of women using game-type language, explaining how guys objectify her the way her lesbian "friends would [sexually] objectify the[se 'straight' girls]." She suggested that, as much as guys want girls to kiss in front of them, lesbians want to "turn out" (i.e., convert to lesbianism) straight girls. "Just like men fantasize about lesbians, lesbians fantasize about straight girls. There's like—you know—the virgin straight girl is for sure like, 10 million bonus points." Women's objectification of other women was a poignant theme among my participants, and its ties to the sexualization and objectification of sexual minority women in the general culture (especially by men) were evident.

Positive Possibilities

Thus far, the focus of this section has been primarily on the negative consequences of sexualization, specifically as they relate to sexual minority women. Whereas the negative implications seemingly far outweigh the positive ones, it is important to point out that some positive outcomes are also possible. With increased representation of sexual minority women in the media, albeit in a very sexualized way, and opportunities to "experiment" in peer culture, some young women may be more likely to question compulsory heterosexuality or come to realize or confirm their sexual identities in a much more agentic way. For example, almost one-third of the participants in my study (Thompson, 2009) reported that their involvement with or exposure to the sexualization of sexual minority women in popular peer culture resulted in their identity questioning, realization, and confirmation. Although most of the women who questioned their identities as a result of these experiences were sexual minorities, many heterosexual women suggested these experiences led them to contemplate other possibilities before settling on a heterosexual identity. These findings highlight the need to consider all possible outcomes of sexualization in future research, both positive and negative.

How Do We Address the Sexualization of Sexual Minority Women?

The lack of research to date in this area and with this population may be related to a heterosexist bias that characterizes research in general. This bias may lead researchers to assume that sexual minority women are somehow less affected by sexualization and much of its negative outcomes because they are not interested in men as partners or seeking the male gaze, and/or their community serves to protect them from mainstream norms surrounding beauty and the body. Researchers addressing the sexualization of women must begin to ask questions about young women's sexuality and sexual identity histories, as this is inherently relevant information to the ways in which psychological and bodily consequences of sexualization can manifest. Researchers must seek to understand how the internalization of sexualization affects women of all sexual identities and must incorporate more sensitive and specific measures that are able to shed light on how sexualization may affect sexual minority women differently.

Future research needs to document the frequency of sexualization of sexual minority girls/women compared to the frequency of nonsexualized appearances in the media, and this analysis could include an examination over time. To date, there have been no strategic or systematic content analyses of these images in various forms of media, and no dedicated uncovering of what messages the images convey, the intended audience, and the actual audience. In addition, more extensive surveys of young women's same-sex experiences might shed light on the frequency of peer sexualization of sexual minority women. It is vital to examine sexualization/objectification in the contexts in which it is occurring as this can provide rich data regarding the actual experiences of sexualization of sexual minority women. Listening to women's experiences, reactions, and feelings can further the development of more relevant, reliable measures of the effects of sexualization for all women.

Additionally, researchers need to more sensitively examine the effects of sexualization on sexual minority girls'/women's health and identities. It will be important to ask whether certain forms of sexualization are more harmful than others in affecting the physical, mental, and sexual health, as well as the identity development, of sexual minority girls/women. Both the effects of the sexualization of girls/women in general and the effects of the sexualization of sexual minority girls/women in particular need to be parsed apart and explored. This can be accomplished through examining the effects of exposure to sexualized images in the experimental context and also studying the effects on young women over time using longitudinal designs. Not only should the commonly measured outcomes of sexualization be examined in this overlooked population, but researchers in this field need to think more carefully about relevant and specific outcomes pertaining to the development of sexual minority girls.

An example of a more specific and relevant experience for sexual minority women may include an examination of the differential effects of sexualization via the male gaze and/or the "female gaze." In this effort, researchers should examine more closely bisexual and other alternative sexual identities (e.g., Diamond, 2008; Thompson & Morgan, 2008). This is especially important because these young women are less likely to have attractions toward and experiences with one sex exclusively. One of the most apparent and startling themes that emerged from my dissertation study was the internalization of sexism and heterosexism resulting in women's objectification of other women. Future research could examine more closely if and how experiences with and exposure to sexualization results in greater likelihood to objectify women. Are there certain women who are more likely to objectify other women? Does sexual identity matter? Does feminist identity matter? Does a history of sexualization predict objectification of other women? Future research could also examine more closely whether women recognize they are objectifying other women and uncover the purposes or benefits of doing so. Further, assuming that gaining power is one goal, it could be important to identify other ways for young women to gain power and agency in our culture without perpetuating the sexualization and objectification that they themselves have experienced.

Along these lines, it is vital to develop interventions for girls centered on their healthy gender and sexual identity development. These interventions must include critiques of both sexism and heterosexism, and could help girls make meaning of the sexualization of sexual minority girls in particular. In this effort, girls must develop critical media skills, find ways to escape the pressure of sexualizing themselves and others, learn to debunk limited stereotypes about what it means to be a sexual minority, and explore the diversity through which they can name and express their sexuality. These strategies for girls' empowerment must foster sexual agency in girls, teaching them how to attend to and understand their own feelings, emotions, and desires (Fine, 1988, 2005; Fine & McClelland, 2006; Tolman, 2002), as access to these skills is often limited for girls raised in a sexist and heterosexist society. This education about what a healthy sexuality entails (see Lamb 2013; Chapter 14, this volume and Bay-Cheng, Livingston, & Fava, 2013; Chapter 13, this volume) must focus on girls and women of all backgrounds, including sexual minority girls who face the added suppression of their sexuality due to compulsory heterosexuality and a lack of societal acceptance.

Interventions must also consider multiple minority stressors impeding girls' healthy sexual development. The experience of being sexualized as both a woman and a sexual minority in a culture that values maleness and heterosexuality results in an additional layer of oppression not currently considered or conceptualized in the (objectification) literature. For sexual minority women of color, these risks and concerns are amplified by rejection from one's own family/community that usually serves to buffer against or facilitate coping strategies with discrimination (Hughes et al., 2006; Scott, 2004; Ward, 1996). Future research must do what it can to uncover the effects of multiple minority stressors (e.g., the role of both internalized sexism and internalized heterosexism and experiences of racism), as well as the ways in which certain oppressed identities might operate as a buffer against effects of sexualization. Further, researchers must consider the unique stressors and differential effects for sexual minority girls/women of color, impoverished sexual minority women, and poor sexual minority women of color. This emphasis on multiple intersecting and oppressed identities is essential to and has implications for the psychological and sexual freedom for all women. As the Combahee River Collective (1977/1982), a black lesbian feminist group, so eloquently explained: "If [we] were free, it would mean that everyone else would have to be free since our freedom would necessitate the destruction of all the systems of oppression" (p. 278).

References

American Psychological Association. (2007). *Report of the APA Task Force on the sexualization of girls* (Chair: E. L. Zurbriggen). Washington, DC: Author. Retrievable from www.apa.org/pi/wpo/sexualization.html

Amos, J. D. (2008). *Katy Perry kisses a girl and makes Billboard history: I Kissed a Girl hits number one.* Retrieved January 23, 2010, from http://www.sheknows.com/articles/804503

Balsam, K. F., Rothblum, E. D., & Beauchaine, T. P. (2005). Victimization over the life span: A comparison of lesbian, gay, bisexual, and heterosexual siblings. *Journal of Consulting and Clinical Psychology, 73,* 477–487.

Bartky, S. L. (1990). *Femininity and domination: Studies in the phenomenology of oppression.* New York: Routledge.

Bay-Cheng, L. Y., Livingston, J. A., & Fava, N. M. (2013). "Not always a clear path": Making space for peers, adults, and complexity in adolescent girls' sexual development. In E. L. Zurbriggen & T.- A. Roberts (Eds.), *The sexualization of girls and girlhood: Causes, consequences, and resistance* (Chapter 13). New York: Oxford University Press.

Benson-Allot, C. (2005). The "mechanical truth" behind *Cruel Intentions:* Desire, AIDS, and the MTV Movie Awards' "Best Kiss." *Quarterly Review of Film and Video, 22,* 341–358.

Beren, S. E., Hayden, H. A., Wilfley, D. E., & Grilo, C. M. (1996). The influence of sexual orientation on body dissatisfaction in adult men and women. *International Journal of Eating Disorders, 20,* 135–141.

Beren, S. E., Hayden, H. A., Wilfley, D. E., & Striegel-Moore, R. H. (1997). Body dissatisfaction among lesbian college students: The conflict of straddling mainstream and lesbian cultures. *Psychology of Women Quarterly, 21*, 431–445.

Berenson, C. (2002). What's in a name? Bisexual women define their terms. *Journal of Bisexuality, 2*(2/3), 9–21.

Bergeron, S. M., & Senn, C. Y. (1998). Body image and sociocultural norms: A comparison of heterosexual and lesbian women. *Psychology of Women Quarterly, 22*, 385–401.

billboard.com (2009). *Katy Perry: Biography & awards.* Retrieved on January 23, 2010, from http://www.billboard.com/artist/katy-perry/958673/artist/katy-perry/bio/958673

Bower, J., Gurevich, M., & Mathieson, C. (2002). (Con)Tested identities: Bisexual women reorient sexuality. *Journal of Bisexuality, 2*(2/3), 23–52.

Bradford, M. (2004). The bisexual experience: Living in a dichotomous culture. *Journal of Bisexuality, 4*(1–2), 7–23.

Brand, P. A., Rothblum, E. D., & Solomon, L. J. (1992). A comparison of lesbians, gay men, and heterosexual on weight and restrained eating. *International Journal of Eating Disorders, 11*, 253–259.

Brown, L. S. (1987). Lesbians, weight, and eating: New analyses and perspectives. In Boston Lesbian Psychologies Collective (Eds.), *Lesbian psychologies: Explorations and challenges* (pp. 294–309). Chicago: University of Illinois Press.

Clarke, V., & Turner, K. (2007). Clothes maketh the queer? Dress, appearance and the construction of lesbian, gay and bisexual identities. *Feminism & Psychology, 17*, 267–276.

Combahee River Collective. (1977/1982). The Combahee River Collective statement. In B. Smith (Ed.), *HOMEGIRLS: A Black feminist anthology* (pp. 272–282). New York: Kitchen Table: Women of Color Press.

Diamond, L. M. (2002). "Having a girlfriend without knowing it": Intimate friendships among adolescent sexual-minority women. *Journal of Lesbian Studies, 6*(1), 5–16.

Diamond, L. M. (2005a). A new view of lesbian subtypes: Stable versus fluid identity trajectories over an 8-year period. *Psychology of Women Quarterly, 29*, 119–128.

Diamond, L. M. (2005b). From the heart or the gut? Sexual-minority women's experiences of desire for same-sex and other-sex partners. *Feminism and Psychology, 15*, 10–14.

Diamond, L. M. (2005c). "I'm straight, but I kissed a girl": The trouble with American media representations of female-female sexuality. *Feminism and Psychology, 15*, 104–110.

Diamond, L. M. (2008). *Sexual fluidity: Understanding women's love and desire.* Cambridge, MA: Harvard University Press.

Downs, D. M., James, S., & Cowan, G. (2006). Body objectification, self-esteem, and relationship satisfaction: A comparison of exotic dancers and college women. *Sex Roles, 54*, 745–752.

Drechsler, C. (2003). We are all others: An argument for queer. *Journal of Bisexuality, 3*(3/4), 265–275.

Dworkin, S. H. (1988). Not in man's image: Lesbians and the cultural oppression of body image. *Women and Therapy, 8*, 27–39.

Engeln-Maddox, R., Miller, S., & Doyle, D. (2009, May). *Mixed evidence for objectification theory in gay, lesbian, and heterosexual community samples.* Poster presented at the annual Meeting of the Association for Psychological Science, San Francisco, CA.

Fine, M. (1988). Sexuality, schooling, and adolescent females: The missing discourse of desire. *Harvard Educational Review, 58*, 29–53.

Fine, M. (2005). Desire: The morning (and 15 years) after. *Feminism and Psychology, 15*, 54–60.

Fine, M., & McClelland, S. (2006). Sexuality education and desire: Still missing after all these years. *Harvard Educational Review, 76*, 297–338.

Forcella, L. (2008, October). Song "I kissed a girl" raises issue of bisexuality. *The Orange County Register.* Retrieved on November 25, 2008, from http://www.ocregister.com/articles/girls-school-bisexuality-2175184-high-girl

Fredrickson, B. L., & Roberts, T. -A. (1997). Objectification theory: Toward understanding women's lived experiences and mental health risks. *Psychology of Women Quarterly, 21*, 173–206.

Gill, R. (2003). From sexual objectification to sexual subjectification: The resexualisation of women's bodies in the media. *Feminist Media Studies, 3*, 100–108.

Gill, R. (2008). Empowerment/sexism: Figuring female sexual agency in contemporary advertising. *Feminism and Psychology, 18*, 35–60.

Golden, C. (1996). What's in a name? Sexual self-identification among women. In R. C. Savin-Williams, & K. M. Cohen (Eds.), *The lives of lesbians, gays, and bisexuals: Children to adults* (pp. 229–249). Fort Worth, TX: Harcourt Brace.

Golden, C. (2006, March). *Constructions of gender by lesbians and queers: What does sexuality and womanhood have to do with it?* Paper presented at the annual meeting for the Association for Women in Psychology, Ann Arbor, MI.

Haines, M. E., Erchull, M. J., Liss, M., Turner, D. L., Nelson, J. A., Ramsey, L. R., et al. (2008). Predictors and effects of self-objectification in lesbians. *Psychology of Women Quarterly, 32*, 181–187.

Hall, A. C., & Bishop, M. J. (Eds.). (2007). *Pop-porn: Pornography in American culture.* Westport, CT: Praeger.

Hill, M. S. (2002). Examining objectification theory: Sexual objectification's link with self-objectification and moderation by sexual orientation and age in White women (Doctoral dissertation, University of Akron, 2002). *Dissertation Abstracts International, 63*, 3515.

Hill, M. S., & Fischer, A. R. (2008). Examining objectification theory: Lesbian and heterosexual women's experiences with sexual- and self-objectification. *The Counseling Psychologist, 36*, 745–776.

Hughes, D., Rodriquez, J., Smith, E. P., Johnson, D. J., Stevenson, H. C., & Spicer, P. (2006). Parents' ethnic–racial socialization practices: A review of research and directions for future study. *Developmental Psychology, 42*, 747–770.

Jackson, S., & Gilbertson, T. (2009). "Hot lesbians": Young people's talk about representations of lesbianism. *Sexualities, 12*, 199–224.

Jensen, R. (1995). Pornographic lives. *Violence Against Women, 1*, 32–54.

Kirby, M. (2008, September). Megan Fox was a teenage lesbian! Plus other confessions from the lips of Hollywood's new favorite temptress. *GQ.* Retrieved on December 1, 2009, from http://www.gq.com/women/photos/200809/actress-model-transformers-sexiest-woman-in-the-world

Kitzinger, C., & Wilkinson, S. (1995). Transitions from heterosexuality to lesbianism: The discursive production of lesbian identities. *Developmental Psychology, 31*, 95–104.

Kozee, H. B., & Tylka, T. L. (2006). A test of objectification theory with lesbian women. *Psychology of Women Quarterly, 30*, 348–357.

Lamb, S. (2013). Toward a healthy sexuality for girls and young women: A critique of desire. In E. L. Zurbriggen & T.- A. Roberts (Eds.), *The sexualization of girls and girlhood: Causes, consequences, and resistance* (Chapter 14). New York: Oxford University Press.

Lasher, A. (Writer), & McLean, A. (Director). (2009, November 9). They shoot Humphreys, don't they? [Television series episode]. In *Gossip girl.* The CW Television Network.

Leitenberg, H., & Henning, K. (1995). Sexual fantasy. *Psychological Bulletin, 117*, 469–496.

Levy, A. (2005). *Female chauvinist pigs: Women and the rise of raunch culture.* New York: Free Press.

Lo, M. (2005, December). *2005 year in review: Lesbian and bisexual women on TV.* Retrieved on February 18, 2006, from http://www.afterellen.com/TV/2005/12/2005.html

Malernee, J. (2003, December 30). South Florida teen girls discovering "bisexual chic" trend [Electronic version]. *Sun Sentinel.* Retrieved on December 30, 2003, from www.sun-sentinel.com/

McKinley, N. M., & Hyde, J. S. (1996). The objectified body consciousness scale: Development and validation. *Psychology of Women Quarterly, 20,* 181–215.

Morgan, E. M., & Thompson, E. M. (2006). Young women's sexual experiences within same-sex friendships: Discovering and defining bisexual and bi-curious identity. *Journal of Bisexuality, 6*(3/4), 7–34.

MTV. (2003). *MTV video music awards.* Retrieved on February 29, 2004, from http://www.mtv.com/onair/vma/2003/

nick.com (2009). *Nickelodeon kids choice awards 2009.* Retrieved on January 23, 2010 from http://www.nick.com/kids-choice-awards/nominees.jhtml

Pharr, S. (1988). *Homophobia: A weapon of sexism.* Little Rock, AR: Chardon Press.

Rich, A. (1980). Compulsory heterosexuality and lesbian existence. *Signs, 5,* 631–660.

Rothblum, E. D. (1994). Lesbians and physical appearance: Which model applies? In B. Greene, & G. M. Herek (Eds.), *Lesbian and gay psychology: Theory, research, and clinical applications* (pp. 84–97). Thousand Oaks, CA: Sage.

Rust, P. C. (1993). "Coming out" in the age of social constructionism: Sexual identity formation among lesbian and bisexual women. *Gender and Society, 7,* 50–77.

Savin-Williams, R. C. (2005). *The new gay teenager.* Cambridge, MA: Harvard University Press.

Savin-Williams, R. C., & Diamond, L. M. (2000). Sexual identity trajectories among sexual-minority youths: Gender comparisons. *Archives of Sexual Behavior, 29,* 607–627.

Scott, L. D., Jr. (2004). Correlates of coping with perceived discriminatory experiences among African American adolescents. *Journal of Adolescence, 27,* 123–137.

Siever, M. D. (1994). Sexual orientation and gender as factors in socioculturally acquired vulnerability to body dissatisfaction and eating disorders. *Journal of Consulting and Clinical Psychology, 62,* 252–260.

Striegel-Moore, R. H., Tucker, N., & Hsu, J. (1990). Body image dissatisfaction and disordered eating in lesbian college students. *International Journal of Eating Disorders, 9,* 493–500.

Szymanski, D. M., Kashubeck-West, S., & Meyer, J. (2008). Internalized heterosexism: Measurement, psychosocial correlates, and research directions. *The Counseling Psychologist, 36,* 525–574.

Thompson, E. M. (2006). Girl friend or girlfriend? Same-sex friendship and bisexual images as a context for flexible sexual identity among young women. *Journal of Bisexuality, 6*(3/4), 47–67.

Thompson, E. M. (2008, March). *(Internalized) bi-negativity: The problem of the "male gaze" and (il)legitimacy of young women's bisexual identity.* Paper presented at the annual meeting of the Association for Women in Psychology, San Diego, CA.

Thompson, E. M. (2009). Young women's same-sex experiences under the "male gaze": Listening for both objectification and sexual agency (Doctoral dissertation, University of California, Santa Cruz). *ProQuest Dissertation and Theses Database.* (UMI No. 3367757)

Thompson, E. M., & Morgan, E. M. (2008). "Mostly straight" young women: Variations in sexual behavior and identity development. *Developmental Psychology, 44,* 15–21.

Tolman, D. L. (2002). *Dilemmas of desire: Teenage girls talk about sexuality.* Cambridge, MA: Harvard University Press.

Tolman, D. L. (2006). In a different position: Conceptualizing female adolescent sexuality development within compulsory heterosexuality. *New Directions for Child and Adolescent Development, 112,* 71–89.

Ward, J. V. (1996). Raising resisters: The role of truth telling in the psychological development of African American girls. In B. J. Leadbeater, & N. Way (Eds.), *Urban girls: Resisting stereotypes, creating identities* (pp. 85–99). New York: New York University Press.

Warn, S. (2003a, July). *Bi with a boyfriend: The latest Hollywood trend.* Retrieved on August 26, 2005, from http://www.afterellen.com/People/bicelebs.html

Warn, S. (2003b, August). *Ally McBeal, heteroflexibility, and lesbian visibility.* Retrieved on August, 26, 2005, from http://www.afterellen.com/TV/allymcbeal – print.html

Warn, S. (2003c, September). *VMA's Madonna-Britney-Christina kiss: Progress or publicity stunt?* Retrieved on August, 26, 2005, from http://www.afterellen.com/TV/vmakiss.html

Warn, S. (2005, January). *The O.C.'s Alex boosts bisexual visibility on TV.* Retrieved on August 26, 2005, from http://www.afterellen.com/TV/2005/1/theoc.html

Wells, B. E., & Twenge, J. M. (2005). Changes in young people's sexual behavior and attitudes, 1943–1999: A cross-temporal meta-analysis. *Review of General Psychology, 9,* 249–261.

Weprin, A. (2008, January). MTV bringing back A Shot at Love with Tila Tequila. *Broadcasting & Cable.* Retrieved on December 1, 2009, from http://www.broadcastingcable.com/article/111781-MTV_Bringing_Back_A_Shot_at_Love_with_Tila_Tequila_Orders_Spinoff.php

Wilkinson, S. (1996). Bisexuality "a la mode." *Women's Studies International Forum, 19,* 293–301.

8

The Sexualization of Girls and Gendered Violence

Mapping the Connections

NATALIE J. PURCELL AND EILEEN L. ZURBRIGGEN

In North America, many commodities and media programs marketed to girls send a message that they should be "sexy" and should be so in particular ways (American Psychological Association [APA], 2007). These products and media tacitly proclaim that girls should conform to certain standards of sexual attractiveness, that they are valued primarily for their sex appeal, that they should be sexually available to boys or men, and, finally, that they should cherish their role as object of a lustful masculine gaze. Together, such cultural messages exemplify the (hetero)sexualization of girlhood—a phenomenon that we distinguish (to the extent possible) from forms of sexual exploration, expression, or interest that are not coercive, limiting, or imposed.

The sexualization of girls is associated with a variety of troubling consequences, including depression, low self-esteem, and eating disorders (APA, 2007). Several commentators have speculated that sexualization could be connected with the sexual abuse, prostitution, and trafficking of girls, as well as with other forms of gendered violence. In this chapter, we take up that question and explore several ways that the sexualization of girlhood may be related to violence. Of particular interest are the effects of exposure to sexualizing media and other cultural forms, and how these might shape the attitudes, beliefs, and behaviors of consumers. We describe the few studies that specifically investigate how the sexualization of girls contributes to aggression and to the sexist attitudes and beliefs that facilitate aggression. We then analyze this evidence in light of more established and extensive research on the sexualization of adult women and on the effects of mainstream, sexually explicit, and violent media. In the process, we offer speculative insights into how the sexualization of girls may contribute to the aggression of potential offenders and how it may enhance the vulnerability of potential victims. Finally, we consider how the production of media and other cultural products that sexualize girls could contribute to their direct abuse in the production process and could work in the service of a sexist sociocultural system that facilitates widespread sexual and gendered violence.

Exposure to Sexualization and Potential Aggressors

Although many of the products and programs that sexualize girls are marketed primarily to teenagers and younger girls, these messages, images, and themes reach most adults and children in societies where they are prevalent. As such, we should explore how a culture that sexualizes girls may influence some people (particularly adult men and older boys, but potentially others as well) to be more aggressive or violent, and/or to direct that aggression at sexualized girls. We begin with some general comments on the social psychology of aggression and its relationship to sexualization and objectification.

Today, a dominant model for understanding the social psychology of violence is the "dehumanization" or "objectification" model (Arendt, 1964; Moshman, 2005; Opotow, 2005; Schwartz & DeKeseredy, 1997). According to this model, violent aggressors must render their victims unrecognizable as kindred subjects in order to harm, kill, or be cruel to them. An aggressor typically accomplishes this feat by maintaining a certain physical or psychological distance from the victim. By ignoring or denying the humanity of their victims, aggressors *objectify* them. This makes it far easier to harm them: there is no need for moral quandary, no wrestling with the thought of harming another conscious, sentient person because there is no "harmable" person present. Defined this way, objectification is a psychological mechanism achieved by an individual aggressor. But objectification can also become a common social practice or even a cultural imperative under some circumstances. Prominent strategies of widespread objectification include the dissemination of propaganda or ideological messages that mark certain people as "other"; that describe them as strange, unrecognizable, or threatening; and that, ultimately, present them as vermin or rubbish rather than people. There is substantial evidence that objectification, endorsed in everyday discourse and in propaganda, has been widely and successfully deployed to make masses of people accept or turn a blind eye toward the otherwise indigestible and unthinkable violence of war and genocide (Arendt, 1964; Moshman, 2005).

Sexual objectification is one of the key components of sexualization (APA, 2007). Given the central role that objectification plays in the perpetration of violence in general, it is plausible that sexual objectification will feature prominently in the perpetration of sexual violence (Schwartz &

DeKeseredy, 1997). By rendering women and girls somehow less than and alien to men, sexual objectification can decrease potential aggressors' empathy toward women and girls, removing an important psychological inhibitor of violence. The objectification of women also suggests that they are incapable of consent, choice, or willed action. Because they are sex objects, sex is what they are *for*; if they refuse, it is coyness, not a real refusal. This belief ranks high among the familiar and widely held "rape myths" supported by the dehumanization of women and girls (Burt, 1980). Myths of this sort facilitate rape by undermining the inhibitions of aggressors; denying the credibility of victims; and biasing criminal, legal, and judicial opinion in cases of sexual or gendered violence (Burt, 1980; National Research Council's Panel on Research on Violence Against Women, 1996; Radford & Russell, 1992). For these reasons, viewing women and girls as sexual objects and portraying them as less human than men is, many believe, one of the factors that enables men to rape, molest, and abuse without guilt and to interpret their victims' pain as pleasure.

With this theoretical framework in mind, we can evaluate the hypothesis that the sexualization of girls, and especially their sexual *objectification*, can lead to increased violence against them. As mentioned, research in this area is limited. At present, no studies directly link exposure to material that sexualizes girls with propensity to aggress against them or against women. There are, however, numerous studies that link exposure to material that sexualizes women with sexual aggression or attitudes associated with sexual aggression. We review this research and explore its relevance to the question of how the sexualization of girls could affect potential aggressors.

Many studies (both correlational and experimental) have investigated the impact of exposure to violent and nonviolent *pornographic* material. These studies, for the most part, suggest a positive correlation between sexual aggression and both short-term and habitual pornography exposure (Allen, D'Alessio, & Brezgel, 1995; Malamuth, Addison, & Koss, 2000; McKenzie-Mohr & Zanna, 1990). Violent pornography is associated with greater effects, but material that is sexually explicit and not overtly violent is also implicated in enhancing aggression (Allen, D'Alessio, & Brezgel, 1995; Malamuth et al., 2000; McKenzie-Mohr & Zanna, 1990). Experimental results suggest that this finding cannot be exhaustively explained by the theory that those who are already aggressive seek more pornographic (and more violent) media; although this is probably the case, it does not account for the increases in aggression that appear after experimental exposure (Allen, D'Alessio, & Brezgel, 1995). Pornography, it seems, does have an impact on levels of reported aggression. It also affects attitudes toward women, toward sexual violence, and toward rape victims: several studies have linked exposure to pornography with greater acceptance of "rape myths" or victim-blaming attitudes and beliefs that trivialize rape (Allen, Emmers, Gebhardt, & Giery, 1995; Corne, Briere,

& Esses, 1992; Malamuth & Check, 1981; McKenzie-Mohr & Zanna, 1990). The most disturbing studies on exposure to sexually explicit media suggest that self-reported level of pornography exposure is related to self-reported history of rape and propensity to rape (Malamuth et al., 2000). Media that are violent but not sexually explicit have also been linked to aggressive behavior: extensive research indicates that exposure to media violence increases the risk of aggression perpetration, and that its effects on youthful viewers are both significant and long-term (Anderson et al., 2003; Huesmann, Moise-Titus, Podolski, & Eron, 2003; Kunkel & Zwarun, 2006).

How does this relate to the sexualization of girls? The findings of studies on media violence and pornography have a direct bearing on this topic when the cultural materials that sexualize girls are pornographic and/or violently themed. Prime examples include child pornography and pseudo-child pornography (e.g., the highly popular "barely legal" genre, in which adult women just over the age of 18 are portrayed to look as young as possible). In these cases, we can hypothesize with some confidence that exposure to sexually explicit and/or violent media that sexualize girls will trivialize their abuse and increase the likelihood of viewers' aggressive behaviors toward them. Russell and Purcell (2006) have argued that this is the case and have presented a causal model linking exposure to child pornography and pseudo-child pornography with child sexual victimization (this model is discussed in more detail below).

But most of the mainstream media and products that sexualize girls are neither violently themed nor sexually explicit. Could they nonetheless affect potential aggressors' propensity to act violently against girls or women? Several studies on nonviolent and nonexplicit media suggest a correlation between level of exposure to mainstream media that sexualize women or girls and the sexist attitudes and beliefs that facilitate sexual/gendered violence. For instance, traditional sex-role ideologies, gender stereotypes, and attitudes that are less critical of gendered/sexual violence are more likely among both men and women with higher levels of sexualized-media consumption (Lanis & Covell, 1995; MacKay & Covell, 1997; Ward, 2002; Ward, Merriwether, & Caruthers, 2006; Zurbriggen & Morgan, 2006). In general, existing experimental evidence suggests that exposure to mainstream media with sexualizing and/or objectifying material leads to greater acceptance of rape myths, child sexual abuse myths, sexist stereotypes, sexual harassment, and some forms of gendered violence (Lanis & Covell, 1995; Machia & Lamb, 2009; MacKay & Covell, 1997; Rudman & Borgida, 1995; Ward, 2002; Ward & Friedman, 2006; Ward, Hansbrough, & Walker, 2005; Ward & Rivadeneyra, 1999). These results apply mostly to research on adults or college students, but some apply to youth as well (Strouse, Goodwin, & Roscoe, 1994; Ward, 2003; Ward & Friedman, 2006; Ward et al., 2005; Ward & Rivadeneyra, 1999). It may be the case that exposure from an earlier age results in more significant and indelible effects because young viewers are still developing their core values and beliefs and are less likely to have cognitive strategies for deconstructing and processing media messages (Gruber & Grube, 2000). Thus, exposing youth to sexualizing and objectifying media may result in the cultivation of more sexism and rape-friendly attitudes than would be the case with adults.

In some studies, men's exposure to nonviolent, nonexplicit media that sexualize women has been shown to alter their behavior toward the women they encounter shortly afterward (Angelone, Hirschman, Suniga, Armey, & Armelie, 2005; McKenzie-Mohr & Zanna, 1990; Rudman & Borgida, 1995). In one experiment, men exposed to sexualized media paid greater attention to a female job applicant's appearance and perceived her as less competent than did a control group (Rudman & Borgida, 1995). Exposure to sexualized media or the sexist behavior of peers may also cause some men to perceive women as less intelligent and to perceive their behaviors as sexual or sexually inviting when they are neither (McKenzie-Mohr & Zanna, 1990; Quinn, 2002). The correlation between sexist attitudes and sexualized media is especially troubling because those with sexist attitudes and beliefs—especially acceptance of rape myths—are more likely to aggress sexually (Greendlinger & Byrne, 1987; Koss, Leonard, Beezley, & Oros, 1985; Malamuth, 1986; 1989a; 1989b; Muehlenhard & Linton, 1987; Murnen, Wright, & Kaluzny, 2002; Osland, Fitch, & Willis, 1996; Truman, Tokar, & Fischer, 1996). We hypothesize that exposure to sexualized images of girls will have similar effects as exposure to sexualized images of adult women: it will increase the risk of sexist and rape-supportive attitudes and of actual sexual aggression. In addition, there may be special risks associated only with the sexualization of girls.

Because only minimal research exists on this topic, we turn again to research on the impact of child pornography—the most extreme and explicit form of girls' sexualization. Russell and Purcell (2006) have argued that exposure to child pornography facilitates and encourages the sexual abuse of children because "merging sexual images of girls and women" makes it more likely that men will use children as "sexual substitutes for women" (p. 67). When girls are sexualized, it is implied that they are mature, sexual beings. Because of this, adults may be more likely to believe that young girls can consent to sexual activity, and that they *want* to engage in sex, perhaps not only with others their age, but also with adults (APA, 2007, p. 35). Citing evidence of successful masturbatory conditioning therapies, Russell believes that sexual attraction to children is a propensity than can develop over time and can be enhanced through exposure to sexualized images of children or adults posed to look like children. Paul and Linz's (2008) experimental work partially supports Russell's hypothesis. In their study, participants exposed to "barely legal" pornography were more likely to associate children (portrayed in a nonsexual way) with sex. In other words, viewing sexualized images of children may, under some circumstances, lead viewers to think of children in a sexual way.

In addition to increasing sexual interest in children, Russell has argued that the extreme sexualization of girls found in child pornography undermines potential aggressors' internal (self-imposed) and external (socially imposed) inhibitions against abuse and violence (Russell & Purcell, 2006). It does so by normalizing or legitimizing the notion of children as sexual beings and by reducing fear of legal or social sanctions for child abuse. Child pornography also tends to trivialize any harm done to children through sexual activity and to desensitize viewers to the pain and trauma of victims. By reinforcing myths about children's will to have sex with adults, exposure to the extreme sexualization of girls (and boys as well), reduces psychological barriers to child abuse.

It is likely that the dismantling of inhibitions against violence that Russell described would be far less extensive and severe with less extreme and explicit forms of sexualization. However, the extent to which the commonplace sexualization of women in mainstream media can affect attitudes, beliefs, and even behaviors suggests that less extreme forms of the sexualization of girls could also have an impact on potential perpetrators of abuse and violence. One recent experiment found that exposure to sexualized images of women portrayed either as adults or as girls led to increased acceptance of child abuse myths (Machia & Lamb, 2009). The sexualization of girls may also reinforce other myths about the sexuality of underage girls (Merskin, 2004).

Additional research is needed on whether, how, and to what extent exposure to violent and nonviolent, as well as sexually explicit and nonexplicit, material that sexualizes girls could contribute to support for rape/abuse myths or other abuse-friendly ideologies. Above all, there is a need for both experimental and epidemiological research that examines the relationship between exposure to media that sexualize girls and the perpetration of actual violence against them.

Exposure to Sexualization and Potential Victims

Sexualization and objectification affect girls themselves and, as such, may shape their vulnerability to sexual or gendered violence. Below, we review the demonstrated and hypothesized intrapsychic effects of sexualization on girls and compare them to the psychic and behavioral factors correlated with enhanced risk of sexual victimization. (This research on girls' *vulnerability* to sexual violence should not be confused with *responsibility* or *culpability* for violence; the latter belong to the aggressors and not to the victims.)

Recent research indicates that experiences of sexualization have intrapsychic effects that may increase vulnerability to violence or abuse. Much of this research is guided by Fredrickson and Roberts' (1997) objectification theory. This theory explains the psychic consequences of enduring and internalizing objectification in a culture that regularly presents women and girls as bodies that exist primarily for the pleasure of others. By turning to Fredrickson and Roberts' work, we shift our focus away from the psychological and behavioral effects of objectification on people who objectify others (e.g., potential aggressors) and focus instead on the psychological consequences of objectification for its victims or for those who experience objectification directed toward themselves. According to Fredrickson and Roberts, to be objectified is to be made into the object of another's gaze; it is to be made, fundamentally, into a body that is ripe for examination and available for judgment. Experiences of objectification are provoked by the constant situating of women's bodies, in their daily lives and especially through exposure to varied media, as objects of sexual interest *apart from* their own needs, desires, personality, and abilities. Society encourages women to pay constant attention to their appearance, and women recognize that others will evaluate and judge their sex appeal regardless of their wishes. Over time, the pressure to conform to dominant standards of sexuality and of beauty comes from within and from without.

Girls, like anyone else, tend to adopt and internalize the standards and norms that they perceive to be dominant or beneficial in their culture, including mainstream standards of sexual attractiveness and behavior (Levy, 2005). According to the APA Task Force Report, a culture rife with objectifying messages/images will encourage "girls to evaluate and control their own bodies more in terms of their sexual desirability to others than in terms of their own desires, health, wellness, achievements or competence" (APA, 2007, p. 21). Frederickson and Roberts (1997) argue that the imperative to monitor one's appearance continuously can be a drain on attentional resources and can thus "profoundly disrupt a woman's [or girl's] flow of consciousness" (p. 180). The inescapability of social and often personal evaluation, paired with the fact that cultural ideals of attractiveness are largely impossible to attain, is a source of shame and anxiety for many women and girls. For some, this can lead to a sense of hopelessness and powerlessness. Frederickson and Roberts suggest that these feelings and experiences are implicated in a variety of the mental and physical health problems that women and girls endure in disproportionate numbers—from eating disorders to low self-esteem and depression.

Emerging research supports the hypotheses that sexualization and objectification are associated with depression and low self-esteem and body esteem in both girls and women (e.g., Durkin & Paxton, 2002; Grabe, Hyde, & Lindberg, 2007; Harrison & Frederickson, 2003; Hawkins, Richards, Granley, & Stein, 2004; Hebl, King, & Lin, 2004; Szymanski & Henning, 2007; Tolman, Impett, Tracy, & Michael, 2006). Girls who are fixated on their appearance and who believe that others are evaluating them on the basis of their appearance are more likely to experience "a host of negative emotional consequences, such as shame, anxiety, and even self-disgust" (APA, 2007, p. 23). Some studies have also identified cognitive effects associated with sexualization. Even a brief or temporary experience of sexualization, like being asked to wear more revealing clothing in a scenario where this is not common or expected, can result in diminished performance on administered exams (Fredrickson, Roberts, Noll, Quinn, & Twenge, 1998; Gapinski, Brownell, & LaFrance, 2003; Hebl et al., 2004). This decline in cognitive performance may take place because a woman's or girl's attention is drawn not only to the task at hand, but also to her appearance and attractiveness in the eyes of others (Fredrickson & Roberts, 1997).

Finally, experiences of sexualization/objectification and exposure to media that sexualize girls can shape girls' attitudes, beliefs, and behaviors when it comes to gender, sex, and sexuality. Many youth turn to media as a source of education and information on sexuality (Gruber & Grube 2000; Ward, 2003). Existing research indicates that traditional gender ideologies, sexual stereotypes, and (for some populations) less critical attitudes toward gendered violence are more common among girls and women who have higher levels of exposure to sexist or sexualizing media of many varieties (MacKay & Covell, 1997; Strouse et al., 1994; Ward 2002, 2003; Ward & Friedman 2006; Ward et al., 2005; Ward & Rivadeneyra 1999).

Many of the psychological problems identified in studies of objectification parallel those of child abuse victims, who are at increased risk for future victimization. In a discussion of victims of child abuse, Zurbriggen and Freyd (2004) argued that changes to "consensual sex decision mechanisms" (mental functions that are necessary to freely choose to engage in a sexual behavior) can lead to high-risk sexual behavior and subsequent victimization (p. 150). Harmful changes to consensual sex decision mechanisms may arise from dissociative tendencies, low self-esteem, and other psychic outcomes associated with the experience of abuse. Additionally, experiences of abuse may generate beliefs about oneself that are inimical to resisting or standing up for oneself in potentially harmful or hurtful situations. In essence, when one experiences dissociation, low self-esteem, or negative beliefs about the self, decision-making about consensual sex in a high-risk or traumatic situation may be hindered.

Notably, some of the cognitive factors that facilitate high-risk behavior in abused or traumatized girls may be present to a lesser but still significant degree in less severely sexualized or objectified girls. These include the low self-esteem and short-term cognitive problems identified in studies on the effects of objectification. Although the cognitive distraction and mental fragmentation associated with sexualization are much less severe than the dissociation experienced by abuse or trauma victims, there are some parallels. Lesser forms of mental fragmentation, like the third-person perspective on the body that results from self-objectification, may affect cognitive functioning in a manner sufficient to produce higher-risk behavior, poorer defense mechanisms, and enhanced vulnerability. Also, any self-esteem problem could potentially hinder one's capacity to reject rape-myths and to stand up for oneself in potentially abusive situations: researchers have found that low self-esteem is correlated with high-risk sexual behavior in some (but not all) contexts (Fritz, 1998; Hollar & Snizek, 1996). Thus, we hypothesize that the cognitive problems and esteem issues correlated with sexualization could diminish assertiveness and facilitate high-risk sexual behavior, which is associated with increased likelihood of sexual victimization (APA, 2007, p. 18; Silbert & Pines, 1981).

These cognitive and self-esteem problems cannot be viewed in isolation from emotional factors that affect behavior and vulnerability. These include persistent feelings of shame, anxiety, and self-dissatisfaction. Such emotions are fundamentally draining and distracting (Fredrickson & Roberts, 1997). The APA Task Force on the Sexualization of Girls worries that "body shame may inhibit women's ability to advocate for, or even acknowledge, their own sexual feelings" (APA, 2007, p. 27). When paired with enhanced acceptance of sexist stereotypes and rape myths, feelings of shame, anxiety, and self-loathing are likely to decrease a victim's assertiveness during and after an experience of abuse or violence. These beliefs and feelings not only reduce a girl's ability to develop the sexual identity and experiences she wants; they also reduce her willingness to resist unwanted sexual activity and to report it afterward. They are, in effect, disempowering and silencing. Indeed, girls who report greater self-objectification are more likely to feel less sexual agency, to have more negative attitudes toward sexuality, and to report more regret about their sexual experiences than girls who experience less sexual (self-)objectification (Hirschman, Impett, & Schooler, 2006). This could partially explain the increased levels of high-risk sexual behavior found among girls with more exposure to sexualized media (Wingood et al., 2003).

The effects of objectification on vulnerability to abuse could be more severe if exposure to sexually explicit and/or violent themes or images is involved. For instance, regular exposure to explicit child pornography may result in more serious psychological effects than regular exposure to mainstream media messages that sexualize girls in less severe ways. Diana Russell has argued that, in certain contexts, exposure to child pornography or pseudo-child pornography "undermines some children's abilities to avoid, resist, or escape sexual victimization" (Russell & Purcell, 2006, p. 77). It does so in several ways:

"1. By arousing children's sexual curiosity and/or desire" (p. 78);
"2. By legitimizing and/or normalizing...sexual victimization for children" (p. 78);

"3. By desensitizing or disinhibiting children" (p. 79);

"4. By creating feelings of guilt and complicity, thereby silencing children" (p. 79).

Russell cites extensive anecdotal evidence from abused children and from child molesters explaining how sexualizing media were deployed to "groom" children for abuse. Specifically, molesters would display child pornography to normalize adult–child sex or to teach their victims that it is both normal and expected for children to cooperate with adults' sexual requests (Russell & Purcell, 2006). Viewing child pornography diminishes victims' beliefs that resistance is possible, justified, or warranted, and reduces their propensity to report what an abuser has done to them. Thus, exposure to extreme forms of childhood sexualization may be especially shaming, silencing, and disempowering, resulting in enhanced vulnerability to victimization.

A Social-Psychological Feminist Perspective

Cultural trends that shape individuals' feelings, attitudes, beliefs, and behaviors also create broader social patterns. The sexualization of girls is one such trend, and thus it is important to consider the broader sociological impact of the psychological phenomena discussed above. If the sexualization of girls persists and grows more extensive, what social changes can we expect, and how do they relate to violence against women and girls?

One potential effect of the increased sexualization of girls is an increase in aggregate demand for media and other products that feature sexualized girls. It goes without saying that girls are sometimes (not always) abused and exploited in the production of cultural materials that sexualize them. This is especially true in the production of child pornography, which is a documentary of actual child abuse (except in special cases such as technologically altered or computer-generated images). It is likely that demand for child pornography can be cultivated within the population of "normal" men, that its appeal is not restricted to the small population of pedophiles who are exclusively interested in sex with children (Russell & Purcell, 2006). If the sexualization of girls becomes more widespread, more people could develop a sexual interest in children. This could result not only in enhanced demand for and production of child pornography, but perhaps also more widespread sexual abuse of girls by those who have developed a sexual interest in teenagers or younger children. For this reason, the APA Task Force worries that "the sexualization of girls may...contribute to the trafficking and prostitution of girls by helping to create a market for sex with children through the cultivation of new desires and experiences" (APA, 2007, p. 35). It seems plausible that the sexualization of girlhood, should it become a persistent cultural norm, will increase aggregate rates of childhood sexual abuse, child pornography production, child prostitution, statutory rape, and other forms of sexual violence. Systematic research focusing on individual responses to sexualized portrayals of girls would be useful in supporting or refuting this hypothesis.

In the long term, the sexualization of girls is likely to have other, less direct effects on rates of violence and abuse. Gendered violence is an act of aggression on the part of a troubled individual, but it is also a form of aggression with social roots. Across places and eras, gendered violence can and does become more and less acceptable, more and less taken for granted, more and less prevalent (Archer & McDaniel, 1995; Burt, 1980; Lottes, 1988; Reiss, 1986; Sanday, 1981). Shifts in attitudes toward gendered violence, as well as in rates of gendered violence, are patterned rather than arbitrary; they are closely related to a culture's values concerning sex and gender. For this reason, feminists have long argued that sexual violence is rooted in a broader social system of sexual and gender-based inequality (Brownmiller, 1975/1994). Within this system, sexual violence represents the extreme end of a continuum of institutionally embedded behaviors and attitudes that promote masculine privilege and afford women only a restricted and secondary status.

The sexualization of women has long been recognized as one of the tools employed to maintain this system (de Beauvoir, 1949/1971; Friedan, 1963; MacKinnon, 1987; Millett, 1970/1994). Presenting women as beings defined through their sexuality—and specifically their sexual usefulness to men—narrowly circumscribes their social and personal value. Historically, the sexual and gendered "nature" of women has been deployed as an apology for their limited work roles and their exploitation within these roles, as a rationale for their diminished legal and social status, and as a myth that justifies sexual violence against them (de Beauvoir, 1949/1971; Friedan, 1963; MacKinnon, 1987). For this reason, the extreme sexualization of women has long been a target of feminists' attention, and second-wave Western feminists challenged it extensively (Bergen, Edleson, & Renzetti, 2005; Dworkin, 1991; MacKinnon, 1987; Radford & Russell, 1992; Russell, 1993a,b, 1998). Their efforts have dramatically changed the sociocultural landscape for women in the Western world, but clearly the sexualization of women is not a relic of the past. Many feminists recognize it as a continued basis of women's oppression and of sexual violence, both in the Western world and elsewhere.

What does it mean that we currently see a proliferation rather than retreat of cultural messages and images that sexualize not only women but also *girls*? As cultural materials that sexualize girls become more commonplace and taken-for-granted, we are likely to see the cultivation of certain beliefs and assumptions—certain ideologies—that are more friendly to sexist institutions and to norms that sustain gendered inequality and violence. As mentioned, several studies on sexualized media have suggested a correlation between level of exposure to images and messages that sexualize and objectify women or girls and sexist attitudes or beliefs. Traditional ideologies that are unsupportive of feminist advances are more likely to be espoused among those with higher levels of sexualized-media consumption (Ward, 2002, 2003; Ward & Friedman, 2006; Ward et al., 2005, 2006; Ward & Rivadeneyra, 1999). These ideologies are, in turn, associated with higher levels of gendered and sexual violence (Malamuth, 1986, 1989a,b; Muehlenhard & Linton, 1987; Murnen et al., 2002; Osland et al., 1996; Truman et al., 1996). All else being equal, there is ample reason to believe that the increased production, dissemination, and consumption of cultural products that sexualize girls will contribute to the development of a more sexist society—one that is more likely to take for granted the abuse and exploitation of women and girls, more likely to forgive and to foster sexual and gendered violence.

Of course, the proliferation of cultural materials that sexualize girls is a phenomenon embedded in a complex social context rife with other factors that could mitigate, amplify, or confound its impact. An analysis of the many interlocking and overlapping social, cultural, and psychological phenomena that shape rates of sexual and gendered violence is beyond the scope of this chapter. Many questions remain: in the aftermath of second-wave Western feminism, what social impact does the sexualization of girls have? Because girls today have greater access to images and examples of women in diverse (sexual and *non*-sexual) roles and have enhanced social and economic opportunities that their grandmothers did not have, are its potential harms mitigated? Are they exacerbated because they are directed at young girls as much as adult women—girls who, as a result of their age and maturity level, may be equipped with less developed strategies of resistance and fewer resources to construct alternative identities or make different life choices? We leave further analysis of these questions to future research.

Conclusion

This chapter has explored how the sexualization of girls may be related to gendered and sexual violence. Our review of existing literature and theory suggests that the sexualization of girls could indeed facilitate additional sexual and gendered violence, and could make girls a more likely target of this violence. It could do so by motivating and disinhibiting potential aggressors and by increasing the vulnerability of disempowered, self-objectifying girls. The increased production of sexualized media may result in the direct abuse of girls, and it could cultivate more widespread sexual interest in underage girls—in other words, it could create a larger pool of potential abusers and victims. The sexualization of girlhood is also likely to have indirect, long-term effects. Above all, it is a contributor to sexism in an already sexist culture, a culture that fuses sex and violence in innumerable ways (Bader, 2002; Jensen, 2007; Kahr, 2008; Kramer, 1997; Wosnitzer, Bridges, & Chang, 2007; Zurbriggen, 2000). Habitual exposure to material that sexualizes and objectifies girls is likely to generate more sexist attitudes and greater acceptance of rape myths among men, women, girls, and boys. This, in turn, could encourage aggression among potential offenders, suppress resistance among the targets of their attacks, silence victims after the fact, and bias the population of potential law enforcement officers, judges, and juries in cases of sexual and gendered violence.

Because existing research on this topic is limited, we developed these hypotheses on the basis of more established bodies of work on the effects of violent, pornographic, and mainstream media, and on the sexualization of adult women. Future researchers can evaluate and elaborate on these hypotheses by conducting research that (a) addresses the specific impact of cultural themes, images, and messages that sexualize girls; (b) differentiates among violent, non-violent, sexually explicit, and nonexplicit material; (c) isolates the differential effects of sexualizing material on girls, women, boys, and men; (d) explores the possibility that these effects might vary not only by age and gender but also by race, ethnicity, sexual orientation, class, and other social roles and identities; and (e) identifies strategies for resisting or transforming the negative effects of sexualization. Finally, future researchers studying the long-term effects of the sexualization of girls can attempt to situate this phenomenon in its broader sociohistorical context by (a) studying the sociohistorical dynamics that gave rise to this trend; (b) exploring how it affects and is affected by other psycho-social factors and historical trends; and (c) revising theory on the sociocultural bases of sexual and gendered violence to incorporate evolving contributors, like the sexualization of girlhood. We hope that, through these and related research agendas, we can attain a better grasp of why sexual and gendered violence persists in the aftermath of significant advances toward gender equality, and how we can collectively resist and transform this dynamic.

References

Allen, M., D'Alessio, D., & Brezgel, K. (1995). A meta-analysis summarizing the effects of pornography: II. Aggression after exposure. *Human Communication Research 22*, 258–283.

Allen, M., Emmers, T., Gebhardt, L., & Giery, M. A. (1995). Exposure to pornography and acceptance of rape myths. *Journal of Communication, 45*, 5–26.

American Psychological Association. (2007). *Report of the APA task force on the sexualization of girls.* Washington, DC: American Psychological Association.

Anderson, C. A., Berkowitz, L., Donnerstein, E., Huesmann, L. R., Johnson, J. D., Linz, D., et al. (2003). The influence of media violence on youth. *Psychological Science in the Public Interest, 4*(3), 81–110.

Angelone, D. J., Hirschman, R., Suniga, S., Armey, M., & Armelie, A (2005). The influence of peer interactions on sexually oriented joke telling. *Sex Roles, 52,* 187–199.

Archer, D., & McDaniel, P. (1995). Violence and gender: Differences and similarities across societies. In R. B. Ruback & N. A. Weiner (Eds.), *Interpersonal violent behaviors: Social and cultural aspects* (pp. 63–88). New York: Springer Publishing.

Arendt, H. (1964). *Eichmann in Jerusalem: A report on the banality of evil.* New York: Viking.

Bader, M. J. (2002). *Arousal: The secret logic of sexual fantasies.* New York: Thomas Dunne/Saint Martin's Press.

Bergen, R. K., Edleson, J. L., & Renzetti, C. M. (2005). *Violence against women: Classic papers.* Boston: Pearson/Allyn & Bacon.

Brownmiller, S. (1975/1994). Against our will: Men, women, and rape. In M. Schneir (Ed.), *Feminism in our time: The essential writings, World War II to the present* (pp. 272–282). New York: Vintage. (Original work published 1975)

Burt, M. R. (1980). Cultural myths and supports for rape. *Journal of Personality and Social Psychology, 38,* 217–230.

Corne, S., Briere, J., & Esses, L. M. (1992). Women's attitudes and fantasies about rape as a function of early exposure to pornography. *Journal of Interpersonal Violence, 7,* 454–461.

de Beauvoir, S. (1949/1971). *The second sex* (H. Parshley, Trans.). New York: Alfred A Knopf. (Original work published 1949)

Durkin, S. J., & Paxton, S. J. (2002). Predictors of vulnerability to reduced body image satisfaction and psychological wellbeing in response to exposure to idealized female media images in adolescent girls. *Journal of Psychosomatic Research, 53,* 995–1005.

Dworkin, A. (1991). *Pornography: Men possessing women.* New York: Plume.

Fredrickson, B. L., & Roberts, T.-A. (1997). Objectification theory: Toward understanding women's lived experiences and mental health risks. *Psychology of Women Quarterly, 21,* 173–206.

Fredrickson, B. L., Roberts, T.-A., Noll, S. M., Quinn, D. M., & Twenge, J. M. (1998). That swimsuit becomes you: Sex differences in self-objectification, restrained eating, and math performance. *Journal of Personality and Social Psychology, 75,* 269–284.

Friedan, B. (1963). *The feminine mystique.* New York: W.W. Norton.

Fritz, R. B. (1998). AIDS knowledge, self-esteem, perceived AIDS risk, and condom use among female commercial sex workers. *Journal of Applied Social Psychology, 28,* 888–911.

Gapinski, K. D., Brownell, K. D., & LaFrance, M. (2003). Body objectification and "fat talk": Effects on emotion, motivation, and cognitive performance. *Sex Roles, 48,* 377–388.

Grabe, S., Hyde, J. S., & Lindberg, S. M. (2007). Body objectification and depression in adolescents: The role of gender, shame, and rumination. *Psychology of Women Quarterly, 31,* 164–175.

Greendlinger, V., & Byrne, D. (1987). Coercive sexual fantasies of college men as predictors of self-reported likelihood to rape and overt sexual aggression. *Journal of Sex Research, 23,* 1–11.

Gruber, E., & Grube, J. W. (2000). Adolescent sexuality and the media: A review of current knowledge and implications. *Western Journal of Medicine, 172,* 210–214.

Harrison, K., & Fredrickson, B. L. (2003). Women's sports media, self-objectification, and mental health in black and white adolescent females. *Journal of Communication, 53,* 216–232.

Hawkins, N., Richards, P. S., Granley, H. M., & Stein, D. M. (2004). The impact of exposure to the thin-ideal media image on women. *Eating Disorders: The Journal of Treatment & Prevention, 12,* 35–50.

Hebl, M. R., King, E. B., & Lin, J. (2004). The swimsuit becomes us all: Ethnicity, gender, and vulnerability to self-objectification. *Personality and Social Psychology Bulletin, 30,* 1322–1331.

Hirschman, C., Impett, E. M., & Schooler, D. (2006). Dis/embodied voices: What late-adolescent girls can teach us about objectification and sexuality. *Sexuality Research and Social Policy, 3,* 8–20.

Hollar, D. S., & Snizek, W. E. (1996). The influences of knowledge of HIV/AIDS and self-esteem on the sexual practices of college students. *Social Behavior and Personality, 24,* 75–86.

Huesmann, L. R., Moise-Titus, J., Podolski, C. -L., & Eron, L. D. (2003). Longitudinal relations between children's exposure to TV violence and their aggressive and violent behavior in young adulthood: 1977–1992. *Developmental Psychology, 39,* 201–221.

Jensen, R. (2007). *Getting off: Pornography and the end of masculinity.* Cambridge, MA: South End Press.

Kahr, B. (2008). *Who's been sleeping in your head? The secret world of sexual fantasies.* New York: Basic Books.

Koss, M. P., Leonard, K. E., Beezley, D. A., & Oros, C. J. (1985). Nonstranger sexual aggression: A discriminant analysis of the psychological characteristics of undetected offenders. *Sex Roles, 12,* 981–992.

Kramer, L. (1997). *After the lovedeath: Sexual violence and the making of culture.* Berkeley, CA: University of California Press.

Kunkel, D., & Zwarun, L. (2006). How real is the problem of TV violence? Research and policy perspectives. In N. E. Dowd, D. G. Singer, & R. F. Wilson (Eds.), *Handbook of children, culture, and violence* (pp. 203–224). Thousand Oaks, CA: Sage.

Lanis, K., & Covell, K. (1995). Images of women in advertisements: Effects on attitudes related to sexual aggression. *Sex Roles, 32,* 639–649.

Levy, A. (2005). *Female chauvinist pigs: Women and the rise of raunch culture.* New York: Free Press.

Lottes, I. L. (1988). Sexual socialization and attitudes toward rape. In A. W. Burgess (Ed.), *Rape and sexual assault II: A researcher's handbook* (pp. 193–220). New York: Garland.

Machia, M., & Lamb, S. (2009). Sexualized innocence: Effects of magazine ads portraying adult women as sexy little girls. *Journal of Media Psychology, 21,* 15–24.

MacKay, N. J., & Covell, K. (1997). The impact of women in advertisements on attitudes toward women. *Sex Roles, 36,* 573–583.

MacKinnon, C. (1987). *Feminism unmodified: Discourses on life and law.* Cambridge, MA: Harvard University Press.

Malamuth, N. M. (1986). Predictors of naturalistic sexual aggression. *Journal of Personality and Social Psychology, 50,* 953–962.

Malamuth, N. M. (1989a). The Attraction to Sexual Aggression Scale: Part one. *Journal of Sex Research, 26,* 26–49.

Malamuth, N. M. (1989b). The Attraction to Sexual Aggression Scale: Part two. *Journal of Sex Research, 26,* 324–354.

Malamuth, N. M., Addison, T., & Koss, M. (2000). Pornography and sexual aggression: Are there reliable effects and can we understand them? *Annual Review of Sex Research, 11,* 26–91.

Malamuth, N. M., & Check, J. V. P. (1981). The effects of mass media exposure on acceptance of violence against women: A field experiment. *Journal of Research in Personality, 15,* 436–446.

McKenzie-Mohr, D., & Zanna, M. P. (1990). Treating women as sexual objects: Look to the (gender schematic) male who has viewed pornography. *Personality and Social Psychology Bulletin, 16,* 296–308.

Merskin, D. (2004). Reviving Lolita? A media literacy examination of sexual portrayals of girls in fashion advertising. *American Behavioral Scientist, 48,* 119–129.

Millett, K. (1970/1994). Sexual politics. In M. Schneir (Ed.), *Feminism in our time: The essential writings, World War II to the present* (pp. 229–244). New York: Vintage. (Originally published in 1970)

Moshman, D. (2005). Genocidal hatred: Now you see it, now you don't. In R. J. Sternberg (Ed.), *The psychology of hate* (pp. 185–209). Washington, DC: American Psychological Association.

Muehlenhard, C. L., & Linton, M. A. (1987). Date rape and sexual aggression in dating situations: Incidence and risk factors. *Journal of Counseling Psychology, 34,* 186–196.

Murnen, S. K., Wright, C., & Kaluzny G. (2002). If "boys will be boys," then girls will be victims? A meta-analytic review of the research that relates masculine ideology to sexual aggression. *Sex Roles, 46,* 359–375.

National Research Council's Panel on Research on Violence Against Women. (1996). *Understanding violence against women.* Washington, DC: National Academy Press.

Opotow, S. (2005). Hate, conflict, and moral exclusion. In R. J. Sternberg (Ed.), *The psychology of hate* (pp. 121–153). Washington, DC: American Psychological Association.

Osland, J. A., Fitch, M., & Willis, E. E. (1996). Likelihood to rape in college males. *Sex Roles, 35,* 171–183.

Paul, B., & Linz, D. G. (2008). The effects of exposure to virtual child pornography on viewer cognitions and attitudes toward deviant sexual behavior. *Communication Research, 35,* 3–38.

Quinn, B. A. (2002). Sexual harassment and masculinity: The power and meaning of "girl watching." *Gender and Society, 16,* 386–402.

Radford, J., & Russell, D. E. H. (1992). *Femicide: The politics of woman killing.* New York: Twayne.

Reiss, I. L. (1986). *Journey into sexuality: An exploratory voyage.* Englewood Cliffs, NJ: Prentice-Hall.

Rudman, L. A., & Borgida, E. (1995). The afterglow of construct accessibility: The behavioral consequences of priming men to view women as sexual objects. *Journal of Experimental Social Psychology, 31,* 493–517.

Russell, D. E. H. (1993a). *Against pornography: The evidence of harm.* Berkeley, CA: Russell Publications.

Russell, D. E. H. (1993b). *Making violence sexy: Feminist views on pornography.* New York: Teachers College Press.

Russell, D. E. H. (1998). *Dangerous relationships: Pornography, misogyny, and rape.* Thousand Oaks, CA: Sage.

Russell, D. E. H., & Purcell, N. J. (2006). Exposure to pornography as a cause of child sexual victimization. In N. E. Dowd, D. G. Singer, & R. F. Wilson (Eds.), *Handbook of children, culture, and violence* (pp. 59–83). Thousand Oaks, CA: Sage.

Sanday, P. R. (1981). The socio-cultural context of rape: A cross-cultural study. *Journal of Social Issues, 37,* 5–27.

Schwartz, M. D., & DeKeseredy, W. S. (1997). *Sexual assault on the college campus: The role of male peer support.* Thousand Oaks, CA: Sage.

Shute, R., Owens, L., & Slee, P. (2008). Everyday victimization of adolescent girls by boys: Sexual harassment, bullying or aggression? *Sex Roles, 58,* 477–489.

Silbert, M. H., & Pines, A. M. (1981). Sexual child abuse as an antecedent to prostitution. *Child Abuse and Neglect, 5,* 407–411.

Strouse, J. S., Goodwin, M. P., & Roscoe, B. (1994). Correlates of attitudes toward sexual harassment among early adolescents. *Sex Roles, 31,* 559–577.

Szymanski, D. M., & Henning S. L. (2007). The role of self-objectification in women's depression: A test of objectification theory. *Sex Roles, 56,* 45–53.

Tolman, D. L., Impett, E. A., Tracy, A. J., & Michael, A. (2006). Looking good, sounding good: Femininity ideology and adolescent girls' mental health. *Psychology of Women Quarterly, 30,* 85–95.

Truman, D. M., Tokar, D. M., & Fischer, A. R. (1996). Dimensions of masculinity: Relations to date rape supportive attitudes and sexual aggression in dating situations. *Journal of Counseling and Development, 74,* 555–562.

Ward, L. M. (2002). Does television exposure affect emerging adults' attitudes and assumptions about sexual relationships? Correlational and experimental confirmation. *Journal of Youth and Adolescence, 31,* 1–15.

Ward, L. M. (2003). Understanding the role of entertainment media in the sexual socialization of American youth: A review of empirical research. *Developmental Review, 23,* 347–388.

Ward, L. M., & Friedman, K. (2006). Using TV as a guide: Associations between television viewing and adolescents' sexual attitudes and behavior. *Journal of Research on Adolescence, 16,* 133–156.

Ward, L. M., Hansbrough, E., & Walker, E. (2005). Contributions of music video exposure to black adolescents' gender and sexual schemas. *Journal of Adolescent Research, 20,* 143–166.

Ward, L. M., Merriwether, A., & Caruthers, A. (2006). Breasts are for men: Media, masculinity ideologies, and men's beliefs about women's bodies. *Sex Roles, 55,* 703–714.

Ward, L. M., & Rivadeneyra, R. (1999). Contributions of entertainment television to adolescents' sexual attitudes and expectations: The role of viewing amount versus viewer involvement. *Journal of Sex Research, 36,* 237–249.

Wingood, G. M., DiClemente, R. J., Bernhardt, J. M., Harrington, K., Davies, S. L., Robillard, A., et al. (2003). A prospective study of exposure to rap music videos and African American female adolescents' health. *American Journal of Public Health, 93,* 437–439.

Wosnitzer, R., Bridges, A., & Chang, M. (2007). *Mapping the pornographic text: Content analysis research of popular pornography.* Panel session presented at the National Feminist Antipornography Conference, Boston, MA.

Zurbriggen, E. L. (2000). Social motives and cognitive power-sex associations: Predictors of aggressive sexual behavior. *Journal of Personality and Social Psychology, 78,* 559–581.

Zurbriggen, E. L., & Freyd, J. J. (2004). The link between child sexual abuse and risky sexual behavior: The role of dissociative tendencies, information-processing effects, and consensual sex decision mechanisms. In J. L. Koenig, A. O'Leary, L. S. Doll, & W. Pequegnat (Eds.), *From child sexual abuse to adult sexual risk: Trauma, revictimization, and intervention* (pp. 117–134). Washington, DC: American Psychological Association.

Zurbriggen, E. L., & Morgan E. M. (2006). Who wants to marry a millionaire? Reality dating television programs, attitudes toward sex, and sexual behaviors. *Sex Roles, 54,* 1–17.

9

Prostitution: An Extreme Form of Girls' Sexualization

MELISSA FARLEY

The American Psychological Association's (APA) Report (2007) and most other chapters in this book have focused on cultural forms of the sexualization of girls that only indirectly involve physical or sexual violence and abuse. For example, narrowing the social definition of acceptable female appearance to one that requires starvation can have adverse physical consequences, just as selling girls clothing that defines them as sexually available can increase both their attractiveness to and vulnerability to predators. Understanding the prevalence and consequences of less extreme forms of sexualization is crucially important. Equally important is an awareness of extreme forms of girls' sexualization, such as sexual abuse and prostitution.

Today, the cultural sexualization of girls increasingly overlaps with and merges into prostitution. As Purcell and Zurbriggen (2013) point out, the prevalence of cultural materials that sexualize girls is likely to result in a greater prevalence of beliefs and ideologies that are "friendly to sexist institutions." Prostitution is here understood as a sexist institution, a culturally promoted institution that creates and reflects profound inequality between men and women.

Girls are sexualized when they are sent the message that they "should always be sexually available, always have sex on their minds, be willing to be dominated and even sexually aggressed against" (Merskin, 2004). Although Merskin was describing the cultural sexualization of girls, this statement also describes what is expected of women and girls in prostitution. Much of what has been termed the *sexualization of girls* is the promotion of prostitution-like activities for children (and for adult women). And there is common ground between the pretend and actual prostitution of girls.

It is emotionally challenging to face the reality of sexual violence as an organized criminal enterprise—prostitution—that operates freely in every community, hidden in plain sight (Herman, 2003). Prostitution of a child (a person under age 18 in most countries) is the sexual abuse of a child who has been sexualized. Despite the fact that money is paid, sexual assault remains the child's (and most women's) experience of prostitution. Thus, sexual exploitation or sexual abuse of children, sexual assaults or rapes of children, and prostitution of children are essentially the same phenomenon from the child's point of view. They result in many of the same psychological sequelae, as will be discussed below.

In this chapter I will summarize the literature on the prostitution of children. A strong association between childhood sexual abuse and subsequent prostitution has been documented. Since 2000, researchers and service providers note that there is an increase in gang-affiliated prostitution, an increased use of the Internet to traffic children, and increasingly younger children in prostitution, especially 13- and 14-year-olds (Boyer, 2008). Prostitution of children may be hidden as child labor or sex work or even sexual freedom. The language of feminist empowerment has sometimes been deliberately employed to confuse sexual objectification and sexual freedom (Walter, 2010).

Sexual Objectification and the Prostitution of Girls

When racially objectified, people are defined mostly or exclusively by their ethnic characteristics, especially specific physical features. The stage is then set for racist violence because objects have no feelings, no matter what is done to them. Similarly, once a girl is "made into a thing for others' sexual use" as the APA Task Force on the Sexualization of Girls (American Psychological Association, 2007) and others have defined sexual objectification, then the stage is set for sexual violence. Men's dominance over women is established and enforced by the dehumanizing process of sexual objectification that is at the psychological foundation of men's violence against women (Leidholdt, 1980).

According to the APA Task Force (2007) sexualization occurs *when a person's value comes only from his or her sexual appeal or behavior, to the exclusion of other characteristics*; and *when a person is sexually objectified*—that is, made into a thing for others' sexual use, rather than seen as a person with the capacity for independent action and decision making; and/or *when sexuality is inappropriately imposed upon a person*. Girls are sexually objectified when they are defined by their sex, for example underpants that say "Who needs Santa when you've got this," "hottie" or "juicy" sweatpants, or breasts marked by shirts saying "hooters" or t-shirts labeling them as "pornstar" (see Downes, 2006).

Prostitution is an extreme form of sexualization in which sexual objectification is institutionalized and monetized. In prostitution, women and girls are valued for the sexual use of their vaginas, mouths, anuses, and breasts.

"Prostitution is renting an organ for 10 minutes," explained a man who bought women in prostitution (Farley, 2006).

In prostitution, johns and pimps transform certain women and girls into objects for sexual use. Johns categorize girls according to their appearance on the basis of race/ethnicity, their ages, and according to their poverty or their presumed social and economic status. For example, pimps create for johns the masturbation fantasy of girls and young women who are assumed to be geishas-in-training or high-class escorts. Other johns are aroused by undocumented immigrants who don't speak English or by drug addicts or by women who have a physical disability. Whatever quality in women johns have sexualized for themselves, such as skin color, poverty, size—whatever/whoever they want to buy for sexual use—pimps find, create, and offer for sale. In prostitution, girls are simply "sex" and nothing else about them matters.

The pimp-manufactured image of the john who is a nice guy and would never "force" anyone to engage in a nonconsenting sex act is belied by research documenting the experiences of young people in prostitution (Boyer, 2008; Curtis, Terry, Dank, Dombrowski, & Khan, 2008; Farley et al., 2003), none of whom was offered a couch for the night or a free meal *without the exchange of permitting sexual assault* for those necessities. There are also many accounts by johns that are variations on the theme, "Well, I did see a few bruises on her leg, and yes, there was a certain look of fear in her eyes but, she didn't complain and um, I already paid for it so..." (Farley, 2006).

Childhood Sexual Assault and Prostitution

Brannigan and Gibbs Van Brunschot (1997) described prostitution as a process of *victimization across the life cycle*. Family abuse and neglect initiate the cycle. For example, one woman stated that by the time she was 17,

> all I knew was how to be raped, and how to be attacked, and how to be beaten up, and that's all I knew. So when he put me on the game [pimped her] I was too down in the dumps to do anything. All I knew was abuse. (Phoenix,1999)

Most studies of prostitution of children document a strong association between childhood sexual abuse and prostitution that usually begins at adolescence (Abramovitch, 2005). Newton-Ruddy and Handelsman (1986) found that 90% of teenagers in prostitution had been sexually abused by caregivers or neighbors. Simons and Whitbeck (1991) considered childhood sexual assault a necessary precipitating factor, although not by itself a sufficient cause of adolescent prostitution.

Familial sexual abuse functions as a training ground for prostitution. The early victimization puts girls at risk for later abuse (James & Meyerding, 1977). Girls learn behaviors that normalize prostitution. They appear to accept their own sexual objectification and exploitation. The widespread sexualization of girls in the culture further reinforces the perpetrator's message that her role is to be sexually used. The child is taught to make herself available to the family perpetrator. Dworkin (1997) described sexual abuse of children as "boot camp" for prostitution. One young woman told Silbert and Pines (1982a), "I started turning tricks to show my father what he made me."

In the 1980s, Silbert, Pines, and colleagues published a number of studies that documented an extremely high level of childhood abuse and trauma in the lives of women who were prostituted, including 96% who had run away from home and 78% who entered prostitution under the age of age 18 (Silbert & Pines, 1981, 1982a,b, 1983). Seventy-three percent had also suffered rapes outside of prostitution (Silbert & Pines, 1983). In a noteworthy finding, 70% of the prostituted young women said that the childhood sexual abuse influenced their decision to later enter prostitution (Silbert and Pines, 1983).

Sexual abuse during adolescence and being an ethnic minority tended to increase the risk of sexual revictimization (Classen, Palesh, & Aggarwal, 2005). Having been sexually abused in childhood not only increased Black women's risk of sexual violence as adults, it also increased their risk of prostitution according to West, Williams, and Siegel (2000). These researchers also found that African American sexual abuse survivors who were revictimized as adults were three times more likely to have been involved in prostitution than African American women who had not been revictimized as adults.

In a prospective study, Widom and Kuhns (1996) found that physical abuse and sexual abuse were associated with subsequent prostitution and that children who had been sexually abused were 28 times more likely to be arrested for prostitution later in their lives. Bagley and Young (1987) associated childhood sexual abuse both with subsequent psychopathology and with subsequent prostitution, and found that 73% of 45 prostitution survivors had been sexually abused as children, in contrast to 28% of nonprostituted controls. Sixty-two percent of those in prostitution had been physically abused as children.

Two studies investigated childhood sexual abuse and subsequent prostitution among women in the criminal justice system. In a sample of 1,240 jailed women, Foti (1995) found that women who had been sexually victimized in childhood engaged in prostitution more than twice as often as nonabused detainees did. Simmons (2000) interviewed 122 women who were either living in halfway houses or were incarcerated. Those who had been involved in prostitution were significantly more likely to have been sexually abused in childhood than were women who had never engaged in prostitution.

An international study found that 63% of women in prostitution had been sexually abused in childhood by an average of four perpetrators; 59% had been physically brutalized in childhood (Farley et al., 2003; see also Schissel and Fedec, 1999).

Psychological Consequences of the Sexual Objectification of Girls Through Incest and Prostitution

Incest and prostitution cause similar physical and psychological symptoms in the victim. When a child is incestuously assaulted, the perpetrator's objectification of the child victim and his rationalization and denial are like those of the john in prostitution (Putnam, 1990; Farley, 2003). When girls are subjected to childhood sexual abuse and/or prostitution, the resulting psychological symptoms include a sense of degradation and self-loathing (Bagley &Young, 1987). Like adult women in prostitution, prostituting youth in New York City reported an entrenched self-hatred. Like adults, children hated and feared buyers, and 87% told the researchers that they wanted to escape prostitution (Curtis et al., 2008).

Andrea Dworkin wrote about prostitution's profound impact on the psyche of the prostituted:

> When men use women in prostitution, they are expressing a pure hatred for the female body. It is as pure as anything on this earth ever is or ever has been. It is a contempt so deep, so deep, that a whole human life is reduced to a few sexual orifices, and he can do anything he wants (Dworkin, 1997).

It is painful for children and young women to articulate the impact of sexualization, in part because they are in the process of internalizing these objectifying beliefs about themselves. The internalized sexual objectification that occurs with incest is likely to increase girls' vulnerability to sexual violence. Other symptoms resulting from incest, such as dissociation and self-contempt, impair girls' ability to protect themselves from sexual assault (Zurbriggen & Freyd, 2004) or from prostitution. A woman explained the gradual development of a sexually objectified identity in strip club prostitution:

> You start changing yourself to fit a fantasy role of what they think a woman should be. In the real world, these women don't exist. They [johns] stare at you with this starving hunger. It sucks you dry; you become this empty shell. They're not really looking at you, you're not you. You're not even there. (Farley, 2003)

The APA Task Force Report (2007) noted that the cultural sexualization of girls was linked to their low self-esteem, depression, and eating disorders, which are also sequelae of childhood sexual abuse and prostitution. West (2009) described the effects of sexualization specifically on African American girls: poor body image unless the girl met specific narrowly defined porno-graphic criteria, viewing one's sexuality as a commodity, adversarial relation-ships with men, tolerance of violent sexuality, and sexual risk-taking. Smith and colleagues (2005) summarized behavioral consequences of the sexualiza-tion of girls including earlier age of sexual activity, risky sexual behavior, and viewing prostitution as humorous and enjoyable.

Symptoms that are known to result from prostitution include eating dis-orders, depression, anxiety disorders including posttraumatic stress disorder (Farley et al., 2003), dissociative disorders (Ross, Farley, & Schwartz, 2003), self-mutilation, substance abuse, suicidal thoughts and attempts (Schissel & Fedec, 1999; Ling, Wong, Holroyd, & Gray, 2007), and complex PTSD (Mayfield-Schwartz, 2006). The malignant identity needed in order to survive prostitution is fragmented and dissociated and requires the pathological regu-lation of emotions (Herman, 1994).

Childhood sexual abuse may result in reenactment of sexual abuse or pro-miscuity or prostitution (Kendall-Tackett, Williams, & Finkelhor, 1993), with different behaviors at different stages of the child's development. For example, sexualized behaviors may first become apparent among sexually abused pre-school aged children, then may submerge during the latency years and reemerge during adolescence as promiscuity, prostitution, or sexual aggression.

Traumatic sexualization is the inappropriate conditioning of the child's sexual responsiveness and the socialization of the child into faulty beliefs and assumptions about sexuality that leave her vulnerable to additional sex-ual exploitation (Browne & Finkelhor, 1986). Traumatic sexualization is an essential component of the grooming process for subsequent prostitution. The sexually abused child may incorporate the perpetrator's perspective into her identity, eventually viewing herself as good for nothing but sex—which is to say she may adopt his view that she is a prostitute (Putnam, 1990). Pimps are heard to say that the women they recruit into prostitution were first trained by their fathers. A pimp explained, "Most of them have been abused sexually by their parents...they been raped so many times they feel they might as well get money for it. Well, it's my job to teach them that it's better to get paid for it than do it for free" (Hansen, 2003).

The constricted sense of self of the sexually abused child and the coercive refusal of the perpetrator to respect the child's physical boundaries may result in subsequent difficulties in asserting boundaries, in impaired self-protection, and a greater likelihood of being further sexually victimized, including prostitution (Briere, 1992). The powerlessness of having been sexually assaulted as a child may be related to the frequent discussions of control and power by women who are prostituting. The emotional and physical helplessness of the sexually abused child may be reenacted in the prostitution transaction with vigilant attention to the tiniest shard of control. Payment of money for an unwanted sex act in prostitution may make the girl or woman feel more in control when compared to the same experience with no payment of money. For example, a woman stated that at age 17 she felt safer and more in control turning tricks on the street than she did at home with her stepfather raping her (Farley, 2003).

The dissociation that appears to be a critical survival mechanism for prostitution (Ross et al., 2003) was itself originally a survival response to childhood sexual assault as survivors explain:

> It was easy for me to turn a trick because I could just take myself
> out—like with my dad. It was like I took myself out of the situation
> and just focused on something else and it was like I wasn't even there.
> (Dalla, 2006)

Although the chronically sexually abused child's dissociative capacity may facilitate physical and emotional survival, it undermines the child's capacity to form attachments with nonabusive caregivers, for example, in foster care (Carr, 2009). Kindness or nurturing can become triggers for dissociation. The sexually abused, homeless, or prostituted child's manipulativeness is another adaptive response to an interpersonal environment that is chaotic and dangerous. The resulting mistrust and manipulation can result in caregivers' frustration or hostility, further disrupting the child's attachments (DiPaolo, 1999).

Homelessness Is Associated with Prostitution of Children

Children's homelessness is preceded by running away or being thrown out of homes. Most youth who are homeless have suffered previous chronic sexual, emotional, and/or physical abuse and neglect (Gwadz, Nish, Leonard, & Strauss, 2007; Whitbeck, Hoyt, & Ackley, 1997a,b; MacLean, Embry, and Cauce, 1999; Stewart, Steigman, Cauce, Cochran, Whitbeck, & Hoyt, 2004). One girl told her probation officer that she was treated very well because her pimp allowed her to have Subway sandwiches when she was hungry (Friedman, 2005). Female homeless youth experience significantly higher levels of sexual trauma than do male homeless youth both before and after their homelessness (Gwadz, 2007; Tyler, Hoyt, Whitbeck, & Cauce, 2001). Molnar, Shade, Kral, Booth, and Watters (1998) studied 775 12- to 19-year-olds who were homeless. Forty-eight percent of the young women had attempted suicide an average of six times, with 70% reporting childhood sexual abuse and 35% reporting childhood physical abuse.

Running away from home is a primary risk factor for youth prostitution (Chesney-Lind & Sheldon, 2004; Seng, 1989). Running away is significantly associated with prostitution as a factor separate from childhood sexual abuse (Nadon, Koverola, & Schludermann, 1998; Potterat, Phillips, Rothenberg, & Darrow, 1985). The links between the sexual abuse of girls in their homes, running away, homelessness, out-of-home-placements such as foster care, and recruitment to prostitution (which may be performed by other exploited youth) are still underresearched, according to Cooper (2009). In addition to homelessness and running away, additional mediating factors have been proposed to explain the links between sexual abuse and prostitution. Brannigan and Gibbs Van Brunschot (1997) suggested that the link between sexual trauma and prostitution is mediated by attachment failure, parental conflict, substance abuse, and physical and verbal abuse. These children's psychological distress is then further exacerbated by disrupted or inadequate attachments in foster care (Carr, 2009).

As with adult women, homelessness in children is a significant risk factor for prostitution. After only 36–48 hours of homelessness, young people are likely to be solicited for sex in exchange for money, food, or shelter (Clayton, 1996). Their risk for ongoing sexual exploitation is increased by the lack of an adequate social safety net. Pimps exploit the vulnerability of runaway or thrown-out children. In Vancouver, 46% of homeless girls had received offers of "assistance to help them work in prostitution." A 13-year-old who had run away from home was given housing by a pimp, but only in exchange for prostituting (Farley, 2003).

An international study of prostitution documented a 75% rate of previous homelessness among prostituted women (Farley et al., 2003). A study of prostituted youth also found a 75% rate of homelessness (Yates, MacKenzie, Pennbridge, & Swofford, 1991). Ninety-six percent of the adults interviewed by Silbert and Pines (1983) had been runaway children and therefore were likely homeless before entering prostitution. Of women who began prostituting between the ages of 12 and 15, 72% had run away from home as children. Half of these women had grown up in a home with other family members who were prostituting (Raphael & Shapiro, 2002).

It is uncomfortable for children to acknowledge their own prostitution. Children name prostitution "survival sex." A survey of 500 homeless youths in Indianapolis reported that, at first, only 14% acknowledged that they were prostituting (Lucas & Hackett, 1995). When the Indiana adolescents were subsequently asked nonjudgmental questions about specific behaviors, 32% said that they had sex to get money; 21% said they had sex for a place to stay overnight; 12% exchanged sex for food; 10% exchanged sex for drugs; and 6% exchanged sex for clothes. It is unclear how much or little these categories overlapped but, at a minimum, 32% of these homeless youths prostituted since prostitution includes the exchange of sex for cash, drugs, food, or shelter.

There is a growing need to address vulnerability to prostitution in immigrant families where traditional practices from the home country may clash with U.S. culture. In New York, the largest increase in runaway children in 2001 was from immigrant communities (Spangenberg, 2001). More than half of 50 prostituting Asian girls aged 11 to 16 said that they had run away from home because of family conflict (Louie, Luu, & Tong, 1991).

Adolescence Is the Most Frequently Documented Age of Entry into Prostitution

Early adolescence is the most frequently reported age of entry into prostitution. The average age of entry into prostitution was age 12–13, according to a study conducted by international organization End Child Prostitution and Trafficking (ECPAT) (Spangenberg, 2001). Of 200 adult women in prostitution, 78% began prostituting as minors, with 68% entering prostitution when they were younger than 16 (Silbert, 1982a). Eighty-nine percent of adult women in prostitution began prostituting when they were younger than 16 (Nadon et al., 1998). Among 45 women in legal Nevada brothels, 23% had begun prostituting as children (Farley, 2007).

These U.S. findings are consistent with reports from other countries. Cusick (2002) found that a majority of British women in prostitution had begun prostitution as minors. Across nine countries 47% of 854 people in prostitution began prostituting as children (Farley et al., 2003).

No Reliable Data on the Number of Children Engaged in Prostitution

At this time, there are no studies that provide an accurate estimate of the numbers of children in prostitution in the United States or elsewhere. There has been great variation in figures reported regarding the prevalence of prostitution of children. Rather than cite numbers that vary by the hundreds of thousands, I refer readers to two discussions of the problems encountered in estimating the number of children in prostitution. Ennew and colleagues (1996) provided an annotated bibliography of the difficulties in measuring the prevalence of the prostitution of children. For example, estimates were made at conferences that were later cited as more credible than the educated guesses that they actually were. Urging those in the field to refrain from offering estimates, Stransky and Finkelhor (2008) provided a Fact Sheet on Juvenile Prostitution, noting that all numbers *and estimates* were suspect. They concluded, "The reality is that we do not currently know how many juveniles are involved in prostitution. Scientifically credible estimates do not exist." Obviously, there is a need for research on the prevalence of prostitution of children.

We do however know *where* children are trafficked into prostitution. As with adults, children today are primarily sold via Internet websites that advertise escort prostitution, erotic encounters, or dates. Children are prostituted in strip clubs, massage parlors, live web cam prostitution, phone sex, and in other locations where adult prostitution takes place. On the ground, it is impossible to differentiate the prostitution of adults from that of children. In most cities, children are sold in certain zones familiar to those who buy them (Boyer, 2008; Spangenberg, 2001).

Racism is an Integral Part of Sexual Objectification and Systems of Prostitution

Marginalization because of race/ethnicity or poverty increases the likelihood that a girl will be prostituted. Young women of color, especially Latinas and African Americans, are overrepresented among prostitution-involved trafficked youth compared to their numbers in the overall U.S. population. Priebe and Suhr (2005) described the demographics of populations at risk for trafficking for prostitution in Atlanta and found that the majority of children in prostitution were African American girls whose average age was 14. Those at greatest risk were not immigrants or refugees, although, unfortunately, when trafficking is addressed, internationally trafficked children may be more likely to be viewed as victims are than African American girls who have been stereotyped as "hardened" or "overly sexualized" and worthy of incarceration (Kittling, 2006).

In the 1990s, African American girls in San Francisco were frequently arrested and incarcerated (Center on Juvenile and Criminal Justice, 2007). African American youth were approximately three times as likely as white European American youth to be detained upon arrest. A decade later, Latino youth were approximately six times more likely than white European American youth to be detained upon arrest (Macallair and Males, 2003). In 2007, San Francisco's Center for Juvenile and Criminal Justice noted a "shocking overuse of detention for Latino youth."

African American homeless young adults were significantly more likely to be prostituted than white European Americans (Tyler, 2009). Noting that African American homeless youth use significantly fewer services than white

European Americans, Tyler speculated that a lack of accessible and culturally relevant services was a factor. There is an urgent need for trauma-informed services, especially for young women of color.

Although the sexual objectification of girls occurs in many forms of music, not exclusively in hip-hop (APA, 2007), it is especially toxic in hip-hop's misogynist and racist lyrics, where women are "ho's" and "bitches" deserving of men's contempt and violence (Armstrong, 2001). African American girls have been especially harmed by rap culture, which glorifies pimping and stereotypes girls as hypersexual, sexually irresponsible, and uninterested in intimate relationships (Davis, 2004). A study of 1,461 12- to 17-year-olds found that degrading lyrics (but not sexual lyrics that were not degrading) were associated with a range of increased adolescent sexual behaviors. The study's authors described prostitution-like roles for girls as degraded "ho's" and roles for boys that were pimp-like or john-like in popular teen music (Martino et al., 2006).

Where there is cultural tolerance of the exploitation of women and people of color, then the most extreme poverty results in girls' greatest risk for prostitution and other sexual violence. The destructive legacy of colonialism creates cultural and familial disruption, resulting in extremely high rates of domestic violence and abuse of children. Hecht (1998) analyzed the situation of prostituting street children in Brazil partly as resulting from that country's history of slavery and colonialism. Although rarely analyzed as such, colonialism is one of the causal factors in the prostitution of indigenous girls and women (Farley, Lynne, & Cotton, 2005). Schissel and Fedec (1999) found that Aboriginal youth in Canadian prostitution were subjected to more violence than were non-Aboriginal youth. The Aboriginal youth were more likely to run away from home, and they had experienced significantly more of the risk factors in childhood for prostitution than non-Aboriginal youth: neglect, physical abuse, verbal abuse, sexual abuse.

Prostitution of Girls Is Characterized by Pimp Control

Service providers and survivors of prostitution agree that almost all children in prostitution are under the control of pimps, usually a series of pimps since they are bought, traded, and sold if they are in prostitution for longer than a very brief time. Studying prostitution of children in California, Carr (2009) found that most had been coerced into prostitution by pimps posing as boyfriends, by friends or classmates, by older women, and by men who were strangers to them. In another study, a young woman explained,

> It was in December and it was really cold. I couldn't stand to be on the street. And this guy saw me, and he was like, "Are you homeless?"

I said, "Yes." And he asked me, "I'm willing to take you in; what are you willing to do for me?" And at the moment, I couldn't answer the question, but I knew what he meant. So I just I went along with it. He took me to his house. He fed me, gave me clothes to change in and everything. And at the end of the night, it was pretty much that I had to do something sexual to him to stay. And I had to give him oral sex. (Curtis et al., 2008, p. 49)

A 15-year-old girl in New York explained how she was recruited by a pimp:

I was in a group home. And he was like, you know, the little leeches that linger around. And I was sittin' on my steps and I was cryin' ... And the things that he was sayin' to me, it sounded good. So, it was like, "Hmm, you know, maybe I can do this." But once I started seein' certain things and certain actions, it was like, I might as well have stayed in the hell I was in, because now, I'm doin' things that I really don't wanna do.' (Curtis et al., 2008, p. 47)

Children may be recruited by their friends, as this child explained:

I got kicked out at 14, and I had nowhere to go. And when I found one a my friends, at first, she referred me to be at a strip club. It's called Oasis, in the Bronx. So I stripped for a couple a months and I didn't like the pay. I tried to look for a job, but I was too young. So, then she referred me to :...do this. And I don't consider myself a prostitute, but an escort. My friends told me their clients...and then their clients...and it just goes up from there. (Curtis et al., 2008, p. 50)

Pimps recruit vulnerable young women who need affection, food, and shelter through a process that is an extremely controlled courtship like the love-bombing recruitment used by cults. Her need for an attachment requires that the girl develop an intimate relationship with someone who is fundamentally untrustworthy, unpredictable, and dangerous (Herman, 1994).

The violent control used by pimps causes feelings of terror, helplessness, and dependence in prostituted girls. Silbert and Pines (1983) described a PTSD-like "psychological paralysis" among prostituted youth and a syndrome they described as *learned helplessness*. A trafficking victim in the United Kingdom explained, "Sometimes I don't see the point in doing anything. It seems useless. When someone has controlled you and made decisions for you for so long, you can't do that for yourself anymore" (Zimmerman et al., 2006).

Prostituted children live under conditions of domestic terrorism. The techniques of control used by batterers with wives, girlfriends, and children

parallel those used by pimps (Stark & Hodgson, 2003). Pimps, like other batterers, make certain that the women are too terrified and too psychologically
and physically beaten down to contemplate escape, using social isolation, economic control, minimization and denial of violence, threats, intimidation, and
emotional, sexual, and physical violence (Giobbe, 1992, 1993).

Unless human behavior under conditions of captivity is understood, the
emotional bond between prostituted girls and pimps is difficult to compre-
hend. Emotional bonding to an abuser under conditions of captivity has been
described as *Stockholm syndrome* (Graham, 1994). Attitudes and behaviors that
are part of this syndrome include intense gratefulness for small favors when
the captor holds life and death power over the captive, denial of the extent
of violence and harm that the captor has inflicted or is obviously capable of
inflicting, hypervigilance with respect to the pimp's needs and identification with the pimp's perspective on the world (an example of this was Patty
Hearst's identification with her captors' ideology), perception of those trying
to assist in escape as enemies and perception of captors as friends, and extreme
difficulty leaving one's captor/pimp even after physical release has occurred.
Paradoxically, girls in prostitution may feel that they owe their lives to pimps
(Graham, 1994).

Herman (2003) noted that the sex industry can be understood as "a primary vector for socialization in the practices of coercive control, and the
pimp might be among the world's most common instructors in the arts of
torture." Coercive subjugation by pimps always contains the threat of violence, which is periodically inflicted under conditions that maximize its
effects: unpredictability, and with a high intensity that overwhelms the
senses and deliberately activates the victim's specific fears, aversions, and
anxieties. Whenever the violence is *not* inflicted on her, the woman in prostitution is immensely grateful. This coerced gratitude is an essential element
of the prostitute–pimp dynamic (Schwartz, 2000).

Pimps' Use of Mind Control Against Children in Prostitution

An abused and frightened 15-year-old girl does not have the skills to outmaneu-
ver a 26-year-old pimp who's offering love, money, and shelter (Boyer, 2008).
Fortunately, new information is now available to better understand how pimps
use mental coercion to control prostituted children.

Pimps gradually remove a child's previous set of values and replace it
with the pimp's own worldview. The girl's attachments to others are carefully undermined and ultimately destroyed, leaving the pimp as the only

available source of support, protection, or validation. Parents and family members may be presented to the girl as the enemy. Society is held in contempt. Subversion of the social order becomes one of many forms of "pulling-one-over" by which the pimp feeds his inflated, narcissistic sense of himself. The pimp's way of thinking is slowly and systematically downloaded into the psyche of the girl in prostitution. As in cults, the pimp and his community ultimately replace any previously existing social system (Schwartz, Williams, & Farley, 2007).

Mind control is facilitated by social isolation and sensory deprivation, which can include being locked up for long periods of time in windowless rooms to keep victims disoriented about time and place, deprived of sunlight, and more vulnerable to the pimp's influence. The social isolation may be so profoundly stressful and disorganizing that the victim will acquiesce to any form of contact, even rape. This coerced choice is then used by the pimp to confuse the girl about her own motivations and to cement his subjugation of her (Schwartz et al., 2007).

Pimps deliberately traumatize prostituted girls in order to establish control over them. They also use starvation, sleep deprivation, protein deprivation, conditioned physiologic hyperarousal, unexpected sexual violence, and learned helplessness (Schwartz et al., 2007). Pimps induce exhaustion and physical debilitation in order to establish control or inflict punishment. They assume psychological, biological, social, and economic control over the lives of the women they sell to johns through chronic terror, captivity, and isolation from others who might offer support and validation. The pimp's total control over young women in prostitution includes what she wears, when and where she can sleep, and what and how much she can eat, whether she can use a toilet or access menstrual supplies, if and how much emergency medical care she receives, even how much air and light she is allowed to have.

Capricious rules degrade, confuse, and reinforce complicity, as in the case of a girl whose pimp required her to lay down in a particular spot on the floor whenever he commanded "Down!" (Schwartz et al., 2007). Pimps threaten to kill girls and their families. Girls are forced to witness extreme violence against others, including death. Pornography is used for blackmail and as "proof" of the victim's complicity in her own sexual abuse by establishing her identity as a prostitute. Any move toward autonomy on her part, any attempt to exert more control over her body or even to use her own critical thinking, is viewed as insubordination by the pimp, a viewpoint that is gradually internalized by the young woman herself (Herman, 1994; Schwartz, 2000; Schwartz et al., 2007).

Girls are permitted no dignity in prostitution. Degradation is at the core of the incapacitating shame and mind control used by pimps. Verbal sadism is psychologically disorganizing and emotionally debilitating, while at the same time it enhances girls' dependence on pimps. A 14-year-old girl wrote about a pimp's use of these techniques.

> We just got in the car and drove to Chicago leaving everything behind. It was dark when we got there. He brought me to this kind of apartment warehouse with a lot of young girls there—black, white, everything. I asked who they were and he said, "these are my girls." He sat me down and told me, either I am with him this way or not at all. Then Tommy began treating me badly. He locked me in a room and left me without food or water. All he left me was some coke [cocaine]. He said this was my punishment, but I didn't know for what. All I heard were the trains going by. I thought about jumping out, but it was so high. Then after maybe 3 days he came back and got me. All the way home, we would stop and go with truckers and then go back in his motel room.
>
> The day before Thanksgiving, Thomas told me his brother died and threw me in the car like it was my fault. *He brought me to a guy's house and told me I was a bad girl and don't deserve to live.* He threw me in the room and tried to assault me. But I didn't want him to touch me. I yelled, "Get away!" He knocked me unconscious and I blacked out. *I woke up to Tommy whispering in my ear: I'm a bad girl; I have no purpose in life; I'm just a sex toy. He just kept whispering these things over and over.* Then he passed out on top of me, after having sex with me. I stayed so still, just lying there, and waited for hours. (Friedman, 2005, p. 11, author's italics)

These techniques are interspersed with special favors, promises of relief, and sometimes affection, all of which create a powerful trauma bond. The psychological and neurobiological reactions generated by alternating terrorism with gratuitous and unpredictable rewards deepens traumatic bonding and reinforces the girl's twisted attachment (Schwartz et al., 2007). The complex psychobiology of trauma, attachment, and survival (brilliantly manipulated by the pimp) leaves the girl ensnared by her own adaptation responses. Outsiders see them as partners rather than dominator and subordinate. This misinterpretation of their relationship further cements her bond to the pimp (Schwartz et al., 2007).

Pimps facilitate the creation of dissociated parts of the self who happily prostitute. In extreme cases, sensory deprivation and torture result in highly compartmentalized "prostitute personalities" in chronically traumatized and dissociative women and children. A young woman who was filmed in sadomasochistic prostitution reported that the cameramen/pimps taught her to use hypnotic techniques to dissociate specific parts of her body for pain control. The pimps/

pornographers convinced vulnerable girls that they were "bondage sluts," who demonstrated their strength based on their tolerance for violent abuse.

Online Sexualization, Sexual Exploitation, and Prostitution

Pimps use the same tactics online that they use elsewhere: enticement, persuasion, grooming, coercion, denial and minimization of harm, social isolation, intimidation, and violent threats (Klien, 2008). Targeting vulnerable or homeless girls, pimps recruit and instruct them in the use of a cell phone and a publicly available computer where the girls are advertised for sexual use.

Children are sold on prostitution websites such as redbook.com, eros.com, or Craigslist. Craigslist originated as an online community bulletin board but has released 25,000 new advertisements every 10 days for "erotic services" which is code for prostitution (Farley, 2006). In Sacramento, a crossroads for organized criminals who traffic girls in the western United States, hundreds of ads for prostitution a day were posted on Craigslist (Branson, 2006).

Children are not specifically advertised as "children" or "girls," although this is clearly implied in much prostitution advertising. In August 2009, for example, Craigslist advertised "cute little Barbie doll" and "INEXPERIENCED, Beautiful, Petite Ballerina-Asian college student" who is described as "I look young but I'm over 18" on adult services (Craigslist, 2009a,b,c). Web searches for hot young girls (2009) produced "first time teeny anal training" and "hot young teen plays with her pussy on bed" (Hottest Teen Videos, 2009a,b). In a 2009 web search for "incest videos," more than 18 computer screens were produced. It is unclear whether the images are of adults who appear childlike or if they are filmed sexual abuse of children who are being trafficked online (Incest Videos, 2009).

In 2008, a 15-year-old ran away from her home in western Wisconsin and was then pimped out on Craigslist, where 15 different advertisements offered her for sale to Milwaukee johns (Diedrich, 2008). In another case a 16-year-old girl was pimped by a man who beat, raped, and photographed her. He posted the photos on Craigslist and was eventually arrested (Diedrich, 2008). In 2008, federal agents arrested two Detroit pimps who had placed 2,800 ads for prostitution on Craigslist, MySpace, and other social networking sites. The pimps were charged with sexual exploitation and sex trafficking of children. The children were transported by organized crime networks across the United States, and their prostitution was photographed and sold as pornography (Snell & Hicks, 2008). An Illinois sheriff has sued Craigslist for trafficking (Coalition Against Trafficking in Women, 2009)

In 2007, there were 29,000 registered sex offenders on MySpace.com (Robertson, 2007). According to his MySpace profile, a 41-year-old man was single, a Sagittarius, a nonsmoker and nondrinker. A database of registered sex offenders offered a different profile of the man. He had convictions for forced sodomy, oral sex, and lewd and lascivious acts with a person under the age of 14. A 22-year-old man created a MySpace college student persona, professing a love for poetry, nature, and coffee house bands, while failing to mention that he was a convicted child molester (Shreve, 2006).

Girls' vulnerability is increased by risky online interactions, such as talking about sex to strangers (Wolak, Finkelhor, Mitchell, & Ybarra, 2004, 2008; Muir, 2005). A review of Internet-initiated sex crimes against minors revealed that 75% of girls between 13 and 15 years of age met adult sex offenders in Internet chat rooms; 64% of offenders communicated online with the victims for 6 months or more; and 77% of the communications were in multiple ways (telephone, mail, pictures, gifts, or money). Fifty percent of the victims felt close to the offender or were in love with the offender (Wolak et al., 2004).

Of the 83 children identified by a U.K. children's advocacy group as having been subjected to Internet or cell phone exploitation, 47% were also prostituted. Eleven children were sold on the Internet, one was sold on a live pay-per-view website, and 27 children were coerced into having pornography made of them. The children gave the following reasons why they either did not tell or why they denied that they had been sexually exploited: first, the photos made it appear that they agreed to the sexual abuse; second, they may have been smiling in the images, as they were directed to do; third, they may have been coerced to recruit other victims (e.g., schoolmates who were invited for sleepovers at the insistence of the sex offender) and therefore felt that they were themselves "responsible bystanders" since friends were sexually abused and often victims of pornography production; fourth, the children were encouraged to be proactive in their own self-exploitation (masturbation) or with other children (mutual sexual abuse), with or without the offender in the images; and finally, children were shown their own images and threatened with the perpetrator's telling nonoffending parents that the child cooperated and did not stop the abuse (Palmer, 2004). These are the same reasons that adult women in prostitution give for blaming themselves for their prostitution.

Mainstreaming Prostitution-like Behaviors

Boundaries between normal adolescent sexual exploration and prostitution-like activity have disappeared on many social networking sites. Sites that are popular with girls, such as MySpace, Facebook, Flickr, Stickam, and Yahoo, host adult pornography, child pornography, and solicitation for prostitution. MySpace, for example, lists thinly veiled prostitution advertising such as "Find a Booty

Call" (Criddle, 2008). Stickam, another socially risky website used by teenagers, encourages the posting of live web cam sexual behaviors (Stone, 2007). *Espin-the-bottle* is advertised as a sexualized "flirting and dating" site for people aged 13–57. The site posts children's responses to sexualized quizzes and accepts advertising from companies that promote ways to help children hide their Internet use from parents (Criddle, 2008). Championing sexual objectification, MissBimbo.com encourages girls to compete to become the "hottest, coolest, most famous bimbo in the whole world."

In 2010, girls' sexualization blends seamlessly with prostitution. Prostitution-like behaviors are part of what it means to be female today. Young women are taught the sexuality of prostitution and pornography (Barry, 1995) and embrace it as their own. They ignore their own sexual feelings (or lack of them) and learn that their role is to service boyfriends who have also learned about sex via pornography.

School-based sex education programs focus on the biology of reproduction, often neglecting sexual behaviors, romance, and intimate relationships (Flood, 2007). Pornography, on the other hand, provides templates for sexual relationships. In 2001, 70% of 15- to 17-year-olds viewed online pornography (Kaiser Family Foundation, 2001). A 2007 Australian survey found that 97% of girls and 100% of boys had viewed pornography before age 15 (Sauers, 2007). Children may be enticed into photographing themselves and transmitting it online (Nyman, 2006). Flirting by sending nude photos of oneself via cellphones (Jayson, 2008) is commonplace, but the photos can easily be passed on and are sometimes posted on the Internet.

Imitating pornography, children enact the sex of prostitution by attempting sex that is casual and nonrelational, learning a sexuality that eroticizes powerlessness. Pornography is mediated prostitution (Catharine A. MacKinnon, personal communication, 2009). Child pornography is indistinguishable from the prostitution/sexual assault of children. Some consider pornography that contains images of the abuse and the prostitution of children to be digital crime scenes (Cooper, 2009).

Learning to present a hypersexualized, prostitution-like version of themselves to the world, girls may unwittingly participate in their own sexual exploitation. Levy described the "imaginary licentiousness" that very young girls enact in order to appear grown up. One girl explained, "Sexually, we didn't really do anything, but you wanted to *look* like you did" (Levy, 2005, p. 150).

Girls are sent the message that they should be available for sex and skilled at it. *Adorable* magazine sent teen subscribers a sex guide entitled *99 Naughty Tricks*. *Seventeen* and *CosmoGirl* magazines offer sex advice, often without mentioning a relationship as the context in which the sex occurs. Casually fellating boys at parties is normative for girls (Azam, 2009). One girl repeated the pimp's argument for prostitution, noting that if she was already fellating two or three boys every weekend at parties for free, she might as well do the same with five or six boys and get paid for it (Hanon, 2009).

Prostitution is normalized for children by "soft" or seemingly amateur pornography like *Girls Gone Wild* and by videos that mainstream prostitution and prostitution-like activities. For *Girls Gone Wild* footage, producer Joe Francis films at clubs where teenagers are partying. After girls are intoxicated, he persuades and entices them into being filmed. Francis pleaded no contest to child abuse and prostitution charges stemming from his pornography production activities (Parrish, 2008).[1]

Children have been encouraged to pursue jobs in the sex industry. Middle school students at a 2005 career day in California were told that stripping and exotic dancing were excellent careers for girls. A smiling job counselor told students that if they had breast enlargement surgery, they could earn excellent salaries as strippers. "For every two inches up there it's another $50, 000," he enthusiastically told the girls (Kim, 2005). An Abercrombie & Fitch marketing catalog promoted stripping as an empowering summer job for students (Smith et al., 2005).

Conclusion: Needs of Prostituted Girls and Needs of Girls at Risk for Prostitution-like Sexualization

"Someplace safe," she said. "Someplace to be a girl. Someplace where I won't have to have sex with men anymore." (Maternowska, 2009) This 16-year-old Swazi girl's answer is as relevant to prostitution of children in the United States as it is to prostitution of children in Swaziland. She needs secure housing in a facility staffed with people who understand her needs not only for physical safety but also for safety from predators who are often caregivers and boyfriends. Before she was sold in prostitution, she was almost certainly sexually assaulted in her family and community, which compounded the harm of the violence in prostitution. She needs long-term residential safety and treatment in order to permit slow and steady healing from childhood trauma and neglect, from the brainwashing of pimps, and from the violent degradation perpetrated on her by johns.

The hold that pimps and the street culture have over prostituted youth is too powerful to be displaced by traditional social services or brief interventions (Boyer, 2008). Health service providers are not yet adequately trained to work with girls whose involvement in prostitution is more Stockholmed and cult-like than is traditionally understood.

Weisberg, in 1985, noted that prostituting adolescents needed crisis housing, medical care, employment, and school counseling. Twenty years later, Friedman (2005) and Boyer (2008) describe the same urgent needs. Prostituting youth are underserved and often unrecognized, even in youth service agencies. They are frequently arrested for nonprostitution offenses, and their prostitution may not be known in the criminal justice system, even though the children are routinely provided with false identification and coached by pimps to lie about their ages.

Children in U.S. prostitution are confronted with a fragmented response from two separate systems, the criminal justice system and the child protective system (Schaffner, 1998). The child protective system's focus on family reunification may be dangerous to children who are sexually abused, prostituted, or pimped by family members. Many services are available to prostituting girls only in juvenile detention programs. This sends a mixed message to girls ("we'll help you deal with the traumatic consequences of paid rape but only after we arrest and incarcerate you"). Finkelhor, Cross, and Cantor (2005) stress the importance of working to better integrate the juvenile justice system's various parts, for example child maltreatment investigations, termination of parental rights, out-of-home placements, court hearings, victim compensation, decisions to prosecute, children's testimony, buyers' and pimps' testimonies, and prosecutions of perpetrators.

To adjudicate prostitution is to criminalize girls' physical, emotional, and psychological strategies, as Chesney-Lind and Sheldon (2004) pointed out. Tragically, many states still arrest, interrogate, prosecute, and incarcerate children in prostitution (Brittle, 2008; Javidan, 2003), which increases traumatic stress (Brown, 2006). In many cases, children under age 18 have been arrested for prostitution as many as 15 or more times.

The prostitution of children is a federal crime since the U.S. definition of trafficking now includes the prostitution of any person under age 18 (William Wilberforce Trafficking Victims Protection Reauthorization Act, 2008). No transportation is required in order to meet the legal requirement of trafficking. The federal law is at odds with local jurisdictions which often continue to arrest and treat minors in prostitution as criminals (Debra Boyer, personal communication, 2009). Beginning in 2010, a number of states have passed "safe harbor laws" that define prostituted children as sexually exploited rather than as criminals. Increased federal resources are slated to assist girls who have been prostituted. It would make logical sense for *noncommercial* sexual assault of a child to also be categorized as a federal crime.[3]

Friedman (2005) summarized the needs of prostituted children: (a) establish and fund safe houses and transitional living facilities for sexually exploited children, (b) develop and fund training programs for all youth workers and social service agencies about early intervention and the physical and emotional needs of sexually exploited children, (c) increase partnerships with and funding for successful agencies now serving the population of sexually exploited children, (d) establish model programs in several cities formalizing existing

linkages between child protective and youth service agencies and criminal justice agencies, and (e) develop recommendations and guidelines for services to
prostituted children for health organizations such as the American Academy
of Pediatrics, the American Psychological Association, the American Public
Health Association and the Society for Adolescent Medicine.

It is not in children's interests to make false distinctions such as the degree
to which a child seems to comply with or resist prostitution, or whether
the child is 16 and therefore has more "agency" than a 12-year-old. A child
advocate told the author that she was disheartened to learn that some viewed
"real" child victims as only those younger than 14, since 16- and 17-year-olds
were considered to have more choice in their prostitution.

Poulin (2009) summarized evidence for the association between the existence of a thriving sex industry and increases in what he termed the pedo-
philization of sex industries. Abolishing the prostitution of children requires
that we abolish the prostitution of everyone since the prostitution of children
is inextricably connected with the prostitution of adults.

The mantra "prostitution's always been with us, you'll never get rid of it" is
a soothing message from perpetrators that urges us to look away from prostitution. When the status of women is equal with men, the status of girls
improves and prostitution is decreased or abolished. Albanese (2007) suggested that the prostitution of children would be decreased by enhancing the
role of women in cultures where they are stereotyped as sex objects. Attending
school for example has been shown to decrease girls' involvement in prostitution (Schissel & Fedec, 1999).

When adults fail to challenge the cultural norms that mainstream prostitution, we are in effect placing the responsibility for prevention of prostitution
on children themselves (Boyer, 2008). Grand Theft Auto (GTA), one of the
most popular video games in the world for 12- to 18-year-old boys, main-
streams violence, rape, and increasingly, prostitution. Several versions of the
game exist, all involving use of a prostitute. In some versions, players can buy
a prostitute, beat her up, run her over, or kill her to earn game points. Players
earn additional points by owning a strip club or a pornography production
studio. In 2008, GTA publishers Take Two Interactive and Rockstar Games
enshrined a trafficker as GTA protagonist (Rockstar Games, 2008). When
adults tolerate graphic depictions of lethally sexist cultural practices, we are
limiting and endangering girls' lives.

Children today need media literacy education so they can counteract toxic
messages about their sexuality. They can learn to assess the sexually exploitive
messages that are lodged in technologies from video games to cell phone applications to Internet pornography. Technical and media consciousness-raising
are essential, first for parents themselves and later for parents to teach children.
Media literacy resource material must include resources on sex stereotyping

and also specific education on the damaging effects of the media's sexualization of children, with recommendations for ways to discuss these issues with children of different ages.[2] Smith et al. (2005) and the Campaign for a Commercial-Free Childhood (2009) proposed that adults challenge corporations that promote the sexualization of children. Other educators have provided models for teaching children to deconstruct common myths about sexuality and love (Galician & Merskin, 2007).

These resources can decrease the toxic media sexualization of girls, encouraging them to grow up with a sexuality that is not imposed on them by pimp- and pornography-dominated cultures. Girls need a culture that defines girlhood as something other than being groomed for prostitution, something other than a culture that teaches them to embrace their own sexual objectification. They need a culture that does not ignore the vulnerability of girls who are poor or who are marginalized because of their race/ethnicity. Girls—and all of us—need to know that there are men in the world who view women as equal to men and who refuse to buy women, girls, or any human for sex.

Acknowledgments

Thanks to Debra Boyer, Catharine A. MacKinnon, and Betsy Salkind for reviewing this paper. Thanks to Jen Coleman and Luciana Huang for research assistance.

Notes

1. See Ariel Levy (2005, pp. 7–17) for an extended description of a Joe Francis shoot. See also Associated Press (2008) "Florida: 'Wild' Girls Founder is Set Free" (Associated Press, 2008); CNN.com (2008) "Spitzer escort's 'Girls Gone Wild' videos surface Via Associated Press," and TMZ.com (2008) "Ashley Dupre Gone 'Wild'—Legal or Jailbait?" Ashley Youmans (known as Ashley Dupre) was filmed at age 17 by Joe Francis. After Eliot Spitzer's arrest for prostitution (Farley & Ramos, 2008), Ashley Youmans was described in most media as a "high-priced escort" and her prostitution by Spitzer and others was glamorized. In real life, she ran away from what she described as an abusive home at the age of 17. For some period of time after running away from home Ms. Youmans was homeless and she became addicted to drugs. "I have been alone," she wrote on her MySpace page. "I have abused drugs. I have been broke and homeless. But, I survived, on my own." After being prostituted and filmed by Francis, Ms. Youmans encountered more pimps. She was recruited into escort prostitution by convicted New York pimp Jason Itzler. Later, Ms. Youmans prostituted for pimps at Emperor's Club VIP, a prostitution ring that sometimes moved women from the United States to Europe on what they called "travel dates" rather than human trafficking. The Emperor's Club presented itself as an elite escort service. Aside from charging more, it worked like any other prostitution business.

2. Resources include Campaign for a Commercial-Free Childhood http://www.commercialexploitation.org/; Media Awareness Network http://www.media-awareness.ca/english/index.cfm provides extensive resources for educating children about pornography and sexual advertising; MediaWatch http://www.mediawatch.com offers a feminist analysis of sexism and violence in the media.
3. Incest and rape can be either commercial or noncommercial sexual assault.

References

Abramovich, E. (2005). Childhood sexual abuse as a risk factor for subsequent involvement in sex work: A review of empirical findings *Journal of Psychology and Human Sexuality, 17*(1/2), 131–146.

Albanese, J. (2007, December). *Commercial sexual exploitation of children: What do we know and what do we do about it?* National Institute of Justice Report NCJ 215733. Available at http://nij.ncjrs.gov/publications/Pub_Search.asp?category=99&searchtype=basic&location=top&PSID=25

American Psychological Association. (2007). *Report of the APA Task Force on the sexualization of girls.* Available at http://www.apa.org/pi/wpo/sexualization.html

Armstrong, E. G. (2001). Gangsta misogyny: A content analysis of the portrayals of violence against women in rap music 1987–1993. *Journal of Criminal Justice and Popular Culture, 8*(2), 96–126.

Associated Press. (2008, March 13). Florida: "Wild" girls founder is set free. *New York Times.* Retrieved from http://www.nytimes.com/2008/03/13/us/13brfs-8216WILD8217_BRF.html?scp=13&sq=&st=nyt

Azam, S. (2009). *Oral sex is the new goodnight kiss:.the sexual bullying of girls.* Los Angeles: Bollywood Entertainment Press

Bagley, C., & Young, L. (1987). Juvenile prostitution and child sexual abuse: A controlled study. *Canadian Journal of Community Mental Health, 6*(1), 5–26.

Barry, K. (1995). *The prostitution of sexuality.* New York: New York University Press.

Boyer, D. (2008). *Who pays the price? Assessment of youth involvement in prostitution in Seattle.* Seattle: Human Services Department, Domestic Violence and Sexual Assault Prevention Division.

Brannigan, A., & Gibbs Van Brunschot, E. (1997). Youthful prostitution and child sexual trauma. *International Journal of Law and Psychiatry, 20*(3), 337–354.

Branson, S. (2006). *Online child prostitution, an alarming trend.* Sacramento Channel 31, a CBS affiliate. Retrieved September 16, 2007 from http://cbs13.com/local/child.prostitution.online

Briere, J. (1992). *Child abuse trauma: Theory and treatment of the lasting effects.* Newbury Park, CA: Sage.

Brittle, K. (2008). Child abuse by another name: Why the child welfare system is the best mechanism in place to address the problem of juvenile prostitution. *Hofstra Law Review, 36*, 1339–1375.

Brown, G. O. (2006, May 24). *Little girl lost: Secondary victimization of teenaged girls treated like enemy combatants: The Las Vegas metro police vice detail and the use of material witness holds.* Paper presented at the annual meeting of the American Society of Criminology. Los Angeles Convention Center, Los Angeles.

Browne, A., & Finklehor, D. (1986). Impact of child sexual abuse: A review of the research. *Psychological Bulletin, 99*, 66–77.

Campaign for a commercial-free childhood. (2009). Available at http://www.commercial-freechildhood.org/

Carr, M. L. (2009, June). *Exploring commercially sexually exploited minors' hopes and goals for their futures: From nightmares to dreams.* Dissertation, Pacific Graduate School of Psychology, Palo Alto, CA.

Center on Juvenile and Criminal Justice. (2007). *Juvenile detention in San Francisco: Analysis and trends 2006.* Available at http://www.cjcj.org/resource/center

Chesney-Lind, M., & Sheldon, R. G. (2004). *Girls, delinquency, and juvenile justice* (3rd ed.). Belmont, CA: Thomson-Wadsworth.

Classen, C., Palesh, O. G., & Aggarwal, R. (2005). Sexual revictimization: A review of the empirical literature. *Trauma, Violence, & Abuse, 6*(2), 103–129.

Clayton, M. (1996, August 30). Sex trade lures kids from burbs. *Christian Science Monitor.* Retrieved from http://www.csmonitor.com/1996/0830/083096.intl.intl.1.html

CNN.com (2008). *Spitzer escort's "Girls Gone Wild" videos surface via Associated Press.* Retrieved April 4, 2008 from http://www.cnn.com

Coalition Against Trafficking in Women. (2009). Amicus Brief in Dart vs. Craigslist, Inc. Available at http://action.web.ca/home/catw/readingroom.shtml?x=126762&AA_EX_S ession=07124ee8f218f6a1137603052fad7464

Cooper, S. W. (2009). The sexual exploitation of children and youth: Redefining victimization. In S. Olfman (Ed.), *The sexualization of childhood* (pp. 88–102). Westport, CT: Praeger.

Craigslist. (2009a, August 20). *"Asian girl crystal massage".* Adult Services, Las Vegas.Retrieved from http://lasvegas.craigslist.org

Craigslist. (2009b, August 20). *"cute little Barbie doll."* Adult Services, Las Vegas. Retrieved from http://lasvegas.craigslist.org

Craigslist. (2009c, August 20). *"INEXPERIENCED, Beautiful, Petite Ballerina-Asian college student".* Retrieved from http://lasvegas.craigslist.org

Criddle, L. (2008, April). *Human trafficking and the internet.* Available at www.look-both-ways.com

Curtis, R., Terry, K., Dank, M., Dombrowski, K., & Khan, B. (2008). *Commercial sexual exploitation of children in New York City, Volume One: The CSEC population in New York City: Size, characteristics, and needs.* Unpublished report by US Department of Justice.

Cusick, L. (2002). Youth prostitution: A literature review. *Child Abuse Review, 11,* 230–251.

Dalla, R. L. (2006). *Exposing the "pretty woman" myth: A qualitative investigation of street-level prostituted women.* Boulder, CO: Lexington Books.

Davis, T. (2004, March 17). New study on hip-hop sexuality finds anti-woman strain even among young women. *Village Voice.* Retrieved May 22, 2005 from http://www.villagevoice.com/issues/0411/davis.php

Diedrich, J. (2008, April 8). Craigslist child sex ads lead to arrests: Investigators follow rising use of web site in prostitution. *Milwaukee Journal-Sentinel.* Retrieved April 8, 2008 from http://www.jsonline.com/story/index.aspx?id=737115

DiPaolo, M. (1999). *The impact of multiple childhood trauma on homeless runaway adolescents.* New York: Garland Publishing.

Downes, L. (2006, December 29). Middle school girls gone wild. *New York Times.* Retrieved from http://www.nytimes.com/2006/12/29/opinion/29fri4.html?scp=1&sq=Middle%20 School%20Girls%20Gone%20Wild&st=cse

Dworkin, A. (1997). Prostitution and male supremacy. In *Life and death.* New York: Free Press. Available at http://www.prostitutionresearch.com/how_prostitution_works/000011.html

Ennew, J., Gopal, K., Heeran, J., & Montgomery, H. (1996). *Children and prostitution: How can we measure and monitor the commercial sexual exploitation of children? Literature review and annotated bibliography* (2nd ed.). With additional material prepared for the Congress Against the Commercial Sexual Exploitation of Children, Stockholm, August 26–31 1996. New York: UNICEF; Children in Especially Difficult Circumstances, Centre for

Family Research, University of Cambridge and Childwatch International. Retrieved from http://childabuse.com

Farley, M. (2003). Prostitution and the invisibility of harm. *Women & Therapy,* 26(3/4), 247–280.

Farley, M. (2006). Prostitution, trafficking, and cultural amnesia: What we must not know in order to keep the business of sexual exploitation running smoothly. *Yale Journal of Law and Feminism, 18,* 109–144.

Farley, M. (2007). *Prostitution and trafficking in Nevada: Making the connections.* San Francisco: Prostitution Research & Education.

Farley, M., Cotton, A., Lynne, J., Zumbeck, S., Spiwak, F., Reyes, M. E., et al. (2003). Prostitution and trafficking in 9 countries: Update on violence and posttraumatic stress disorder. *Journal of Trauma Practice, 2,* 33–74. Available at http://www.prostitutionresearch.com/prostitution_research/000116.html

Farley, M., Lynne, J., & Cotton, A. (2005). Prostitution in Vancouver: Violence and the colonization of first nations women. *Transcultural Psychiatry, 42,* 242–271.

Farley, M., & Ramos, N. (2008, November 10). Why allowing Eliot Spitzer to break the law is a mistake. *Newsweek.* Available at http://www.newsweek.com/id/168395

Finkelhor, D., Cross, T. P., & Cantor, E. N. (2005). The justice system for juvenile victims: A comprehensive model of case flow. *Trauma, Violence, & Abuse, 6,* 83–102.

Flood, M. (2007). Exposure to pornography among youth in Australia. *Journal of Sociology, 43*(1), 45–60.

Foti, S. M. (1995). Child sexual abuse as a precursor to prostitution. *Dissertation Abstracts International: Section B: The Sciences & Engineering, 55*(8-B), 3586.

Friedman, S. A. (2005). *Who is there to help us? How the system fails sexually exploited girls. Examples from four cities in the U.S.* Brooklyn, NY: ECPAT-USA. Retrieved from http://www.ecpatusa.org/resources.html

Galician, M., & Merskin, D. L. (2007). *Critical thinking about sex, love, and romance in the mass media.* Mahwah, NJ: Lawrence Erlbaum.

Giobbe, E. (1992). Juvenile prostitution: Profile of recruitment. In A. W. Burgess (Ed.), *Child trauma: Issues & research.* New York. Garland Publishing.

Giobbe, E. (1993). An analysis of individual, institutional, and cultural pimping. *Michigan Journal of Gender and Law, 1,* 33–57.

Graham, D. L. R., with Rawlings, E., & Rigsby, R. (1994). *Loving to survive: Sexual terror, men's violence and women's lives.* New York: New York University Press.

Gwadz, M. V., Nish, D., Leonard, N. R., & Strauss, S. M. (2007). Gender differences in traumatic events and rates of post-traumatic stress disorder among homeless youth. *Journal of Adolescence, 30,* 117–129.

Hanon, A. (2009, April 1). Teen girls trading sex for favours. *Edmonton Sun.* Available at http://cnews.canoe.ca/CNEWS/Canada/2009/04/01/8959961-sun.html

Hansen, J. (2003, February 1). Flashy pimp shindig outrage in Atlanta. *Atlanta Journal Constitution.*

Hecht, T. (1998). *At home in the street: Street children of northeast Brazil.* New York: Cambridge University Press.

Herman, J. (1994). *Trauma and recovery: The aftermath of violence from domestic abuse to political terror.* New York: Basic Books.

Herman, J. (2003). Introduction: Hidden in plain sight: Clinical observations on prostitution. In M. Farley (Ed.), *Prostitution, trafficking, and traumatic stress* (pp. 1–13). New York: Routledge.

Hottest Teen Videos. (2009a). *First time teeny anal training.* August 20, 2009. Available at http://www.hottestonly.com/search.aspx/hottest_video~teen/

Hottest Teen Videos. (2009b). *Hot young teen plays with her pussy on bed.* August 20, 2009. http://www.hottestonly.com/search.aspx/hottest_video~teen/

Incest videos. (2009). August 20, 2009. http://www.xforums.org/support/viewtopic.php?f=10&t=23825

James, J., & Meyerding, J. (1977). Early sexual experience as a factor in prostitution. *Archives of Sexual Behavior, 7*(1), 31–42.

Javidan, P. (2003). Defining feminism: Invisible targets: Juvenile prostitution, crackdown legislation, and the example of California. *Cardozo Women's Law Journal, 9*, 237–254.

Jayson, S. (2008, December 16). Nude photos: A new way for young people to flirt? *USA Today.* Retrieved from http://www.pnj.com

Kaiser Family Foundation. (2001). *Generation Rx.com: How young people use the internet for health information.* Menlo Park, CA: Henry J. Kaiser Foundation.

Kendall-Tackett, K. A., Williams, L. M., & Finkelhor, D. (1993). Impact of sexual abuse on children: A review and synthesis of recent empirical studies. *Psychological Bulletin, 113*(1), 164–180.

Kim, R. (2005, January 14). Bump, grind your way to riches, students told. *San Francisco Chronicle.* Retrieved from http://www.fradical.com/Pimping_at_school_career_day.htm

Kittling, N. (2006). God bless the child: The United States' response to domestic juvenile prostitution. *Nevada Law Journal, 6*, 913–926.

Klien, G. (2008, April 15). MySpace predator pimps 16 year-old. *Marin Independent Journal.* Retrieved April 15, 2008 from http://www.marinij.com/sanrafael/ci_8939903

Leidholdt, D. (1980). *Some notes on objectification: From objectification to violence.* New York: Women Against Pornography. Document available from author

Levy, A. (2005). *Female chauvinist pigs: Women and the rise of raunch culture.* New York: Free Press.

Ling, D. C., Wong, W. C., Holroyd, E. A., & Gray, A. (2007). Silent killers of the night: An exploration of psychological health and suicidality among female street sex workers. *Journal of Sex & Marital Therapy, 33*, 281–299.

Louie, L., Luu, M., & Tong, B. (1991, August). *Chinese American adolescent runaways.* Paper presented at Annual Convention of the Asian American Psychological Association, San Francisco.

Lucas, B., & Hackett, L. (1995). *Street youth: On their own in Indianapolis.* Indianapolis: Health Foundation of Greater Indianapolis.

Macallair, M. P., & Males, M. A. (2003). *An analysis of San Francisco juvenile justice reforms during the Brown administration: A report to the San Francisco Board of Supervisors.* San Francisco: Center on Juvenile and Criminal Justice. Available at http://www.cjcj.org/files/sfjj.pdf

MacLean, M. G., Embry, L. E., & Cauce, A. M. (1999). Homeless adolescents' paths to separation from family: Comparison of family characteristics, psychological adjustment, and victimization. *Journal of Community Psychology, 27*(2), 179–187.

Martino, S. C., Collins, R. C., Elliott, M. N., Strachman, A., Kanouse, D. E., & Berry, S. H. (2006). Exposure to degrading versus nondegrading music lyrics and sexual behavior among youth. *Pediatrics, 118*(2), 430–441. Available at http://pediatrics.aappublications.org/cgi/content/full/118/2/e430

Maternowska, M. C. (2009, August 23). Lives: Truck-stop girls. *New York Times Magazine.* Retrieved from http://www.nytimes.com/2009/08/23/magazine/23lives-t.html?_r=1

Mayfield-Schwarz, L. (2006). *Severity of trauma exposure and complex posttraumatic stress disorder symptomatology in women who prostitute.* Dissertation submitted in partial fulfillment of Ph.D. California Institute of Integral Studies, San Francisco.

Merskin, D. (2004). Reviving Lolita? A media literacy examination of sexual portrayals of girls in fashion advertising. *American Behavioral Scientist, 48*(1), 119–129.

Molnar, B. E., Shade, S. B., Kral, A. H., Booth, R. E., & Watters, J. K. (1998). Suicidal behavior and sexual/physical abuse among street youth. *Child Abuse & Neglect, 22*(3), 213–222.

Muir, D. (2005). *Violence against children in cyberspace, a contribution to the United Nations study on violence against children*. Bangkok: ECPAT International.

Nadon, S. M., Koverola, C., & Schludermann, E. H. (1998). Antecedents to prostitution: Childhood victimization. *Journal of Interpersonal Violence, 13*, 206–221.

Newton-Ruddy, L., & Handelsman, M. M. (1986). Jungian feminine psychology and adolescent prostitutes. *Adolescence, 21*, 815–825.

Nyman, A. (2006). Risky behavior on the Internet. In *Children and young persons with abusive and violent experiences connected to cyberspace: Challenges for research, rehabilitation, prevention and protection*. Report from an expert meeting sponsored by the Swedish Children's Welfare Foundation and the Working Group for Cooperation of Children at Risk under Council of the Baltic Sea States.

Palmer, T. (2004). Just one click: Sexual abuse of children and young people through the internet and mobile telephone technology. Ilford, UK: Barnardo's.

Parrish, M. (2008, August 18). "Girls Gone Wild" founder faces I.R.S. *New York Times*. Retrieved from http://www.nytimes.com/2008/08/19/business/19francis.html?_r=1& scp=1&sq=Francis+IRS&st=cse&oref=slogin

Phoenix, J. (1999). *Making sense of prostitution*. London: MacMillan Press.

Potterat, J. J., Phillips, L., Rothenberg, R. B., & Darrow, W. (1985). On becoming a prostitute: An exploratory case-comparison study. *Journal of Sex Research, 21*, 329–335.

Poulin, R., with Claude, M. (2009). *Pornographie et hypersexualisation. Enfances dévastées, tome 2*. Ottawa: L'Interligne.

Priebe, A., & Suhr, C. (2005, September). *Hidden in plain view: The commercial sexual exploitation of girls in Atlanta*. Atlanta, GA: Atlanta Women's Agenda. Retrieved from http://www.womensagenda.com

Purcell, N. J., & Zurbriggen, E. L. (2013). The sexualization of girls and gendered violence: Is there a connection? In E. L. Zurbriggen, & T. –A. Roberts (Eds.), *The sexualization of girls*. New York: Oxford University Press.

Putnam, F. (1990). Disturbances of "self" in victims of childhood sexual abuse. In R. Kluft (Ed.), *Incest-related syndromes of adult psychopathology* (pp. 113–131). Washington, DC: American Psychiatric Press.

Raphael, J., & Shapiro, D. L. (2002). *Sisters speak out: The lives and needs of prostituted women in Chicago*. Chicago: Center for Impact Research.

Robertson, G. D. (2007). MySpace.com finds 29,000 sex offenders, more than 4 times previous total, officials say. *Associated Press*, release posted at ABCNews.com. Retrieved from http://www.abcnews.go.com/

Rockstar Games. (2008). See http://www.gamespot.com/xbox360/action/grandtheftauto4/index.html or http://www.rockstargames.com/IV/

Ross, C., Farley, M., & Schwartz, H. L. (2003). Dissociation among women in prostitution. *Journal of Trauma Practice, 2*(3/4), 199–212.

Sauers, J. (2007). *Sex lives of Australian teenagers*. Sydney: Random House.

Schaffner, L. (1998). Female juvenile delinquency: Sexual solutions, gender bias, and juvenile justice. *Hastings Women's Law Journal, 9*, 1–25.

Schissel, B., & Fedec, K. (1999). The selling of innocence: The gestalt of danger in the lives of youth prostitutes. *Canadian Journal of Criminology, 41*, 33–56.

Schwartz, H. (2000). *Dialogues with forgotten voices: Relational perspectives on child abuse trauma and treatment of dissociative disorders*. New York: Basic Books.

Schwartz, H., Williams, J., & Farley, M. (2007). Pimp subjugation of women by mind control. In M. Farley (Ed.), *Prostitution and trafficking in Nevada: Making the connections* (pp. 49–84). San Francisco: Prostitution Research & Education.

Seng, M. J. (1989). Child sexual abuse and adolescent prostitution: A comparative analysis. *Adolescence, 24*, 665–675.

Shreve, J. (2006, April 18). MySpace faces a perp problem. *Wired*. Retrieved from http://www.wired.com/culture/lifestyle/news/2006/04/70675

Silbert, M. H., & Pines, A. M. (1981). Sexual child abuse as an antecedent to prostitution. *Child Abuse & Neglect, 5*, 407–411.

Silbert, M. H., & Pines, A. M. (1982a). Entrance into prostitution. *Youth & Society, 13*, 471–500.

Silbert, M. H., & Pines, A. M. (1982b). Victimization of street prostitutes. *Victimology, 7*, 122–133.

Silbert, M. H., & Pines, A. M. (1983). Early sexual exploitation as an influence in prostitution. *Social Work, 28*, 285–289.

Simmons, R. V. (2000). Child sexual trauma and female prostitution. *Dissertation Abstracts International: Section B: The Sciences & Engineering, 61*(2-B), 1096.

Simons, R. L., & Whitbeck, L. B. (1991). Sexual abuse as a precursor to prostitution and victimization among adolescent and adult homeless women. *Journal of Family Issues, 12*(3): 361–379.

Smith, L.W., Herman-Giddens, M. E., & Everette, V. D. (2005). Commercial sexual exploitation of children in advertising. In S. W. Cooper, R. J. Estes, A. P. Giardino, N. D. Kellogg, & V. I. Vieth (Eds.), *Medical, legal, and social science aspects of child sexual exploitation: A comprehensive review of pornography, prostitution, and internet crimes* (Vols. 1 & 2, pp. 25–57). St Louis: GW Medical Publishing.

Snell, R., & Hicks, M. (2008, March 21). Federal probe breaks up two child prostitution sex rings. *The Detroit News*. Retrieved March 22, 2008 from http://www.detnews.com

Spangenburg, M. (2001). *Prostituted youth in New York City: An overview*. Brooklyn, NY: ECPAT-USA.

Stark, C., & Hodgson, C. (2003). Sister oppressions: A comparison of wife battering and prostitution. In M. Farley (Ed.), *Prostitution, trafficking, and traumatic stress* (pp. 17–32). New York: Routledge.

Stewart, A. J., Steigman, M., Cauce, A. M., Cochran, B. N., Whitbeck, L. B., & Hoyt, D. (2004). Victimization and posttraumatic stress disorder among homeless adolescents. *Journal of the American Academy of Child Psychiatry, 43*(3), 325–331.

Stone, B. (2007, January 2). Using web cams but few inhibitions, the young turn to risky social sites. *New York Times*. Retrieved from http://www.nytimes.com/2007/01/02/technology/02net.html?_r=1&ref=business&oref=slogin

Stransky, M., & Finkelhor, D. (2008). *Juvenile prostitution factsheet*. Durham, NH: Crimes Against Children Research Center. Retrieved from http://www.unh.edu/ccrc/prostitution/Juvenile_Prostitution_factsheet.pdf

TMZ.com. (2008). *Ashley Dupre gone "wild"—legal or jailbait?* Retrieved April 4, 2008 from http://www.tmz.com

Tyler, K. A. (2009). Risk factors for trading sex among homeless young adults. *Archives of Sexual Behavior, 38*, 290–297.

Tyler, K. A., Hoyt, D. R., Whitbeck, L. B., & Cauce, A. M. (2001). The impact of childhood sexual abuse on later sexual victimization among runaway youth. *Journal of Research on Adolescence, 11*(2), 151–176.

Walter, N. (2010). *Living dolls: The return of sexism*. London: Virago Press.

Weisberg, D. K. (1985). *Children of the night: A study of adolescent prostitution*. Lexington: Lexington Books.

West, C. M. (2009). Still on the auction block: The (s)exploitation of black adolescent girls in rap(e) music and hip-hop culture. In S. Olfman (Ed.), *The sexualization of childhood* (pp. 88–102). Westport, CT: Praeger.

West, C. M., Williams, L. M., & Siegal, J. M. (2000). Adult sexual revictimization among black women sexually abused in childhood: A prospective examination of serious consequences of abuse. *Child Maltreatment*, 5(1), 49–57.

Whitbeck, L. B., Hoyt, D. R., & Ackley, K. A. (1997a). Abusive family backgrounds and later victimization among runaway and homeless adolescents. *Journal of Research on Adolescence*, 7(4), 375–392.

Whitbeck, L. B., Hoyt, D. R., & Ackley, K. A. (1997b). Families of homeless and runaway adolescents: A comparison of parent/caretaker and adolescent perspectives on parenting, family violence and adolescent conduct. *Child Abuse & Neglect*, 21(6), 517–528.

Widom, C. S., & Kuhns, J. B. (1996). Childhood victimization and subsequent risk for promiscuity, prostitution, and teenage pregnancy: A prospective study. *American Journal of Public Health*, 86(11), 1607–1612.

William Wilberforce Trafficking Victims Protection Reauthorization Act. (2008). Washington, DC: U.S. Department of Justice. Available at www.usdoj.gov/olp/pdf/wilberforce-act.pdf

Wolak, J., Finkelhor, D., Mitchell, K. J., & Ybarra, M. L. (2008). Online "predators" and their victims: Myths, realities, and implications for prevention and treatment. *American Psychologist*, 63(2),111–128. Available at http://www.apa.org/releases/sexoffender0208. html

Wolak, J., Finkelhor, D., Mitchell, K., & Ybarra, M. (2004). Internet-initiated sex crimes against minors: Implications for prevention based on findings from a national study. *Journal of Adolescent Health*, 35(5), 424–433. Available at http://www.unh.edu/ccrc/ internet-crimes/papers.html

Yates G. L., MacKenzie, R. G., Pennbridge, J., & Swofford, A. (1991). A risk profile comparison of homeless youth involved in prostitution and homeless youth not involved. *Journal of Adolescent Health*, 12, 545–548.

Zimmerman, C., Hossain, M., Yun, K., Roche, B., Morison, L., & Watts, C. (2006). *Stolen smiles: A summary report on the physical and psychological health consequences of women and adolescents trafficked in Europe*. London School of Hygiene and Tropical Medicine. Retrieved from www.lshtm.ac.uk/hpu/docs/StolenSmiles.pdf

Zurbriggen, E. L., & Freyd, J. J. (2004). The link between child sexual abuse and risky sexual behavior: The role of dissociative tendencies, information-processing effects, and consensual sex decision mechanisms. In J. L. Koenig, A. O'Leary, L. S. Doll, & W. Pequegnat (Eds.), *From child abuse to adult sexual risk: Trauma revictimization intervention* (pp. 117–134). Washington, DC: American Psychological Association.

PART FOUR

INTRAPERSONAL CONTRIBUTIONS AND CONSEQUENCES

10

Teens, Pre-teens, and Body Image

MARIKA TIGGEMANN

Teenage girls requesting (and receiving) breast implants for their 18th birthday. Ten-year-old girls reading magazines with "boy trouble" advice. Eight-year-old girls wearing Pussycat Dolls t-shirts with slogans like "Don'tcha wish your girlfriend was hot like me?" and going on diets so they can be sexy. These are some increasingly common examples (Durham, 2008; Reist, 2009) that illustrate the objectification and concern with body image that have become part of the everyday lives of contemporary teenage and pre-teen girls.

This chapter sets out to review the concepts of objectification and self-objectification (as outlined in objectification theory) as they apply to the body image of teenage and pre-teenage girls. Both the general literature on body image, as well as the small amount of existing empirical evidence that has investigated the consequences of self-objectification (as outlined in objectification theory) on girls' attitudes to their body and appearance, will be reviewed. Separate sections will consider the research on teenage girls and younger pre-teen girls. In so doing, the chapter attempts both to summarize what is known and to identify gaps in the literature for future research.

Recap of Objectification Theory

Feminist analyses have long adopted a social constructionist account of the female body. This account holds that, in Western societies, the female body is sexually objectified and construed primarily as an object that exists for the pleasure of others, to be looked at and evaluated. Specific examples include the representation of women in the visual mass media, and interpersonally, the sexualized male gaze or "checking out." Accordingly, sexual objectification forms part of women's daily experience. It also forms part of the sociocultural context into which adolescent and younger girls grow.

One particularly sad and insidious consequence is what is termed *self-objectification* (Fredrickson & Roberts, 1997). This refers to the process whereby women and girls are gradually socialized to adopt an observer's perspective on their physical self, that is, to view *themselves* as primarily an object to be looked at and evaluated on the basis of appearance. Thus, self-objectification represents a form of self-consciousness characterized by habitual and constant monitoring of the body's external appearance. Objectification theory (Fredrickson & Roberts, 1997) argues that this self-objectification then leads logically to a number of negative experiential consequences for women, in particular an increase in both shame and anxiety about the body and appearance, as well as to the consumption of attentional resources. Finally, it is argued that the accumulation of such experiences contributes to three conditions experienced disproportionately by women: eating disorders, unipolar depression, and sexual dysfunction.

In the decade since the formulation of the theory, there has been a great deal of empirical support with respect to adult women's bodies. In particular, the proposed links between self-objectification or body surveillance and body shame and disordered eating have now been reliably demonstrated in samples of undergraduate women (e.g., Fredrickson, Roberts, Noll, Quinn, & Twenge, 1998; McKinley, 1998; McKinley & Hyde, 1996; Noll & Fredrickson, 1998; Tiggemann & Slater, 2001; Tylka & Hill, 2004), in samples of older women (Augustus-Horvath & Tylka, 2009; Greenleaf, 2005; McKinley, 1999; Tiggemann & Lynch, 2001), and in women with clinical eating disorders (Calogero, Davis, & Thompson, 2005). Together, they confirm that self-objectification is an important explanatory concept in the body experience of contemporary adult women.

But objectification and self-objectification are also concepts increasingly relevant to younger women and girls. For example, the 2007 report of the American Psychological Association (APA) Task Force on the Sexualization of Girls concluded that the objectification and sexualization of young women and girls has increased over time, as indicated by the content of mainstream teen magazines, music videos, and music lyrics. To date, however, little research (in the United States and elsewhere) investigates the consequences of objectification in younger women and girls. In fact, the need for such future studies focusing on girls forms part of the APA report's very first recommendation.

Objectification and Body Image in Teenage Girls

The APA (2007) report presents overwhelming and irrefutable evidence that the bodies of adolescent girls are increasingly objectified. This is most clearly seen in portrayals in the general mass media, where the bodies of teenage girls are on display and used to sell products. A casual flick through any teen magazine will also reveal a plethora of thin, idealized, and potentially objec-tified images of teenage girls, along with accompanying text that reinforces the ultimate importance of appearance. Further, girls are avid consumers of such media, which play a major part in their teenage lives. It is estimated that approximately 85% of adolescent girls read fashion magazines (Field et al., 1999), and virtually every home has at least one television set switched on for an average of 7 hours per day, with individuals watching 3–4 hours per day (Levine & Smolak, 1996). Not only do the media present thin ideals, but they also contribute to the conversations of adolescent girls around top-ics like clothes and the lives of celebrities. This influence is likely to increase with the even greater access to the every movement of the celebrities now obtainable via social networking sites like Facebook and Twitter. Thus, the media contribute in developing what Jones, Vigfusdottir, and Lee (2004) have described as an "appearance culture" for teenage girls, in which media ideals and peer conversations reinforce each other. This focus on appearance is not surprising, in that it returns considerable rewards for girls in terms of popu-larity (Tiggemann, 2001), as well as subsequent social and economic success (Fredrickson & Roberts, 1997).

Objectification, however, may be particularly problematic when it happens to teenage girls. Adolescence is a time of remarkable transition, when changes occur in each of the physical, cognitive, and social domains. Most theories of human development (e.g., Erikson, 1968) posit the development of a coherent sense of identity as the major task of adolescence. In addition, it is a time when self-awareness, self-consciousness, introspectiveness, and preoccupation with self-image all dramatically increase (Harter, 1999). Thus, adolescents are likely to be especially susceptible to media messages and images. Unfortunately for adolescent girls, at this same time that there is an enormous focus on physi-cal appearance, the developmental changes associated with puberty (including increased fat deposition on the hips and thighs) move them further away from rather than closer to current societal ideals of female beauty, which inordi-nately emphasize thinness. Finally, there is a likely disjunction between ado-lescent girls' presentation and their knowledge. Tolman (2002) has argued that teenage girls are encouraged to look good (which equates with "sexy"), even though they have little knowledge of what it means to be sexual and little experience in intimate relationships. As a result of a sexually appealing appear-ance, adolescent girls may be subject to sexual attention that they neither want nor understand.

In this light, it is not surprising that the majority of adolescent girls are wor-ried, preoccupied, dissatisfied with their bodies, and wish to be thinner (e.g., Attie & Brooks-Gunn, 1989; Grigg, Bowman, & Redman, 1996; Thompson,

Coovert, Richards, Johnson, & Cattarin, 1995). The recent 2007 Mission Australia Report found that body image was the most highly ranked issue of concern (ahead of family conflict or alcohol and drug issues) among a national sample of 29,000 young Australians (11 to 24 years old). The desire to be thinner may lead to unhealthy dieting and other compensatory behaviors such as excessive exercise. We know that dieting behavior is not uncommon during early adolescence (O'Dea & Abraham, 2000), and it becomes increasingly common during middle adolescence (Neumark-Sztainer, Butler, & Palti, 1995; Paxton, 1993; Stice, Killen, Hayward, & Taylor, 1998). More generally, Stice's (2002) meta-analytic review identifies body dissatisfaction as a consistent risk factor for eating disorders such as anorexia and bulimia nervosa, which both typically have their onset during late adolescence (Touyz & Beumont, 1985). Body dissatisfaction during adolescence may also play a role in low self-esteem and depression (Jones, 2004). For example, a number of studies (e.g., DuBois, Tevendale, Burk-Braxton, Swenson, & Hardesty, 2000) have demonstrated that satisfaction in the appearance domain is the best predictor of global self-esteem. More specifically, Tiggemann (2005a) found that poor body image prospectively predicted lower self-esteem 2 years later. Meta-analyses document that girls (but not boys) typically suffer a drop in self-esteem in adolescence (Kling, Hyde, Showers, & Buswell, 1999). Putting all this altogether, it is estimated that a substantial percentage, perhaps 20%, of females from age 12 have levels of negative body image and disordered eating high enough to create significant suffering for themselves and others (Levine & Murnen, 2009).

Given that adolescents can be described as "morbidly preoccupied with how they appear in the eyes of others" (Harter, 1998), the concept of self-objectification is one that appears particularly pertinent. Although few studies have actually measured self-objectification, there is much more general evidence consistent with the conceptualization. Sociocultural theory (e.g., Thompson, Heinberg, Altabe, & Tantleff-Dunn, 1999) argues that the thin idealized images presented in the media set up unrealistic ideals that, despite their impossibility, girls then internalize as standards for themselves. Because it is so difficult to match the societally prescribed ideal standard, girls are left dissatisfied. Indeed, internalization of the thin ideal has been shown to be a prospective predictor of body dissatisfaction and eating pathology (Stice, 2002; Thompson & Stice, 2001). Conceptually, it seems to reflect one aspect of self-objectification.

Media Effects in Teenage Girls

Consistent with this perspective, a large amount of evidence demonstrates an association between media exposure and poor body image among teenage girls. An earlier meta-analysis of experimental manipulations of the thin beauty ideal as portrayed in fashion magazines (Groesz, Levine, & Murnen, 2002) came to the conclusion that women's body image was significantly more negative after viewing media images and, importantly, that the effect was strongest for participants younger than 19 years of age. The recent meta-analysis by Levine and Murnen (2009) of correlational studies of naturally occurring exposure to fashion magazines found significant positive relationships with thin ideal internalization, body dissatisfaction, and disordered eating. Particularly for thin ideal internalization, the effect was again strongest for adolescent girls under age 18.

A number of other studies have shown poor body image to be associated with the watching of television. Although the overall effect for television is small (Grabe, Ward, & Hyde, 2008; Levine & Murnen, 2009), effects are much stronger for particular kinds of television, notably soap operas (Tiggemann, 2005b; Tiggemann & Pickering, 1996) and music videos (Borzekowski, Robinson, & Killen, 2000; Tiggemann & Pickering, 1996), which are correlated with body dissatisfaction, drive for thinness, and internalization of the thin ideal. Soap operas present a sense of "realness" (Barbatsis & Guy, 1991) that make them uniquely positioned to offer the more complex cultural scripts that equate appearance and thinness to success. And adolescent girls, more than boys, use television for social learning purposes and as a source of behavioral and appearance standards, a habit which is itself associated with more negative body image and symptoms of disordered eating (Tiggemann, 2005b).

Music television programs, on the other hand, provide very explicit appearance ideals. They represent one of the most popular forms of entertainment for young people, targeting audiences between the ages of 12 and 34. In an Australian study (Tiggemann, 2005b), on average, adolescent girls reported watching more than 2 hours of these programs per week. Content analyses of music videos have shown that, like other forms of popular culture, the portrayal of women is decidedly sexist in orientation, with high levels of sex-role stereotyping (Kalof, 1993). In particular, the physical appearance of women is emphasized (Gow, 1996), and they are commonly depicted as thin and attractive, usually provocatively or scantily clad, and often involved in implicitly sexual or subservient behavior (e.g., Sommers-Flanagan, Sommers-Flanagan, & Davis, 1993). In short, women are portrayed as "adornments, decorations and sexual playthings" (Reist, 2009).

Existing Research on Objectification Theory in Adolescent Girls

As indicated above, only a few studies have examined the components of objectification theory in samples younger than undergraduate students. However, the increased self-consciousness and increased concern with both external appearance and social acceptance that accompany adolescence suggest that it might present a critical period for the development of self-objectification. This section reviews the existing research on adolescent girls (from around age 11). The next section deals with research on younger preadolescent girls.

In the first study to actually measure self-objectification in adolescents, Slater and Tiggemann (2002) observed levels of self-objectification comparable to adult women in their small sample of adolescent girls (n = 83; aged 12–16 years, M = 14). We found that, just as is the case in undergraduate women, self-objectification was correlated with body shame, appearance anxiety, and disordered eating, and that the relationship between self-objectification and disordered eating was partially explained by body shame. We concluded that objectification theory was indeed applicable to adolescent girls.

Aspects of these results have now been replicated with much larger samples. For example, Harrison and Fredrickson (2003) found that self-objectification became more marked between early and mid-adolescence. Specifically, it increased with grade in their sample (n = 374), covering preadolescent and adolescent girls from the sixth to the twelfth grades (aged 10–19 years, M = 13.4). However, self-objectification was correlated with body shame and disordered eating across all grades. They also found that participation in "lean" sports (e.g., gymnastics, diving) correlated positively with self-objectification and disordered eating, whereas nonlean sports participation correlated negatively with self-objectification. Similarly, in a different culture, Knauss, Paxton, and Alsaker (2008) found that self-objectification was related to body shame, body dissatisfaction, and internalization of the thin ideal among a Swiss sample of 791 girls aged 14–16 years. It was also related to perceived pressure to achieve the thin media ideal. Other studies have indicated that self-objectification is related to diminished motor ability (Fredrickson & Harrison, 2005), and depression and low self-esteem in adolescent girls (Tolman, Impett, Tracy, & Michael, 2006).

In a slightly younger sample of 10- to 12-year-old girls (M = 11.2 years), Lindberg, Hyde, and McKinley (2006) reported that self-objectification was likewise related to body shame and body esteem. It was also related to pubertal development, appearance-related teasing, and reported peer sexual harassment (Lindberg, Grabe, & Hyde, 2007). Finally, Grabe, Hyde, and Lindberg (2007) reported links between self-objectification, body shame, and depression, while also showing that girls experienced higher levels of these constructs than do boys.

Although these studies have demonstrated links between self-objectification, body shame, disordered eating, and depression in adolescent girls, they largely have not sought to test the components and steps of the model put forward in objectification theory. Slater and Tiggemann (2010) attempted to explicitly test the model in a sample of 332 adolescent girls ranging in age from 12 to 16 years (as well as in a comparison group of boys). We found that girls displayed higher levels of self-monitoring, body shame, appearance anxiety, and disordered eating than boys, and that the model proposed by objectification theory was largely supported. Specifically, path analyses indicated that self-objectification led to self-monitoring, which led to both body shame and appearance anxiety, which in turn led to disordered eating. These pathways are consistent with the mediational findings reported for adult women (Greenleaf, 2005; Noll & Fredrickson, 1998; Tiggemann & Lynch, 2001; Tiggemann & Slater, 2001; Tylka & Hill, 2004). In the same sample, we found that time spent exercising at a gym or fitness center was positively correlated with self-objectification (Slater & Tiggemann, 2011), as was teasing while playing sport. Interestingly, the major source of this teasing was "boys."

Thus, it appears that self-objectification and its consequences are already pertinent to girls as young as 11 or 12 years old, a sad reflection of the values in our society. Taken together, the studies indicate that the consequences of self-objectification for adolescent girls are much the same, and indeed appear to operate in much the same way as they do for adult women.

Future research needs to address these consequences in more detail. For example, only one study (Harrison & Fredrickson, 2003) has explicitly tested for ethnic or cultural differences. Interestingly, there were no significant differences found in levels of self-objectification, body shame, or disordered eating between white girls and girls of color (mostly African American). Nor was there any difference in the strength of observed relationships, indicating that objectification theory seems equally applicable to both groups.

Importantly, in addition to outlining the consequences of self-objectification, some of the studies have begun the task of considering possible antecedents to this perspective. Thus far, potential predictors identified include pubertal development (Lindberg et al., 2007), participation in lean sports (Harrison & Fredrickson, 2003), exercising at a gym or fitness center (Slater, 2006), perceived media pressure to achieve the thin ideal (Knauss et al., 2008), and appearance-related teasing and peer sexual harassment (Lindberg et al., 2007; Slater, 2006). The identification of factors and experiences that lead to self-objectification is vital for both our understanding of the phenomenon, as well as for the development of appropriately targeted interventions for adolescent girls.

Objectification and Body Image in Preadolescent Girls

It is quite clear from the APA (2007) report that the phenomena of objectification and sexualization have increasingly extended to increasingly younger girls.

Anecdotal evidence suggests that it is not uncommon to find 10-year-old (or even 8-year-old) girls wearing sexually provocative clothing, padded bras, and make-up, and in other ways striving to look "hot" (Hamilton, 2008). Certainly advertisers have targeted the "tween" market (usually defined as between 8 and 12 years of age, although sometimes starting as young as 6), in an attempt to use so-called "pester-power" to influence the purchasing decisions of parents. There are also an increasing number of "fashion" magazines (e.g., Barbie, Total Girl) dedicated to this age group.

Two comprehensive reviews of the existing literature on the body image of children (Ricciardelli & McCabe, 2001; Smolak & Levine, 2001) have come to the conclusion that a significant minority of children aged 8–12 years are dissatisfied with their body shapes or weight. Ricciardelli and McCabe (2001) reported that specific estimates for the number of girls who desire a thinner body size range between 28% and 55%. Estimates for dieting to lose weight range from 20% to 56%. Such body dissatisfaction among children was also implicated as a precursor for lower self-esteem, diminished psychological well-being, and the development of later eating disorders (Ricciardelli & McCabe, 2001; Smolak & Levine, 2001). Indeed, recent anecdotal clinical evidence suggests that children are now presenting with eating disorders in greater numbers at a younger age (Phillips & Leo, 2006). An Australian study conducted over 3 years identified 101 children, aged 5–13 years, with early-onset eating disorders (Madden, Morris, Zurynski, Kohn, & Elliot, 2009). The authors estimated the annual incidence to be 1.4 per 100,000 children.

Furthermore, there is increasing evidence that still younger girls have absorbed many societal appearance ideals, especially the desire to be thinner. Our own research indicates that this desire to be thinner typically arises around age 6. In the main, 5-year-old girls, if anything, wish to be larger, but 6-year-old girls on average wish to be thinner (Dohnt & Tiggemann, 2005, 2006a; Lowes & Tiggemann, 2003). Girls of this age are also well aware of dieting as a means of achieving the thin ideal. In these studies, girls' levels of body dissatisfaction and dieting awareness were correlated with their perception of their peers' body dissatisfaction, consistent with demonstrations of shared peer appearance norms among older (adolescent) girls.

Perhaps because parents are assumed to be the major source of influence on their children, only limited research exists on the influence of the mass media on body dissatisfaction in children. Yet, children are exposed to the media from a very early age (Berk, 2000) and, reportedly, during a single year, on average spend more time watching television than in any other activity besides sleeping (Levine & Smolak, 1996). Like their adolescent counterparts, Clark and Tiggemann (2006) provided evidence for the existence of an "appearance culture" consisting of interrelated media and peer influences among girls as young as 9–12 years of age. In a follow-up study, Clark and Tiggemann (2007) found that reading appearance-focused magazines and watching appearance television (especially music television shows) were related to investment in appearance, body dissatisfaction, and dieting behaviors among 9- to 12-year-old girls.

One piece of evidence that suggests that childhood, as opposed to adolescence, might be particularly important comes from longitudinal studies of media exposure. Although it has generally been assumed that media exposure is causally related to body image in adolescent girls, studies have simply not been able to show this (Levine & Murnen, 2009). In fact, some studies (e.g., Tiggemann, 2006) have explicitly demonstrated that actual media exposure is not temporally antecedent to body image among adolescents. One possible reason for this seemingly surprising finding is that media exposure may have reached saturation point by then. In support, there exist two studies that have shown longitudinal prediction, but both in quite young girls. Dohnt and Tiggemann (2006b) found that appearance television (but not magazine) exposure predicted a decrease in appearance satisfaction 1 year later in their sample of 5- to 8-year-olds. In addition, the desire for thinness predicted subsequent low self-esteem. Similarly, Harrison and Hefner (2006) found that television viewing (but not magazine consumption) predicted increased disordered eating and a thinner future (but not current) ideal 1 year later in their sample of girls ($M = 8.7$ years). Together, these present persuasive evidence that what happens in childhood matters for later body image development.

One final study of relevance using a completely different methodology is that of Dittmar, Halliwell, and Ive (2006), who experimentally manipulated exposure to a Barbie doll. Most (99%, Rogers, 1999) young girls 3–10 years old own at least one Barbie. She is the cultural icon of female beauty that provides an "aspirational role model" for young girls. Yet, Barbie is so exceptionally thin that her weight and body proportions are completely unrealistic. Dittmar and colleagues found that body dissatisfaction was significantly higher among 5- to 8-year-old girls after they had been exposed to Barbie doll images, and this was more so among the younger (5.5–7.5 years) than older (7.5–8.5 years) girls. Future studies might address the consequences of the even more disturbing Bratz dolls, with their thin bodies but oversized heads with heavily made up faces and sexy clothes (often described as "hooker chic"), marketed at girls from age 6 upward.

However, despite its potential relevance, none of the above research with young preadolescent girls has been explicitly conceptualized within the framework of objectification theory. This would be an important next step, not only to advance our knowledge of preadolescent development, but also to test the generalizability of objectification theory across developmental stages. In particular, the question of how and when self-objectification develops is a critical one. At the societal level, there is considerable public debate as to whether or not "sexualized" behaviors (e.g., wearing make-up) among young girls are actually problematic. On the one hand, it is argued that little girls have always played at dressing up and acting grown up. Others argue, however, that sexualized attitudes and behaviors have negative consequences for both the girl (in instilling a particular self-objectified perspective of herself, which may then lead to inappropriate responses from others) and for society as a whole (for example, in contributing to the acceptability of child pornography). Thus, future research needs to demonstrate whether objectification harms young girls' developing body image.

Retrospective Accounts of Objectification

Three other studies examining the retrospective accounts of adult women underline the importance of childhood in the development of body image in general, and of self-objectification in particular. First, Parsons and Betz (2001) asked female undergraduate students to report retrospectively about their high school sport participation. Body shame was found to be related to participation in sports that tended to objectify the female body (such as gymnastics, cheerleading, and synchronized swimming) compared to sports that were less likely to do so.

Second, Tiggemann and Slater (2001) included a sample of former dancers in their study, women who had formerly participated in classical ballet lessons, usually from around age 6–14. We reasoned that dancers (even recreational ones) operate in an environment likely to accentuate an awareness of observers' perspectives on their bodies, that is, to induce self-objectification: they appear on stage and spend innumerable hours practising in front of mirrors. We further reasoned that this might then become the habitual and enduring way of perceiving the self. In support, we found that former dancers scored higher on self-objectification, habitual body monitoring, and disordered eating than did nondancers. Thus, even though former dancers are no longer exposed to a situation virtually demanding self-objectification, it appears that they still view themselves in this way. This suggests that objectifying experiences at a young age may lead to a particular way of perceiving oneself. Future research should address whether there is any specific age or maturational milestone that is critical for the development of self-objectification.

Finally, Slater and Tiggemann (2006) asked female undergraduate students to report retrospectively on how often they had read teen or fashion magazines, how often they had watched music video programs, and how much television they had watched, separately for while they were in primary school (approximate ages 7–12) and in high school (approximate ages 13–17). We found that childhood (primary school) experiences of media use predicted current (adult) levels of body shame, appearance anxiety, body dissatisfaction, and drive for thinness. Importantly, these relationships were stronger for media use while in primary school, than for high school or current media use. It was concluded that early experience of media use during childhood may play an important role in the development of women's body image.

These findings, together with the longitudinal studies of media exposure discussed earlier, suggest that earlier experiences may be the most critical in the development of later self-objectification and body image. In contrast to popular belief, childhood may be the most important stage at which particular experiences may lead to enduring beliefs around body image and the self.

Future Directions

As recommended in the APA Report, there is an urgent need for research investigating the consequences of the increasing sexualization of young girls. In particular, we need empirical data on the impact of self-objectification and "sexualized" behaviors on adolescent and preadolescent girls' well-being. Without such data, we are not able to move on from simply decrying the media treatment of children. A strong empirical base, however, allows the identification of children who might be particularly vulnerable, as well as suitable targets for intervention.

Of course, the conduct of such research is likely to be difficult and challenging. It requires clever age-appropriate methodologies that are ethical and acceptable to the young participants, as well as able to elicit the constructs without "putting words" in girls' mouths. In addition to studying consequences, we also need information on the predictors of self-objectification. Although self-objectification is postulated to be a developmental process, as yet little work has addressed its origins. Further, not only do we need to identify factors and experiences that increase vulnerability, but also those that promote resilience and protect against a self-objectifying perspective in the face of enormous societal pressure.

In this light, a number of studies have demonstrated that media literacy programs that teach young people to critically analyze and deconstruct objectifying media images and messages have positive benefits for the body image of adolescents (Levine & Murnen, 2009). Future research should assess the effectiveness of other interventions that empower girls to metaphorically reclaim their bodies and live embodied lives (Hirschman, Impett, & Schooler, 2006). These might include activities like playing sport or doing yoga or meditation.

Perhaps the biggest limitation of existing objectification research across all age groups is that nearly all studies are cross-sectional and correlational in design. Thus, it is not possible to offer definitive causal conclusions. To my knowledge, the only prospective study is that of Grabe et al. (2007). In their sample of early adolescent girls (initially aged 10–12, $M = 11.2$ years) over 2 years, self-objectification was related to depressive symptoms at both time points. More importantly, initial self-objectification actually predicted body shame and depressive symptoms 2 years later. Further, Time 2 body shame (as well as rumination) mediated this relationship. Thus, the study shows that self-objectification was indeed temporally antecedent to body shame and depressive symptoms, consistent with its postulated causal role in objectification theory. This is the very first such evidence. Future longitudinal research should track self-objectification and its postulated predictors and consequences for longer periods across the developmental stages of childhood and adolescence.

The major practical significance of a greater understanding of the consequences of objectification for teenage and younger girls lies in the grounding of any subsequent interventions in empirical research. Whatever predictors (both vulnerabilities and protective factors) emerge, then present suitable targets for intervention. For example, adolescent girls may be encouraged to continue playing team sports, or the parents of younger girls may be encouraged to co-view particular forms of media with their child.

Parents, schools, and governments alike are crying out for tools and strategies to help young girls resist the enormous pressures they face.

Conclusion

There is no doubt that the objectification of women is extending to teenage and pre-teenage girls. And, clearly, young girls are adopting many of the behaviors of their older peers. If this extreme focus on appearance becomes their habitual way of viewing themselves, then this is liable to have negative consequences for their well-being as teenagers and as adult women. As a society, we have yet to see the consequences of an entire new generation of girls brought up in this environment and largely socialized by the mass media. What is urgently needed is research addressing these issues in young girls. At a practical level, we need strategies to resist self-objectification.

Acknowledgments

Preparation of this chapter was supported by an Australian Research Council Discovery Project Grant (Project no. DP0986623).

References

American Psychological Association Task Force on the Sexualization of Girls. (2007). *Report of the APA task force on the sexualization of girls.* Washington, DC: American Psychological Association. Retrieved from www.apa.org/pi/wpo/sexualization.html

Attie, I., & Brooks-Gunn, J. (1989). Development of eating problems in adolescent girls: A longitudinal study. *Developmental Psychology, 25,* 70–79.

Augustus-Horvath, C. L., & Tylka, T. L. (2009). A test and extension of objectification theory as it predicts disordered eating: Does women's age matter? *Journal of Counseling Psychology, 56,* 253–265.

Barbatsis, G., & Guy, Y. (1991). Analyzing meaning in form: Soap opera's compositional construction of "realness." *Journal of Broadcasting and Electronic Media, 35,* 59–74.

Berk, L. E. (2000). *Child development* (5th ed.). Boston: Allyn and Bacon.

Borzekowski, D. L. G., Robinson, T. N., & Killen, J. D. (2000). Does the camera add 10 pounds? Media use, perceived importance of appearance, and weight concerns among adolescent girls. *Journal of Adolescent Health, 26,* 36–41.

Calogero, R. M., Davis, W. N., & Thompson, J. K. (2005). The role of self-objectification in the experience of women with eating disorders. *Sex Roles, 52,* 43–50.

Clark, L., & Tiggemann, M. (2006). Appearance culture in nine- to 12-year-old girls: Media and peer influences on body dissatisfaction. *Social Development, 15,* 628–643.

Clark, L., & Tiggemann, M. (2007). Sociocultural influences and body image in 9 to 12 year old girls: The role of appearance schemas. *Journal of Child and Adolescent Psychology, 36,* 76–86.

Dittmar, H., Halliwell, E., & Ive, S. (2006). Does Barbie make girls want to be thin? The effect of experimental exposure to images of dolls on the body image of 5–8-year-old girls. *Developmental Psychology, 42,* 283–292.

Dohnt, H., & Tiggemann, M. (2005). Peer influences on body dissatisfaction and dieting awareness in young girls. *British Journal of Developmental Psychology, 23,* 103–116.

Dohnt, H., & Tiggemann, M. (2006a). Body image concerns in young girls: The role of peers and media prior to adolescence. *Journal of Youth and Adolescence, 35,* 141–151.

Dohnt, H., & Tiggemann, M. (2006b). The contribution of peer and media influences to the development of body satisfaction and self-esteem in young girls: A prospective study. *Developmental Psychology, 42,* 929–936.

DuBois, D. L., Tevendale, H. D., Burk-Braxton, C., Swenson, L. P., & Hardesty, J. L. (2000). Self-system influences during early adolescence: Investigation of an integrative model. *Journal of Early Adolescence, 20,* 12–43.

Durham, M. G. (2008). *The Lolita effect: The media sexualization of young girls and what we can do about it.* London: Gerald Duckworth & Co.

Erikson, E. H. (1968). *Identity: Youth and crisis.* Oxford, UK: Norton & Co.

Field, A. E., Cheung, L., Wolf, A. M., Herzog, D. B., Gortmaker, S. L., & Colditz, G. A. (1999). Exposure to the mass media and weight concerns among girls. *Pediatrics, 103,* E361–E365.

Fredrickson, B. L., & Harrison, K. (2005). Throwing like a girl: Self-objectification predicts adolescent girls' motor performance. *Journal of Sport and Social Issues, 29,* 79–101.

Fredrickson, B. L., & Roberts, T. -A. (1997). Objectification theory: Toward understanding women's lived experiences and mental health risks. *Psychology of Women Quarterly, 21,* 173–206.

Fredrickson, B. L., Roberts, T. -A., Noll, S., Quinn, D. M., & Twenge, J. M. (1998). That swimsuit becomes you: Sex differences in self-objectification, restrained eating, and math performance. *Journal of Personality and Social Psychology, 75,* 269–284.

Gow, J. (1996). Reconsidering gender roles on MTV: Depictions in the most popular music videos of the early 1990s. *Communication Reports, 9,* 151–161.

Grabe, S., Hyde, J. S., & Lindberg, S. M. (2007). Body objectification and depression in adolescents: The role of gender, shame and rumination. *Psychology of Women Quarterly, 31,* 164–175.

Grabe, S., Ward, L. M., & Hyde, J. S. (2008). The role of the media in body image concerns among women: A meta-analysis of experimental and correlational studies. *Psychological Bulletin, 134,* 460–476.

Greenleaf, C. (2005). Self-objectification among physically active women. *Sex Roles, 52,* 51–62.

Grigg, M., Bowman, J., & Redman, S. (1996). Disordered eating and unhealthy weight reduction practices among adolescent females. *Preventive Medicine, 25,* 748–756.

Groesz, L. M., Levine, M. P., & Murnen, S. K. (2002). The effect of experimental presentation of thin media images on body satisfaction: A meta-analytic review. *International Journal of Eating Disorders, 31,* 1–16.

Hamilton, M. (2008). *What's happening to our girls?* Camberwell, Vic., AU: Viking.

Harrison, K., & Fredrickson, B. L. (2003). Women's sport media, self-objectification and mental health in black and white adolescent females. *Journal of Communication, 53,* 216–232.

Harrison, K., & Hefner, V. (2006). Media exposure, current and future body ideals, and disordered eating among preadolescent girls: A longitudinal panel study. *Journal of Youth and Adolescence, 35,* 153–163.

Harter, S. (1998). The development of self-representations. In N. Eisenberg (Ed.), *Handbook of child psychology: Social, emotional and personality development* (pp. 553–600). New York: Wiley.

Harter, S. (1999). *The construction of the self: A developmental perspective.* New York: Guilford.

Hirschman, C., Impett, E. A., & Schooler, D. (2006). Dis/Embodied voices: What late-adolescent girls can teach us about objectification and sexuality. *Sexuality Research and Social Policy, 3,* 8–20.

Jones, D. C. (2004). Body image among adolescent girls and boys: A longitudinal study. *Developmental Psychology, 40,* 823–835.

Jones, D. C., Vigfusdottir, T. H., & Lee, Y. (2004). Body image and the appearance culture among adolescent girls and boys: An examination of friend conversations, peer criticism, appearance magazines and the internalization of appearance ideals. *Journal of Adolescent Research, 19,* 323–339.

Kalof, L. (1993). Dilemmas of femininity: Gender and the social construction of sexual imagery. *The Sociological Quarterly, 34,* 639–651.

Kling, K. C., Hyde, J. S., Showers, C. J., & Buswell, B. N. (1999). Gender differences in self-esteem: A meta-analysis. *Psychological Bulletin, 125,* 470–500.

Knauss, C., Paxton, S. J., & Alsaker, F. D. (2008). Body dissatisfaction in adolescent boys and girls: Objectified body consciousness, internalization of the media body ideal and perceived pressure from media. *Sex Roles, 59,* 633–643.

Levine, M. P., & Murnen, S. K. (2009). Everybody knows that mass media are/are not [pick one] a cause of eating disorders: A critical review of evidence for a causal link between media, negative body image, and disordered eating in females. *Journal of Social and Clinical Psychology, 28,* 9–42.

Levine, M. P., & Smolak, L. (1996). Media as a context for the development of disordered eating. In L. Smolak, M. P. Levine, & R. Striegel-Moore (Eds.), *The developmental psychopathology of eating disorders: Implications for research, prevention, and treatment* (pp. 235–257). Hillsdale, NJ: Lawrence Erlbaum.

Lindberg, S. M., Grabe, S., & Hyde, J. S. (2007). Gender, pubertal development, and peer sexual harassment predict objectified body consciousness in early adolescence. *Journal of Research on Adolescence, 17,* 723–742.

Lindberg, S. M., Hyde, J. S., & McKinley, N. M. (2006). A measure of objectified body consciousness for preadolescent and adolescent youth. *Psychology of Women Quarterly, 30,* 65–76.

Lowes, J., & Tiggemann, M. (2003). Body dissatisfaction, dieting awareness and the impact of parental influence in young children. *British Journal of Health Psychology, 8*, 135–147.

Madden, S., Morris, A., Zurynski, Y. A., Kohn, M., & Elliot, E. J. (2009). Burden of eating disorders in 5–13-year-old children in Australia. *Medical Journal of Australia, 190*, 410–414.

McKinley, N. M. (1998). Gender differences in undergraduates' body esteem: The mediating effect of objectified body consciousness and actual/ideal weight discrepancy. *Sex Roles, 39*, 113–123.

McKinley, N. M. (1999). Women and objectified body consciousness: Mothers' and daughters' body experience in cultural, developmental, and familial context. *Developmental Psychology, 35*, 760–769.

McKinley, N. M., & Hyde, J. S. (1996). The Objectified Body Consciousness Scale: Development and validation. *Psychology of Women Quarterly, 20*, 181–215.

Mission Australia. (2007). *National survey of young Australians: Key and emerging issues.* Canberra, AU: Author.

Neumark-Sztainer, D., Butler, R., & Palti, H. (1995). Eating disturbances among adolescent girls: Evaluation of a school-based primary prevention program. *Journal of Nutrition Education, 27*, 24–31.

Noll, S. M., & Fredrickson, B. L. (1998). A mediational model linking self-objectification, body shame, and disordered eating. *Psychology of Women Quarterly, 22*, 623–636.

O'Dea, J. A., & Abraham, S. (2000). Improving the body image, eating attitudes, and behaviours of young male and female adolescents: A new educational approach that focuses on self-esteem. *International Journal of Eating Disorders, 28*, 43–57.

Parsons, E. M., & Betz, N. E. (2001). The relationship of participation in sports and physical activity to body objectification, instrumentality, and locus of control among young women. *Psychology of Women Quarterly, 25*, 209–222.

Paxton, S. (1993). A prevention program for disturbed eating and body dissatisfaction in adolescent girls: A 1 year follow-up. *Health Education Research, 8*, 43–51.

Phillips, K., & Leo, J. (2006, April 26). At risk: The body-image blues. *Advertiser*, p. 9.

Reist, M. T. (2009, September 5–6). For girls, add sex and stir. *Weekend Australian*, pp. 4–5.

Ricciardelli, L. A., & McCabe, M. P. (2001). Children's body image concerns and eating disturbance: A review of the literature. *Clinical Psychology Review, 21*, 325–344.

Rogers, M. F. (1999). *Barbie culture.* Thousand Oaks, CA: Sage.

Slater, A., & Tiggemann, M. (2002). A test of objectification theory in adolescent girls. *Sex Roles, 46*, 343–349.

Slater, A., & Tiggemann, M. (2006). The contribution of physical activity and media during childhood and adolescence to adult women's body image. *Journal of Health Psychology, 11*, 553–565.

Slater, A., & Tiggemann, M. (2010). Body image and disordered eating in adolescent girls and boys: A test of objectification theory. *Sex Roles, 63*, 42–49.

Slater, A., & Tiggemann, M. (2011). Gender differences in adolescent sport participation, teasing, self-objectification and body image concerns.*Journal of Adolescence, 34*, 455–463.

Smolak, L., & Levine, M. P. (2001). Body image in children. In J. K. Thompson, & L. Smolak (Eds.), *Body image, eating disorders, and obesity in youth: Assessment, prevention, and treatment* (pp. 41–66). Washington, DC: American Psychological Association.

Sommers-Flanagan, R., Sommers-Flanagan, J., & Davis, B. (1993). What's happening on music television? A gender role content analysis. *Sex Roles, 28*, 745–753.

Stice, E. (2002). Risk and maintenance factors for eating pathology: A meta-analytic review. *Psychological Bulletin, 128*, 825–848.

Stice, E., Killen, J. D., Hayward, C., & Taylor, C. B. (1998). Support for the continuity hypothesis of bulimic pathology. *Journal of Consulting and Clinical Psychology, 66*, 784–790.

Thompson, J. K., Coovert, M. D., Richards, D. J., Johnson, S., & Cattarin, J. (1995). Development of body image, eating disturbance, and general psychological functioning in female adolescents: Covariance structure modelling and longitudinal investigations. *International Journal of Eating Disorders, 18,* 221–236.

Thompson, J. K., Heinberg, L. J., Altabe, M., & Tantleff-Dunn, S. (1999). *Exacting beauty: Theory, assessment, and treatment of body image disturbance.* Washington, DC: American Psychological Association.

Thompson, J. K., & Stice, E. (2001). Thin-ideal internalization: Mounting evidence for a new risk factor for body image disturbance and eating pathology. *Current Directions in Psychological Science, 10,* 181–183.

Tiggemann, M. (2001). The impact of adolescent girls' life concerns and leisure activities on body dissatisfaction, disordered eating, and self-esteem. *Journal of Genetic Psychology, 162,* 133–142.

Tiggemann, M. (2005a). Body dissatisfaction and adolescent self-esteem: Prospective findings. *Body Image, 2,* 129–135.

Tiggemann, M. (2005b). Television and adolescent body image: The role of program content and viewing motivation. *Journal of Social and Clinical Psychology, 24,* 193–213.

Tiggemann, M. (2006). The role of media exposure in adolescent girls' body dissatisfaction and drive for thinness: Prospective results. *Journal of Social and Clinical Psychology, 25,* 522–540.

Tiggemann, M., & Lynch, J. (2001). Body image across the life span in adult women: The role of self-objectification. *Developmental Psychology, 37,* 243–253.

Tiggemann, M., & Pickering, A. S. (1996). Role of television in adolescent women's body dissatisfaction and drive for thinness. *International Journal of Eating Disorders, 20,* 199–203.

Tiggemann, M., & Slater, A. (2001). A test of objectification theory in former dancers and nondancers. *Psychology of Women Quarterly, 25,* 57–64.

Tolman, D. L. (2002). *Dilemmas of desire: Teenage girls talk about sexuality.* Cambridge, MA: Harvard University Press.

Tolman, D. L., Impett, E. A., Tracy, A. J., & Michael, A. (2006). Looking good, sounding good: Femininity ideology and adolescent girls' mental health. *Psychology of Women Quarterly, 30,* 85–95.

Touyz, S.W., & Beumont, P. J. V. (Eds.). (1985). *Eating disorders: Prevalence and treatment.* Sydney: Williams & Wilkins.

Tylka, T. L., & Hill, S. (2004). Objectification theory as it relates to disordered eating among college women. *Sex Roles, 51,* 719–730.

11

Kiddy Thongs and Menstrual Pads

The Sexualization of Girls and Early Menstrual Life

MARGARET L. STUBBS AND INGRID JOHNSTON-ROBLEDO

The transition to menstrual life is a significant one in girls' development, both physically and psychologically. As a discrete event, menarche, or first menstruation, heralds reproductive maturity, and yet the transition from girl to woman is a much longer process that is influenced by other developmental and cultural factors. At the most basic level, cognitive ability filters cultural messages about what it means to be a woman. As part of that process, girls' early menstrual experiences are influenced by the myriad and mixed sociocultural messages about menstruation they learn from parents, friends, school, the media, and more. For example, they may learn that menstruation is dirty, scary, a source of discomfort or sickness, embarrassing, and something to conceal from others. Yet, they are encouraged simultaneously to view it as a positive, healthy, normal experience, even one to celebrate. They may be especially confused about the connections among menstruation, reproduction, and sexuality, a complex topic that is often avoided by mothers and omitted in formal menstrual education. Yet, menarche, as a symbol of adult womanhood, has been shown to be related to girls' interest in dating, sense of self as sexually differentiated and sexualized, and their concerns about physical appearance. Clearly, early menstrual experience is best understood as a complex biopsychosocial phenomenon that involves the interaction of biology, intraindividual psychological processes, and cultural context.

How might the new, pervasive phenomenon of the sexualization of girls complicate the already loaded and confusing cultural context within which girls experience menstruation? How might it impact girls' experiences with puberty, menarche, and menstruation? As of the writing of this chapter, there was virtually no published scholarship on this new topic. Furthermore, the extant literature on menstruation and menarche often neglects issues related to girls' emerging sexualities. In this chapter, we review the literature on menarche and early menstrual life to consider the potential ways girls' early menstrual experiences may be influenced by the sexualization of girls. We argue that the sexualization of girls in the culture may encourage girls to internalize a sexualized image or identity that excludes an acceptance of menstruation as normative and healthy. Further, we suggest that the sexualization of girls may reinforce and even amplify mixed messages about menstruation and puberty, particularly those relevant to sexuality. These messages may lead girls to feel alienated from their developing bodies, to engage in excessive body discipline and self-sexualization, and to obscure important information about healthy development, embodiment, and sexuality.

Throughout our discussion, we draw on data from our own exploratory study of these issues (Johnston-Robledo, Stubbs, Calleri, & Hepworth, 2009; Stubbs, Johnston-Robledo, Mickel, & White, 2009). We conducted two focus groups with mothers of young girls between the ages of 9 and 13. In one group, five mothers each had one premenarcheal daughter and, for the other of the seven mothers, six of the daughters were pre- and three were postmenarchal. All mothers were European American, middle-income women. We asked mothers about their daughters' pubertal development and whether they had discussed sexuality issues in conjunction with puberty. Mothers were also asked about their views on the sexualization of girls in the culture and their ideas about how this trend might influence girls' experiences with puberty and early menstrual life. To facilitate this portion of the conversation, participants were shown several images reflecting the sexualization of young girls (e.g., clothing, toys, young models in suggestive positions).

Finally, based on our focus group findings and review of the literature, we offer suggestions for future research that explores the relationship between the sexualization of girls and their early puberty and menstruation experiences. This work will inform more comprehensive menstrual and sexual education, and assist in developing strategies to help girls resist negative cultural messages about these bodily functions and experiences. The resulting foundation will encourage a more embodied, agentic understanding of sexuality and the menstrual cycle, and promote girls' well-being as they move forward through development.

Pubertal Development

Menarche is a late event within pubertal development that has been primed since infancy (see Dorn & Rotenstein, 2004; Steingraber, 2007). Briefly, at puberty, a reactivation of gonadotropin-releasing hormone (GnRH) stimulates the ovary to produce estradiol, which first impacts breast development. With an increase in estradiol and other hormones, menarche occurs, and eventually, cyclical menstruation (Dorn & Rotenstein, 2004). In addition, increases in adrenal androgens, which do not produce external physical changes between the ages of 6 and 9, are implied by the development of pubic hair (pubarche), body odor, and acne (Dorn & Rotenstein, 2004). Biologically, the transition to full physical reproductive maturity lasts for several years, typically into the mid teens.

Although it has long been recognized that pubertal timing is variable among girls, some recent research (Herman-Giddens et al., 1997) suggests that girls are experiencing pubertal development earlier than in the past. In order to make sense of this claim, it is important to remember that pubertal development entails several discrete events, not just one. The average age of breast bud development, or thelarche, was reported to be 11.5 years in early research (Marshall & Tanner, 1969), but data from Herman-Giddens and colleagues (1997) indicate earlier breast bud development, for both European American (9.96 years) and African America girls (8.87) years. These data have led some researchers (e.g., Kaplowitz, 2004; Kaplowitz & Oberfield, 1999; Steingraber, 2007), but not all (see Dorn & Rotenstein, 2004, for a critique) to conclude that pubertal *onset*, as indicated by thelarche, is, on average, occurring earlier for U.S. girls.

With respect to menarche, today's girls, both in Europe and the United States, are experiencing the onset of menstruation at an earlier age than their nineteenth- and early twentieth-century sisters, that is, on average at age 12.5 as compared with age 17 (Dorn & Rotenstein, 2004; Hillard, 2002; Steingraber, 2007). However, the average age of onset has not varied much since the 1970s. Ethnic and geographic differences have been observed, both over time and currently. In the United States, African American girls experience onset about 6 months earlier than European American girls, and worldwide, the rate of decline is greatest in newly industrialized countries (Steingraber, 2007). Although the exact mechanism accounting for the onset of menstruation is unknown, increased nutritional status (Frisch, 1983) interacting with economic change (Kaplowitz & Oberfield, 1999; Steingraber, 2007) has been identified as an important explanatory factor. Menarche has been generally thought to occur about 2 years after breast bud development, but it is not clear if this relationship is changing (see Kaplowitz, 2004). At this point, media reports of earlier menarche related to earlier breast development should not be taken as fact. What is known is that the age of onset of menstruation can occur as early as age 8 and as late as 17 (Hillard, 2002).

Perhaps more important than age norms related to pubertal events is that, for those girls who do experience early development, childhood is at the very least biologically truncated. Related questions quickly emerge: how are girls adapting psychosocially to early (in particular) or earlier (in general) physical development? Studies of early development have compared girls designated as early, average/on-time, or late developers based on age at menarche and/or subjective timing (a girl's self-perception of whether she is an early, average, or late maturer) (e.g., Rierdan & Koff, 1985). But as Summers-Effler (2004) points out, these studies do not take into account earlier, more visible aspects of pubertal development (e.g., breast development). Girls can experience early breast development/fat deposition but begin to menstruate at an average age, or begin menstruation without significant breast development. No doubt, as Summers-Effler suggests, these girls differ from one another in terms of adaptation to pubertal change.

In her qualitative study of girls' responses to early breast development, Summers-Effler (2004) found that some felt ashamed, embarrassed, and isolated from peers, both girls and boys, who teased. A common strategy for these girls was to hide their breasts until other girls caught up. Martin (1996) also found that girls viewed their new breasts as a source of increased and unwanted attention from boys and men, which led them to feel anxious and objectified as a result.

It is also possible that girls who experience significant breast development as children will embrace this aspect of puberty, given the value placed on breasts as sexual objects for adult women and the emphasis on a sexualized appearance for girls. Indeed, Summer-Effler (2004) reports that some girls used early breast development to social advantage, once it was clear that breasts brought sexual attention from and popularity with boys, although she notes that this attention was not wholly positive. Although boys were attentive, other girls were jealous of that attention. Moreover, all of the early developers mentioned unwanted sexual attention and thus had early experience with sexual objectification from others well before they may have behaved in ways to invite it. In her recent study of young women's menarche narratives, Lee (2009) found that none of her participants considered breast development humiliating or shameful. In fact, one of her participants even acknowledged the premium placed on sexualized breasts in the culture and noted push-up bras as evidence of this. The availability of bras that are designed to appeal to children through branding with popular characters such as Hannah Montana® or Hello Kitty® may diminish the shame attached to early breast development and/or encourage girls without breasts to obtain and wear bras. Regardless of the timing of breast development, girls may enhance the appearance and size of their breasts through padded bras. In fact, it is difficult to find bras for young girls that are not padded. As Brumberg (1997) notes:

> Because a bra shapes the breasts in accordance with fashion, it acts very much like an interpreter, translating functional anatomy into a sexual or erotic vocabulary. When we dress little girls in brassieres or bikinis, we imply adult behaviors and, unwittingly, we mark them as sexual objects. (p. 118)

The mothers in our study were aware of and concerned about padded bras being marketed to young girls. One mother stated, "My daughter got a few hand-me-down training bras and she is very excited to have and wear them, but she doesn't have breasts." Another added, "You have these little girls with flat chests but they put the [padded training] bra on...and then they have breasts." Mothers also commented on their frustration with their daughters' desire to wear tight and revealing shirts. Said one, "I'm constantly saying, 'pull up your cammy, pull up your cammy...no one needs to see your boobs;'" and another, "I definitely dislike it that my older daughters wear very low-cut shirts...I am always like 'pull it up'"; and a third, "Why did she want to go out and buy tighter fitting t-shirts to start with? We weren't dressing like that at home. Mom's too old, so it had to come from some place [else]."

It seems obvious that girls for whom breast development is a catalyst for sexual objectification confront extra challenge in sorting out what it means to become a woman, and before later-occurring pubertal events prompt additional self-reflection. Further, it makes sense that girls' experiences of early occurring pubertal events (e.g., thelarche) would have some impact on their experience of later occurring events (e.g., menarche). Thus, toward a fuller understanding of pubertal experience, we applaud the broader perspectives of Summers-Effler (2004) and Lee (2009) and urge additional study of the possible interactions among the experiencing of various pubertal events. That said, it is reasonable to look with renewed concern at the relationship between girls' pubertal development and the sexualization of girls, and especially in the context of early development.

Cognitive and Psychosocial Development

How do young girls understand their changing bodies? The mothers in our focus groups grappled with this question throughout their discussions. For example, one asked, "I just wonder, does an 11-year-old see breasts as sexual?" Another offered, "I think it's especially dangerous with the character stuff like Hello Kitty © and the Disney © because for parents and kids alike...if you're into that product line then, and you see that, that is confusing...for kids ...." Knowing what cognitive skills girls *can* apply to this task is a starting point for *our* understanding of what *they* understand about pubertal change.

School-aged children are concrete thinkers who use more complex systems of categorization to understand their world than do younger children (Berger, 2009). Nevertheless, they can be very rigid in their thinking. As they attempt to make sense of the world and their place in it, these children scrutinize various attributes and make judgments about whether any individual person, item, or even a playground activity "fits" within the category of interest. School-aged children are notorious for vigorously defending a rule set, social or conceptual, that they believe has been violated. In addition, when preadolescent girls see a disconnect (or categorization violation) between what they are experiencing and what the culture expects of them, they may be more likely than older girls to subject themselves to self-silencing in order to conform to culture's view of appropriate behavior, a phenomenon that Brown and Gilligan (1992) observed nearly two decades ago in their work on European American girls' development.

Simultaneously, social comparison is a key aspect of development for these children (Berger, 2009). Although younger children are somewhat immune from others' judgments, and tend to view themselves very positively, school-aged children are more socially aware and absorb information from peers and the culture at large to evaluate both themselves and others. Concrete aspects of self, such as appearance, physical ability, social competence (being popular), and academic competence, factor heavily in school-aged children's judgments. Tied as they are to the concrete, it is difficult for these children to assume a critical stance with respect to the cultural messages about growing up that emphasize, for girls, being attractive (to boys); that is, "pretty," thin, and sexy. And the younger they are, the more difficult this critique will be.

The increased focus that pubertal growth necessarily directs to the body helps to set the stage for self-objectification, that is, perceiving oneself as an object, and coming to value the attributes that the "observer" values, such as physical appearance, instead of those associated with personal strength and health (Fredrickson & Roberts, 1997). Breast development usually necessitates buying bras, which draws girls' attention to the size and shape of their breasts; with menses comes learning to watch the calendar, monitoring and managing menstrual flow, and concerns about leaks and the visibility of sanitary pads. Girls who want to fit in may self-sexualize to conform to cultural standards of beauty, and most problematically, come to see the developing female body, especially with respect to menstruation, as at odds with cultural portrayals of what a sexy adult female should be. What, then, are girls thinking about menarche, and how are they experiencing their early menstrual life?

Early Menstrual Attitudes and Experiences

Studies have consistently indicated that girls report mixed, although negatively biased feelings about menstruation (see Stubbs, 2008). Both pre- and postmenarchal girls anticipate negative changes with menstruation (e.g., Clarke & Ruble, 1978; Koff & Rierdan, 1995a,b) and report embarrassment (Kissling, 1996), surprise, and fear (Teitelman, 2004). At the same time, girls affirm menstruation as natural and normative, part of being a woman and growing up, and something that puts you in touch with your body (Kalman, 2003; Koff & Riedan, 1995a; Stubbs, Rierdan, & Koff, 1989). Some studies indicate that premenarcheal girls are more likely to have positive attitudes about the "growing up" aspect of menstruation than are postmenarchal girls, who report more negative symptoms, mood disruptions, and poor school performance (e.g., Clarke & Ruble, 1978). Other studies find that premenarcheal girls are more anxious about menstruation than postmenarchal girls (Whisnant & Zegans, 1975) and anticipate more pain than postmenarchal girls reported experiencing (Ruble & Brooks-Gunn, 1982).

Against the backdrop of enduring negative portrayals of menstruation in Western and other cultures (Delaney, Lupton, & Toth, 1977; Houppert, 1999; Kissling, 2006; Weideger, 1977), it is somewhat heartening to note that girls' attitudes are both negative *and* positive. Positive attitudes toward menstruation per se have been little studied in adults or children. Additional insight into girls' notions of positive aspects of menstruation is needed and could be helpful in devising interventions to facilitate a more positive transition to menstrual life. Indeed, studies of two such interventions found that supportive listening sustained positive attitudes toward menstruation (Frank & Williams, 1999), and body objectification was counteracted for premenarcheal girls who participated in a program designed for that express purpose just prior to menarche (Rembeck & Gunnarsson, 2004).

Girls' attitudes and early menstrual experiences also vary as a function of menarcheal timing. Research indicates that girls who menstruate for the first time before the age of 12 have less positive menarcheal experiences (Ruble & Brooks-Gunn, 1982) and are more worried about menstruation than on-time or late maturers (Stubbs et al., 1989). Stubbs and colleagues (1989) found that more worry about menstruation was related to more depressive symptoms, lower body satisfaction, lower self-esteem, a more external locus of control, and greater anxiety. Similarly, girls who perceive themselves as early maturers relative to their peers remember menarche as more negative (Rierdan & Koff, 1985). McPherson and Korfine (2004) suggest that early menstrual experience may influence how a woman thinks about her period for years to come.

Early menarche has been associated with negative outcomes in the areas of sexuality and body image, two domains highly relevant to the sexualization of girls. Researchers have found a fairly consistent relationship between early menarche and earlier onset of sexual activity (Martin, 1996; Posner, 2006). In a large study of more than 19,000 Finnish girls, those who had menstruated before the age of 11 reported more advanced sexual activities than their on-time peers (Kaltiala-Heino, Kosunen, & Rimpela, 2003). Mendle, Turkheimer, and Emery (2007) reviewed several studies demonstrating a clear relationship between early menarche and dating behavior, early sexual initiation, and more advanced sexual activities. Relationships between early puberty and sexually transmitted disease (STD)/early pregnancy have not been established (Posner, 2006).

In the context of these findings, it is of some concern that a direct discussion of the relationship between menstruation and sexuality is missing from menstrual education. Indeed, the mothers in our focus groups agreed that explicit coverage of issues related to sexuality were not age-appropriate for their pre- and postmenarchal daughters: One admitted, "No, we don't talk sex at all." Another agreed, "We don't have to worry about the sexual aspect of it yet..." but did acknowledge "...you have to think about those things earlier than you used to." These mothers were nervous about having such conversations with their daughters. Said one, "I'm hoping that I can have the sex talk with my daughter before she hears it from anyone else...the news was about the vaccine for cervical cancer and so she wants to know, 'what's the cervix?' I didn't even want to have that conversation." They freely admitted being in denial about their daughters' emerging sexualities. One mother commented, "To think that my daughter is going to be capable of some kind of sexual life is extremely difficult. I think that you just want to bury your head in the sand."

Girls are certainly told that menstruation results when an egg is not fertilized, but little more is offered about how the egg gets to be fertilized. One of the mothers in our focus group reported, "I said 'the egg sheds'...then I did mention sperm and making a baby but I haven't made the jump to how that happens." Another told her daughter, "Women get something on a monthly basis and they have an egg...when mommy and daddy love each other then it becomes a baby in mommy's tummy." Not surprisingly, pre- and young adolescent girls are also not very knowledgeable about the physiology of menstruation itself (Koff & Rierdan, 1995a,b). Although we acknowledge that much careful thought should be given to when and how to educate girls about healthy sexuality, we concur with Koff and Rierdan (1995b), who suggest that the lack of specific information about menstruation and reproductive capacity can contribute to girls' confusion about healthy sexuality. To us, this aspect of menstrual education is even more crucial in the context of media messages about sexuality that young children now encounter, especially for girls who experience menarche before their peers.

With respect to body image, Mendle et al. (2007) concluded in their review of the early menarche literature that early maturation is associated with dieting behavior, bulimia, and poor body image. A longitudinal study of more than 2,000 African American and European American girls (Striegel-Moore et al., 2001) indicated that, for girls of both ethnic groups, a heavier body mass index (BMI) was associated with early menarche, and that girls with an earlier onset of menarche reported higher levels of body dissatisfaction and more attempts to lose weight than girls with on-time or later menarche. The researchers suggest that it is not early menarche per se that contributes to later eating pathology but a higher BMI. As Kaplowitz (2004) suggests, additional research that explores the role of pediatric obesity in early maturing girls' menstruation is needed since studies to date do not reveal whether increased obesity is causing the trend in early puberty, or, earlier puberty is causing the obesity. Results from a more recent study (Mangweth-Matzek, Rupp, Hausmann, Kemmler, & Biebl, 2007) suggest that early menarche is not associated with the development of an eating disorder, but that girls with eating disorders report more negative experiences with menarche than do healthy girls. The authors hold that girls who later develop eating disorders may have a negative body attitude that encompasses menstruation during early puberty.

It is likely that the current emphasis and value placed on a sexualized appearance may influence girls' perceptions of their body size and shape, which, in turn, may contribute to body dissatisfaction and negative attitudes toward menarche, particularly for girls who fall on extreme ends of a weight spectrum. Roberts and Waters (2004) noted that even the normative weight gain at puberty may lead girls to compare themselves to a thin, sexualized body ideal and/or a male body ideal and fall short with either comparison. Several studies have demonstrated that dating behavior moderates the relationship between early menarche and disordered eating (Cauffman & Steinberg, 1996; Smolak, Levine, & Gralen, 1993). Roberts and Waters (2004) argued that dating behavior may lead to girls' self-objectification, which could exacerbate body dissatisfaction and preoccupation, especially for early maturing girls.

Self-Objectification and Menstruation

Self-objectification has been shown to have negative consequences for psychological and sexual well-being (Muehlenkamp & Saris-Baglama, 2002; Szymanski & Henning, 2007; Tylka & Hill, 2004). Feminist researchers have begun to consider the impact of self-objectification on attitudes toward menstruation, a bodily function that is incompatible with the view of the body as a sexual object (Andrist, 2008; Johnston-Robledo, Sheffield, Voigt, & Wilcox-Constantine, 2007a; Roberts, 2004). For example, undergraduate students with stronger tendencies to self-objectify had more negative attitudes toward menstruation (Roberts, 2004; Johnston-Robledo et al., 2007a) and also reported a desire to live without their menses than did young women without these tendencies (Johnston-Robledo, Ball, Lauta, & Zekoll, 2003).

Others have investigated the influence of negative attitudes about menstruation on young women's reproductive health care and sexual behaviors. Schooler, Ward, Merriwether, and Caruthers (2005) found that undergraduate students who had feelings of shame regarding menstruation reported more sexual risk-taking than those who did not score high on measures of menstrual shame. On the contrary, women who have positive attitudes toward menstruation have been found to report higher levels of personal comfort with sexuality than do women with more negative or shameful attitudes toward menstruation (Rempel & Baumgartner, 2003).

In related work, Johnston-Robledo et al. (2007a) suggested that some women may develop a global sense of shame about their reproductive functioning and capacities (e.g., menstruation, pregnancy, childbirth, breastfeeding). In their attempts to capitalize on the social currency associated with sexual availability and attractiveness and/or to avoid feelings of reproductive shame, it is possible that women may distance themselves from these embodied experiences through health behaviors and decisions such as the suppression of monthly menstruation, the avoidance of breastfeeding, and the election of a cesarean delivery (Andrist, 2008; Johnston-Robledo et al., 2007a; Johnston-Robledo, Wares, Fricker, & Pasek, 2007b). It appears as though self-sexualization and shameful attitudes may be mutually reinforcing. To date, research into the interaction of variables affecting this relationship has been conducted on college-aged or slightly older females. We urge researchers to query younger girls about these issues and to explore the extent to which the sexualization of girls might influence this bidirectional relationship. Are self-objectification, menstrual shame, and/or reproductive shame associated with other consequences for adolescent girls' and young women's reproductive and sexual health (e.g., sexual subjectivity, gynecological care, and body discipline practices such as breast augmentation and extensive pubic hair removal)?

Conversely, Lee (2009) has suggested that a sexualized culture might lead girls to have positive or neutral attitudes toward menarche because it symbolizes an adult woman's body and is associated with other desirable changes, although empirical study is needed to evaluate this notion. We argue that positive attitudes toward menarche may not translate into positive attitudes toward ongoing menses. Young girls and adolescents who are heavily influenced by sexualization in the culture may develop negative attitudes toward monthly menstruation. Although menstruation symbolizes adult womanhood, it is a taboo bodily function that is incompatible with a sexualized self-presentation. As girls become more familiar with and assimilate cultural norms about the stigmatized status of menstruation, they may come to believe that, during menstruation, they are unavailable as a sexual or dating partner, or that it may be difficult to wear clothing that is consistent with a sexualized self-presentation (short skirts, fitted clothing, etc.). As such, they may go to great lengths to conceal their menstrual status by changing their appearance and activities. Contemporary menstrual product advertising features convey the concealment imperative by presenting models who portray sexualized ideals through fitted clothing and other indicators of sexual attractiveness (Erchull, 2011). In our focus groups, one mother noted that the sexualization trend might influence girls to have positive attitudes about breast development but negative attitudes toward menstruation: "I would say that the breasts and the body changes would be more likely to be welcomed just from what it means because no one can see you're bleeding...But, I think the outwardly changes would be celebrated more because you can accentuate [them] if you're looking to be sexual."

We note that negative attitudes toward menstruation are abundantly referenced in much of the current advertising of continuous oral contraceptives (e.g., those that eliminate monthly bleeding, also known as *menstrual suppression*). We are concerned about the extent to which young girls are or will be drawn to these products. Although advertising for these contraceptives is not aimed at school-aged girls, they nevertheless avidly read magazines and access websites targeting older females (Merskin, 1999). In their brief position paper, Sucato and Gold (2002) provided tips for clinicians interested in prescribing these contraceptives to adolescents and argued that this may be an option for "all young women" who prefer not to experience monthly menstruation (p. 327). Other feminist researchers and health care providers have argued that continuous oral contraceptive use is being promoted without sufficient data on long-term safety (Society for Menstrual Cycle Research [SMCR], 2007) and that monthly menstruation should be regarded as a vital sign of adolescent girls' health (American Academy of Pediatrics, 2006; Stubbs, 2008).

A content analysis of messages about menstrual suppression in mainstream print media found that readers were persuaded to view menstruation as unhealthy and to view menstrual suppression as a panacea to an inconvenient, bothersome, monthly flow (Johnston-Robledo, Barnack, & Wares, 2006). We are not arguing that menstrual suppression is inappropriate for all adolescent girls, but we are concerned about the impact of this widespread marketing on adolescent girls' attitudes toward and experiences with menstruation. Furthermore, we believe the pressure to conform to a sexualized ideal faced by contemporary adolescents may increase their vulnerability to messages in the media that promote the elimination of monthly menstruation. The mothers in our focus groups were aware of this advertising but believed their daughters would not be affected by it: "those commercials...for the medication that would stop your period. Playing with nature like that is just awful. Thankfully my daughter was too young to be influenced by that." The availability and widespread acceptance of menstrual suppression may also exacerbate their ambivalence toward and confusion about menstruation and its role in their development and identities. These are all fruitful areas for future research with important implications for adolescents and young women's health and well-being.

We must add that, in general, the mothers in our focus group seemed to be at a loss at first to respond to our question about how the sexualization trend might impact their daughters' pubertal development. Indeed, the very question was met first with silence, as if they were perhaps considering this relationship for the first time. One mother commented, "I never really related the two, menstruation and that, ever. So, that was kind of confusing. I don't know what girls are talking about either." Another agreed she wasn't sure "...they'd equate the things that they're seeing with having their first period, really?"

However, as the conversation continued, mothers agreed that the media play a large role in perpetuating sexualized messages about girls, but as one explained, "Now they're just used to it—in a sad sense—they're just bombarded with information—but I don't think they're so much affected by it...they are desensitized...nothing shocks them." Interestingly, although aware of some aspects of sexualization (e.g., the marketing of padded bras to girls), these mothers were themselves somewhat shocked by the marketing of thongs for little children. When we showed them pictures of these products, two replied in disbelief: "Nun uh!!" "No way!" Upon further reflection, they remarked: "It's all about being seen as an object;" and, "Oh my gosh, I get chills just thinking about it. It's sickening. Isn't that strange how none of us are aware of that."

Although slow to warm up to this topic, the mothers eventually offered examples of how their daughters engaged in activities that reflected sexualization. Some discussed the stark contrast between their daughters' child-like behavior and adult appearance and behavior, especially in the context of activities such as dance. For example, one mother stated, "When she goes to dance class, it's like she's another person. I bring her home, and she crawls around and barks like a dog...she's still nine and she's still a kid. Then she puts her dance clothes on and she poses for the camera." Another shared, "She still likes to pretend...but then if Nickelodeon is on and she sees these teenage kids, she really gravitates to that as well."

Girls' self-perceptions related to maturity change during these years of pubertal growth. In a classic study, Koff, Rierdan, and Silverstone (1978) explored a shift in girls' gender identity development associated with the experience of menarche through a longitudinal study of seventh-grade girls' drawings of human figures. The girls were instructed to draw a person on two separate occasions, separated by a 6-month interval. Some of the girls remained either pre- or postmenarchal for the duration of the study, but some girls who were premenarcheal at pretest were postmenarchal at posttest. Girls who were postmenarchal throughout the study tended to draw a woman's body first and drew pictures of women that were more sexually differentiated than those of the premenarcheal girls, and the drawings from the group whose menarcheal status had changed reflected this trend as well (Koff et al., 1978).

It would be fascinating to replicate this study to explore girls' conceptualization of adult womanhood as a function of their menarche status, and to extend it by asking girls to draw girls their own age. It is possible, given the sexualization of girls within the culture, that girls may draw sexually differentiated adults regardless of their own menarcheal status, or that menarche no longer serves as an important or significant marker of identity development. It is also possible that girls might no longer equate menstruation with "being a woman," or think of that characterization as important in early menstrual experience (see Koff & Rierdan, 1995b). Some (albeit adult) fiction (e.g., Weitz, 2008) portrays losing one's virginity as "becoming a woman." Clearly, more research on what girls think signifies "becoming a woman" and how they are integrating physical and psychosocial development would provide important information to adults who want to facilitate girls' healthy development.

Additionally, cross-cultural work with adult women found strong relationships between menarche and sense of self as both different from boys and from children (Chrisler & Zittel, 1998; Uskul, 2004). Girls who reported liking their changing bodies and wanting to be an adult had more positive attitudes toward menstruation than did girls who did not endorse these statements (Rembeck, Moller, & Gunnarsson, 2006). Data from several different qualitative studies suggest that the shame attached to female pubertal development, particularly menstruation, may stem from an awareness of the devaluation of women and ambivalence about adult womanhood. For example, girls have noted that boys' pubertal changes lead to power and pride, whereas girls' lead to shame and anxiety (Burrows & Johnson, 2005; Martin, 1996). Feminist researchers have also argued that girls may feel alienated from or even betrayed by the physical changes in their bodies, as a result of their growing awareness of the sexual objectification of women's bodies and the extent to which others were sexualizing their growing bodies. This awareness may lead to girls' confusion about their own sexual feelings and impending adulthood (Lee & Sasser-Coen, 1996; Martin, 1996). These shifts in identity development may be more confusing to kids and striking to parents than they may have been before the widespread sexualization trend.

A Key Role for Adults

A number of studies have found that preparation for menstruation is related to more positive attitudes and experience (e.g., Koff, Rierdan, & Sheingold, 1982; McPherson & Korfine, 2004; Rierdan, 1983). But even girls who report being well prepared for menstruation also report feeling disgust, shame, and apprehension about it (Koff & Rierdan, 1995b). Further, there is little clarity about what "good" preparation for menstruation entails. Girls name their mothers as their main source of information and rate them as helpful, although not consistently so (Bloch, 1978; Koff, Rierdan, & Jacobson, 1981; Koff & Rierdan, 1995b; Lee, 2008, 2009).

Lee (2008) analyzed the first-period narratives of a sample of young women who experienced menarche between 1999 and 2003 when, presumably, shifts in the cultural scripts about women and girls (e.g., increased sexualization; increased visibility of and openness about menstruation) were occurring. In their narratives, the young women recalled their mothers as supportive and emotionally engaged with them. Nevertheless, such support did not always guarantee a positive menarcheal experience. Indeed, in spite of such support, negative menarcheal experiences were recalled by some. Supportive mothers, who reacted in a matter-of-fact, action-oriented way (e.g., to help with supplies) were acknowledged as most helpful. Least helpful were mothers who "made a big deal" of the daughter's menarche, by announcing it to family relatives or by organizing public celebrations of some kind. Lee (2008) notes that ethnicity and social class were important variables: whites and the affluent were over-represented as celebratory and emotionally engaged, whereas women of color and the less affluent were overrepresented as helpful and less demonstrative.

Mothers' "no big deal" attitude was also reflected in the young women's descriptions of their first periods. Lee (2008) reports that over 50% of her sample described their first periods as overwhelmingly positive or "no big deal," in contrast to reports from earlier studies that featured mostly negative memories of menarche (e.g., Lee & Sasser-Coen, 1996). Although it is possible to conclude from these data that contemporary mothers are less likely than mothers in the past to convey negative messages to their daughters about menstruation, Lee (2009) also entertains the possibility that these reports reflect the way young women *think* they should react to menstruation, particularly given that themes of shame, embarrassment, and fear are still present in the narratives:

> the increased cultural openness about menstruation...may cause pressure for girls to feel that they have to be "cool" about menarche and might mask more nuanced feelings. Cultural pressures may guide perceptions, frame experiences, and encourage a re-narration of stories that flatten negative experiences into a socially expected "no problem." (p. 625)

Lee (2008, 2009) asserts that attitudes and practices about menarche are changing, and that support from an engaged and helpful mother is a powerful buffer to negative cultural messages about menstruation. At the same time, she and others (Costos, Ackerman, & Paradis, 2002; Lee & Sasser-Coen, 1996) acknowledge that mother–daughter dialogues can convey restrictions associated with adult femininity and are linked to negative memories of menarche. Stubbs and Costos (2004) note that negative messages about menstruation in the culture can exacerbate negative mother–daughter dialogues and serve to drive a wedge between mothers and daughters.

The mothers in our focus groups earnestly gave voice to wanting to do a better job of educating their daughters about puberty and healthy sexuality than their mothers had done with them, and believed that they were doing so to some extent. We noticed that, at the beginning of the focus group discussions, mothers were tentative about venturing their thoughts and betraying their own lack of knowledge or comfort in talking about their daughters' becoming more mature and specifically, a sexual person. However, as the discussions continued, the mothers became more involved and interactive, less afraid to ask "stupid" questions, eager to ask each other for advice and trade tips for talking about sensitive issues. All were eager for follow-up meetings together or with some guidance from us as discussion leaders. These mothers evidenced what previous research has shown—that mothers recognized their own lack of knowledge as one barrier in talking to their daughters (Golub & Catalano, 1983). Their reactions lead us to suggest that researchers should examine the current challenges mothers face as they discuss menstruation, pubertal development, and sexuality in a cultural context that promotes self-sexualization of girls. This research would have implications for interventions and resources aimed at enhancing mothers' comfort with and effectiveness in talking to their daughters about these very important aspects of healthy development. Mother–daughter dialogues about menstruation and growing up could be opportunities to begin discussing sexuality, and, as many have previously suggested (e.g., Golub, 1992; Hillard, 2002; Stubbs, 1990), these conversations should be ongoing during the pre-teen and teenage years. Toward that end, data-based psychoeducational interventions could assist mothers in overcoming their resistance to their daughters' development as sexual beings and help them critique, challenge, and resist sexualized messages from the culture.

Such conversations would seem to be especially important given the inadequacy of more formal menstrual education materials and other venues that girls access for information about growing up. Today's menstrual education materials are not much better than those reviewed some 30 years ago at providing more detailed information about physiology, or about puberty in general, and continue to focus on menstruation as a hygienic crisis and promote the ideal of a neat, clean body that doesn't "leak" (Erchull, Chrisler, Gorman, & Johnston-Robledo, 2002). Whisnant, Brett, and Zegans (1975) first disclosed this focus and pointed out how the double messages in menstrual education (e.g., menstruation is normal and natural but must be hidden at all costs) serve to confuse cognitively immature girls. Charlesworth (2001) notes another double message in today's materials—menstruation is important, but one should ignore it, act normal as on any other day. Such a message suggests a distancing of the self from menstruation that is further reinforced by product information that promotes this distance (e.g., applicators as alternatives to having to touch menstrual fluid) (Simes & Berg, 2001) and, more recently, products touting silent wrappers. Simes and Berg (2001) assert that menstrual product advertising relies on exploiting fears about being caught menstruating by assuring girls (and women) that their product best prevents leakage, disguises odor, and allows them to continue to participate as usual in activities so no one will know. In addition, girls who consult magazine articles about menstruation for information will find a reiteration of negative messages about shame and embarrassment (Kalman, 2000).

Some discourse analysts (e.g., Polak, 2006) have noted that in a quest for knowledge about menstruation, girls are engaging in frank question-and-answer discussions with each other in online forums. Although these discussions could signal girls' increasing comfort with talking about menstruation, the accuracy of their information exchange is clearly of concern, as is the absence of caring and knowledgeable adults as participants in these conversations.

One related consideration is that girls do not, and do not *want* to, talk to fathers about menstruation (Kalman, 2003; Koff & Rierdan, 1995b). Kalman (2003) is concerned about this gap, especially for girls in single-father-headed households. She found that although girls reported close relationships with their fathers, they also reported feeling distanced from them after the beginning of menstruation. Kalman advocates for more support for fathers in helping daughters adjust to menstrual life. Lee (2009) also suggests helping boys become more supportive of girls, especially sisters, since in her sample, girls with brothers, especially older brothers, were vulnerable to continued internalization of negative cultural messages about menstruation.

If distance between males and menstruation is a feature of family life, it is also a feature of other male–female relationships. Research into males' attitudes toward menstruation, though scant, indicates that males do not learn much about menstruation while growing up and what they do learn is often inaccurate and reflects negative stereotypes about the process (Allen, Kaestle, & Goldberg; 2011; Chang, Hayter, & Lin, 2011; Gardner, 2009; Stubbs, 1985). One participant from an early study put it well: he remembered being told to be nice to girls during their periods, but was hard pressed to do so because he did not know how to tell when girls were doing it (Stubbs, 1985). His dilemma is further illuminated by more recent data from Fingerson (2005, 2006), who notes that girls use codes to continue talking about menstruation when boys are present. Although she believes that this strategy shows agency and creativity, we wonder if it also (unwittingly) reinforces the separation between males and menstruation. Indeed, Allen, Kaestle, and Goldberg (2011) found from their study of how boys learn about menstruation that boys think menstruation is gross during late childhood and early adolescence. The researchers argue that menstruation serves as a "gender wedge" between boys and girls at this stage of development (p. 129). Such a distinct and early separation of this female experience from males may, then, also contribute to gender intensification for both girls and boys. A fruitful area for future research might be the impact of the sexualization of girls on gender intensification, with respect to adolescents' negotiations of physical development and early sexual experiences. Although boys and girls certainly experience pubertal growth in different ways, there are many similarities that might also be highlighted; for example, both boys and girls sometimes feel self-conscious about changing bodies (Martin, 1996). A focus on similarities rather than unique differences, which are assumed to be impossible to understand without direct experience, might encourage more empathy and connection between boys and girls, and might make it easier for them to later negotiate heterosexual relationship issues related to menstruation, such as perceived or actual premenstrual moodiness, or sexual activity during menstruation.

Conclusion

As our review details, a good deal of information about girls' attitudes toward menstruation and early menstrual experience has been gleaned from previous research. And yet, additional research into contemporary girls' attitudes and experiences about menstruation and other pubertal events is needed. Research on girls' actual experiences has not kept up with the acceleration of sexual messages in the culture. Some of the newer research reviewed does not take into account the current sexualized cultural context in which girls are growing up. Even Lee's (2008, 2009) work, which includes a more contemporary sample, relies on retrospective rather than real-time data. And, while she investigates both ethnicity and income level as important variables, much more research on the experiences of girls from families of low income, of varying ethnicity, and who identify as bisexual or lesbian is needed.

Although research about puberty and adolescent sexuality is difficult to conduct, we hope researchers will work to overcome these logistical barriers. We also hope that parents will acknowledge the importance of this work and support such research by enrolling daughters (and sons) as participants. We suggest the following specific questions for future research with girls: Does the sexualization of girls influence their reactions to menarche and their attitudes toward menstruation and other pubertal events? Does menstruation interfere with or enhance their attempts to view and present themselves as sexual objects? Does menarche and early menstruation make girls more vulnerable to self-sexualization and body discipline practices, such as the elimination of monthly bleeding through hormonal contraceptives? In what ways does the sexualization of girls reinforce the mixed messages about menstruation or transmit new messages about menstruation and being a woman? Most importantly, how does sexualization influence the impact of menstruation on girls' sexual esteem, agency, experiences, responses, relationships, and behavior?

We believe that this research is crucial in the current culture, in which commercial interests are playing such a prominent role in articulating the "norms" for gendered behavior to children and adults alike. Well-meaning but busy parents (and children) need help processing and responding to these messages, and, perhaps more importantly, understanding that a cornerstone of girls' (and women's) well-being is a developing sense of agency with respect to their maturing bodies. What this means is new effort, enlisting data-based resources and interventions that expose girls to a broader conceptualization of the many ways to be a woman in the culture and help them resist cultural messages that associate shame and embarrassment with maturing female physicality. This is no small task, and one that we look forward to undertaking with others.

References

Allen, K. R., Kaestle, C. E., & Goldberg, A.E. (2011). More than just a punctuation mark: How boys and young men learn about menstruation. *Journal of Family Issues, 32*(2), 129–156.

American Academy of Pediatrics. (2006). Menstruation in girls and adolescents: Using the menstrual cycle as a vital sign. *Pediatrics, 118,* 2245–2250.

Andrist, L. C. (2008). The implications of objectification theory for women's health: Menstrual suppression and "maternal request" cesarean delivery. *Health Care for Women International, 29,* 551–565.

Berger, K. (2009). *The developing person through childhood and adolescence.* New York: Worth Publishers.

Bloch, D. (1978). Sex education practices of mothers. *Journal of Sex Education and Therapy, 4,* 7–12.

Brown, L. M., & Gilligan, C. (1992). *Meeting at the crossroads: Women's psychology and girls' development.* Cambridge, MA: Harvard University Press.

Brumberg, J. J. (1997). *The body project: An intimate history of American girls.* New York: Vintage.

Burrows, A., & Johnson, S. (2005). Girls' experiences of menarche and menstruation. *Journal of Reproductive and Infant Psychology, 23,* 235–249.

Cauffman, E., & Steinberg, L. (1996). Interactive effects of menarcheal status and dating on dieting and disordered eating among adolescent girls. *Developmental Psychology, 32,* 631–635.

Chang, Y. T., Hayter, M., & Lin, M. L. (2011). Pubescent male students' attitudes towards menstruation in Taiwan: Implications for reproductive health education and school nursing practice. *Journal of Clinical Nursing.* Advance online publication. doi: 10.1111/j.1365-2702.2011.03700.x

Charlesworth, D. (2001). Paradoxical constructions of self: Educating young women about menstruation. *Women and Language, 24,* 13–20.

Chrisler, J. C., & Zittel, C. B. (1998). Menarche stories: Reminiscences of college students from Lithuania, Malaysia, Sudan, and the United States. *Health Care for Women International, 19,* 303–312.

Clarke, A. E., & Ruble, D. N. (1978). Young adolescents' beliefs concerning menstruation. *Child Development, 41*, 231–234.

Costos, D., Ackerman, R., & Paradis, L. (2002). Recollections of menarche: Communication between mothers and daughters regarding menstruation. *Sex Roles, 46*, 83–101

Delaney, J., Lupton, M. J., & Toth, E. (1977). *The curse: A cultural history of menstruation*. New York: Mentor.

Dorn, L. D., & Rotenstein, D. (2004). Early puberty for girls: The case of premature adrenarche. *Women's Health Issues, 14*, 177–183.

Erchull, M. J., Chrisler, J. C., Gorman, J. A., & Johnston-Robledo, I. (2002). Education and advertising: A content analysis of commercially produced booklets about menstruation. *Journal of Early Adolescence, 22*, 455–474.

Erchull, M. J. (in press). Distancing through objectification? Depictions of women's bodies in menstrual product advertisements. *Sex Roles*. doi:10.1007/s11199-011-0004-7

Fingerson, L. (2005). Agency and the body in adolescent menstrual talk. *Childhood, 12*, 91–110.

Fingerson, L. (2006). *Girls in power: Gender, body and menstruation in adolescence*. Albany, NY: State University of New York.

Frank, D., & Williams, T. (1999). Attitudes about menstruation among fifth-, sixth-, and seventh-grade pre- and post-menarcheal girls. *Journal of School Nursing, 15*, 25–31.

Fredrickson, B. L., & Roberts, T. (1997). Objectification theory: Toward understanding women's lived experiences and mental health risks. *Psychology of Women Quarterly, 21*, 173–206.

Frisch, R. E. (1983). Fatness, puberty, and fertility. In S. Golub (Ed.), *Menarche* (pp. 5–20). Lexington, MA: Lexington Books.

Gardner, M. C. (2009). Understanding men's attitudes about the menstrual cycle. *Dissertation Abstracts International: Section B: The Sciences and Engineering, 69*(11), 7187.

Golub, S. (1992). *Periods: From menarche to menopause*. Newbury Park, CA: Sage.

Golub, S., & Catalano, J. (1983). Recollections of menarche and women's subsequent experiences with menstruation. *Women & Health, 8*, 49–61.

Herman-Giddens, M. E., Wasserman, R. C., Bourdony, C. J., Bhapkar, M. V., Kock, G. G., & Hasemeier, C. M. (1997). Secondary sexual characteristics and menses in young girls seen in office practice: A study from the pediatric research in office settings network. *Pediatrics, 4*, 505–512.

Hillard, P. J. A. (2002). Menstruation in young girls: A clinical perspective. *Obstetrics & Gynecology, 99*(4), 655–662.

Houppert, K. (1999). *The curse: Confronting the last unmentionable taboo—menstruation*. New York: Farrar, Straus, & Giroux.

Johnston-Robledo, I., Ball, M., Lauta, K., & Zekoll, A. (2003). To bleed or not to bleed: Young women's attitudes toward menstrual suppression. *Women & Health, 38*(3), 59–75.

Johnston-Robledo, I., Barnack, J., & Wares S. (2006). "Kiss your period good-bye": Menstrual suppression in the popular press. *Sex Roles, 54*, 353–360.

Johnston-Robledo, I., Sheffield, K., Voigt, J., & Wilcox-Constantine, J. (2007a). Reproductive shame: Self-objectification and young women's attitudes toward their bodies. *Women & Health, 46*(1), 25–39.

Johnston-Robledo, I., Stubbs, M. L., Calleri, S., & Hepworth, A. (2009, June). The Impact of sexualization on girls' early menstruation: Part 2—An exploratory study: Mothers' perceptions of the impact of sexualization on their daughters' early menstrual experiences. In I. Johnston-Robledo (Chair), *From girlhood to girls gone wild: Menstruation and development in a sexually objectifying culture*. Symposium presented at the biennial meeting of the Society for Menstrual Cycle Research, Spokane, WA.

Johnston-Robledo, I., Wares, S., Fricker, J., & Pasek, L. (2007b). "Indecent exposure": Self-objectification and young women's attitudes toward breastfeeding. *Sex Roles, 56*, 429–437.

Kalman, M. (2000). Adolescent lay menstrual literature. *Journal of Multicultural Nursing and Health, 6*, 35–41.

Kalman, M. B. (2003). Adolescent girls, single-parent fathers, and menarche. *Holistic Nursing Practice, 17*, 36–40.

Kaltiala-Heino, R., Kosunen, E., & Rimpela, M. (2003). Pubertal timing, sexual behavior, and self-reported depression in middle adolescence. *Journal of Adolescence, 26*, 531–545.

Kaplowitz, P. (2004). Precocious puberty: Update on secular trends, definitions, diagnosis, and treatment. *Advances in Pediatrics, 52*, 37–62.

Kaplowitz, P. B., & Oberfield, S. E. (1999). Reexamination of the age limit for defining when puberty is precocious in girls in the United States: Implications for evaluation and treatment. *Pediatrics, 104*(4), 936–941.

Kissling, E. A. (1996). Bleeding out loud: Communication about menstruation. *Feminism & Psychology, 6*, 481–504.

Kissling, E. A. (2006). *Capitalizing on the curse: The business of menstruation.* Boulder, CO: Lynne Rienner Publishers.

Koff, E., & Rierdan, J. (1995a). Early adolescent girls' understanding of menstruation. *Women & Health, 22*, 1–19.

Koff, E., & Rierdan, J. (1995b). Preparing girls for menstruation: Recommendations from adolescent girls. *Adolescence, 30*, 795–811.

Koff, E., Rierdan, J., & Jacobson, S. (1981). The personal and interpersonal significance of menarche. *Journal of the American Academy of Child Psychiatry, 20*, 148–156.

Koff, E., Rierdan, J., & Sheingold, K. (1982). Memories of menarche: Age, preparation and knowledge as determinants of initial experience. *Journal of Youth and Adolescence, 11*, 1–9.

Koff, E., Rierdan, J., & Silverstone, E. (1978). Changes in representation of body image as a function of menstrual status. *Developmental Psychology, 14*, 635–642.

Lee, J. (2008). "A Kotex and a smile": Mothers and daughters at menarche. *Journal of Family Issues, 29*(10), 1325–1347.

Lee, J. (2009). Bodies at menarche: Stories of shame, concealment and sexual maturation. *Sex Roles, 60*, 615–627.

Lee, J., & Sasser-Coen, J. (1996). *Blood stories: Menarche and the politics of the female body in contemporary U.S. society.* New York: Routledge.

Mangweth-Matzek, B., Rupp, C. I., Hausmann, A., Kemmler, G., & Beibl, W. (2007). Menarche, puberty, and first sexual activities in eating-disordered patients as compared with a psychiatric and a nonpsychiatric control group. *International Journal of Eating Disorders, 40*, 705–510.

Marshall, W. A., & Tanner, J. M. (1969). Variations in the pattern of pubertal changes in girls. *Archives of Disease in Childhood, 44*, 291–303.

Martin, K. (1996). *Puberty, sexuality, and the self: Boys and girls at adolescence.* New York: Routledge.

McPherson, M. E., & Korfine, L. (2004). Menstruation across time: Menarche, menstrual attitudes, experiences, and behaviors. *Women's Health Issues, 14*, 193–2004.

Mendle, J., Turkheimer, E., & Emery, R. E. (2007). Detrimental psychological outcomes associated with early pubertal timing in adolescent girls. *Developmental Review, 27*, 151–171.

Merskin, D. (1999). Adolescence, advertising, and the ideology of menstruation. *Sex Roles, 40*, 941–957.

Muehlenkamp, J. L., & Saris-Baglama, R. N. (2002). Self-objectification and its psychological outcomes for college women. *Psychology of Women Quarterly, 26*, 371–379.

Polak, M. (2006). From the curse to the rag: Online gURLS rewrite the menstrual narrative. In Y. Jiwani, C. Steenbergen, & C. Mitchell (Eds.,), *Girlhood: Redefining the limits* (pp. 191–207). Montreal: Black Rose Books.

Posner, R. B. (2006). Early menarche: A review of research on trends in timing, racial differences, etiology and psychosocial consequences. *Sex Roles, 54*, 315–322.

Rembeck, G. I., & Gunnarsson, R. K. (2004). Improving pre- and post-menarcheal 12-year-old girls' attitudes toward menstruation. *Health Care for Women International, 25,* 680–689.

Rembeck, G. I., Moller, M., & Gunnarsson, R. K. (2006). Attitudes and feelings towards menstruation and womanhood in girls at menarche. *Acta Pediatica, 95,* 707–714.

Rempel, J. K., & Baumgartner, B. (2003). The relationship between attitudes toward menstruation and sexual attitudes, desires, and behavior in women. *Archives of Sexual Behavior, 32,* 155–163.

Rierdan, J. (1983). Variations in the experience of menarche as a function of preparedness. In S. Golub (Ed.), *Menarche* (pp. 119–125). Lexington, MA: D. C. Heath.

Rierdan, J., & Koff, E. (1985). Timing of menarche and initial menstrual experience. *Journal of Youth and Adolescence, 14,* 237–244.

Roberts, T. (2004). Female trouble: The Menstrual Self-evaluation Scale and women's self-objectification. *Psychology of Women Quarterly, 28,* 22–26.

Roberts, T., & Waters, P. L. (2004). Self-objectification and that "not so fresh feeling": Feminist therapeutic interventions for healthy female embodiment. In J. C. Chrisler (Ed.), *From menarche to menopause: The female body in feminist therapy* (pp. 5–21). New York: Haworth.

Ruble, D. N., & Brooks-Gunn, J. (1982). The experience of menarche. *Child Development, 53,* 1557–1566.

Schooler, D., Ward, M. L., Merriwether, A., & Caruthers, A. S. (2005). Cycles of shame: Menstrual shame, body shame, and sexual decision-making. *Journal of Sex Research, 42,* 324–334.

Simes, M. R., & Berg, D. H. (2001). Surreptitious learning: Menarche and menstrual product advertisements. *Health Care for Women International, 11,* 455–469.

Smolak, L., Levine, M. P., & Gralen, S. (1993). The impact of puberty and dating on eating problems among middle school girls. *Journal of Youth and Adolescence, 7,* 411–427.

Society for Menstrual Cycle Research. (2007). *Menstruation is not a disease.* Retrieved June 21, 2009 from http://menstruationresearch.org/position-statements/menstrual-supression-2007/

Steingraber, S. (2007). *The falling age of puberty in U.S. girls: What we know, what we need to know.* San Francisco: Breast Cancer Fund.

Striegel-Moore, R. H., McMahon, R. P., Biro, F. M., Schreiber, G., Crawford, P. B., & Voorhees, C. (2001). Exploring the relationship between timing of menarche and eating disorder symptoms in Black and White adolescent girls. *International Journal of Eating Disorders, 30,* 421–433.

Stubbs, M. L. (1985). *Attitudes towards menstruation across the life span: The development of the Menstrual Attitudes and Experience Questionnaire.* Unpublished doctoral dissertation, Brandeis University, Waltham, MA.

Stubbs, M. L. (1990). *Body talk for parents of girls.* Wellesley, MA: Centers for Research on Women.

Stubbs, M. L. (2008). Cultural perceptions and practices around menarche and adolescent menstruation in the United States. *Annals of the New York Academy of Sciences, 1135,* 58–66.

Stubbs, M. L., & Costos, D. (2004). Negative attitudes toward menstruation: Implications for disconnection within girls and between women. *Women & Therapy, 27,* 37–54.

Stubbs, M. L., Johnston-Robledo, I., Mickel, S., & White, M. (2009, June). The impact of sexualization on girl's early menstrual experiences: Part 1—Congratulations, now you are a Woman!? In I. Johnston-Robledo (Chair), *From girlhood to girls gone wild: Menstruation and development in a sexually objectifying culture.* Symposium presented at the biennial meeting of the Society for Menstrual Cycle Research, Spokane, WA.

Stubbs, M. L., Rierdan, J., & Koff, E. (1989). Developmental differences in menstrual attitudes. *Journal of Early Adolescence, 9,* 480–489.

Sucato, G., & Gold, M. A. (2002). Extended cycling of oral contraceptive pills for adolescents. *Journal of Pediatric Adolescent Gynecology, 15*, 325–327.

Summers-Effler, E. (2004). Little girls in women's bodies: Social interaction and the stigmatizing of early breast development. *Sex Roles, 51*, 29–44.

Szymanski, D. M., & Henning, S. L. (2007). The role of self-objectification in women's depression: A test of objectification theory. *Sex Roles, 56*, 45–53.

Teitelman, A. M. (2004). Adolescent girls' perspectives of family interactions related to menarche and sexual health. *Qualitative Health Research, 14*, 1292–1308.

Tylka, T. L., & Hill, M. S. (2004). Objectification theory as it relates to disordered eating among college women. *Sex Roles, 51*, 719–730.

Uskul, A. (2004). Women's menarche stories from a multicultural sample. *Social Science & Medicine, 59*, 667–679.

Weideger, P. (1977). *Menstruation and menopause.* New York: Delta.

Weitz, P. (2008). *College girl.* New York: Riverhead Books.

Whisnant, L., Brett, E., & Zegans, L. (1975). Implicit messages concerning menstruation in commercial educational materials prepared for young adolescent girls. *American Journal of Psychiatry, 132*, 815–820.

Whisnant, L., & Zegans, L. (1975). A study of attitudes towards menarche in white middle-class American adolescent girls. *American Journal of Psychiatry, 132*, 809–814.

12

"I'd Rather Be a Famous Fashion Model than a Famous Scientist"

The Rewards and Costs of Internalizing Sexualization

SARAH K. MURNEN AND LINDA SMOLAK

"I sometimes act sexy to get what I want from a man," "I have broken dates with female friends when a guy has asked me out," and "I would rather be a famous fashion model than a famous scientist." These items from the hyperfemininity scale (Murnen & Byrne, 1991) measure women's agreement with the idea that they should value themselves primarily as sexual objects in heterosexual relationships. In this chapter, we discuss the dilemma that girls and women in U.S. culture face about whether to treat themselves as sexual objects, to self-sexualize. Consider the teenage girl whose friends are wearing tight, midriff-baring shirts. Should she wear one or not? On the one hand, her friends will think she looks "cool," and the older guy she is attracted to might pay attention to her. Thus, as she had hoped, she may feel special, grown up, and even more powerful because of her sexiness. On the other hand, the guy on the bus who comments on her body to make his friends laugh will likely say something to embarrass or frighten her, and her teachers might think she is not a serious student if she dresses in such a "sexy" way. This is a side of looking sexy that she did not expect. Although girls are encouraged to self-sexualize, and there are rewards associated with being "sexy," there are also costs that are less clearly "advertised." In this chapter, we discuss these rewards and costs. We begin by defining sexualization and its relationship to objectification. This is followed by a discussion of how the patriarchal society encourages gendered expectations for behavior related to sexuality and self-sexualization; how women's sexualization is encouraged in the consumer culture; and, finally, the rewards and costs associated with self-sexualization.

Sexualization and Objectification

The American Psychological Association (APA) Task Force on the Sexualization of Girls (APA Task Force, 2007, p. 2) defines sexualization as having four forms, any one of which indicates that sexualization has occurred. Sexualization is evident when: (a) sexual appeal is the sole determinant of a person's value; (b) sexual appeal is wholly based on physical attractiveness, which is narrowly defined; (c) someone is sexually objectified; or (d) sexuality is forced on a person, a criterion that is particularly applicable to children and adolescents. Sexualization is distinct from healthy sexuality. Healthy sexuality involves mutual responsibility, respect, control, and pleasure within the context of an intimate relationship. There is no mutuality in sexualization. One person is "using" the other for his or her own gratification, without regard for the other's needs, interests, or desires.

It is noteworthy that objectification is one form of sexualization. Objectification theory (Fredrickson & Roberts, 1997; McKinley & Hyde, 1996) has received substantial empirical attention (Moradi & Huang, 2008). Within this framework, objectification is sexualized. Women's bodies are treated as objects for the sexual pleasure of men. Gradually, girls and women come to internalize the sexualized gaze of men, leading them to monitor their own appearance to make sure they are sufficiently sexy. This self-monitoring has been experimentally, cross-sectionally, and longitudinally related to depression, body image and eating disturbances, and sexual dysfunction (Moradi & Huang, 2008). Piran and Cormier (2005) suggest that the lack of connection with their bodies that girls and women develop due to objectification is related to various self-harm behaviors, including smoking, cutting, and disordered eating. Thus, at least this form of sexualization has clearly been related to a variety of problems in girls and women and will be the emphasized type of sexualization in this discussion.

Although women's sexuality could be seen as a source of power that women have over men (an issue we return to later), there are social constraints on the expression of women's sexuality. Women are taught that their sexuality is not valuable in itself; instead, its primary purpose is to attract a man who will provide status and possible protection against other dominant men. Rigid prescriptions about appropriate sexual behavior are provided by the "heterosexual script." Kim and colleagues (2007) defined the heterosexual script to include a set of gendered expectations for sexual behavior that support the patriarchal structure of society. Men are stereotyped as the initiators of sexual activity, who have uncontrollable sex drives, whereas women are the "good girl" gatekeepers of male desire. Masculine courtship strategies encourage men to display wealth and power to attract women, who are sexual objects valued for their attractiveness. Feminine strategies include passive and indirect methods to indicate romantic interest and women's exploitation and disciplining of their own bodies to attract male attention. Women are expected to desire a committed relationship whereas men should want sex without commitment. This means that women will need to attract men into relationships while men's constant interest in sexy, new women is viewed as "natural." Male-oriented homophobia and an appropriation of female homosexuality are also part of the heterosexual script. Mahalik and colleagues' work on the measurement of contemporary gender role norms is quite consistent with the idea of a heterosexual script (Mahalik et al., 2003, 2005). Kim and colleagues provided evidence that elements of the heterosexual script are portrayed prevalently on prime-time television shows that are popular among adolescents (Kim et al., 2007).

Further, some of the largest gender differences in behavior occur in the realm of sexuality, with women indicating a much lower likelihood of masturbation than men and less acceptance of casual sex (Hyde, 2005). These findings suggest that the most socially appropriate expression of women's sexuality occurs within a committed, romantic relationship in which women are expected to be fairly passive and submissive. Consistent with this idea, Sanchez, Kiefer, and Ybarra (2006) found that college women (but not college men) implicitly associated sex with submissiveness. Further, women who showed a strong association between sex and submissiveness were more likely to report engaging in submissive sexual behavior and to report lower sexual arousal. Thus, the socially defined role for adolescent girls and women includes sexiness but not healthy sexuality.

The enactment of the heterosexual script logically means that women's sexual role is limited and potentially under men's control. Further ramifications of the script include the idea that men are naturally sexually aggressive and should not be blamed for sexually impositional behavior. Instead, women can be blamed since they are put in the position of gatekeepers of men's uncontrollable desire. Women are reminded in a variety of ways that men have sexual control over their (women's) bodies. Girls and women are likely to experience men staring at them (e.g., "ogling," "leering,"), men commenting on their bodies, men touching them without their consent, and possibly men raping them. The majority of middle and high school girls report being sexually harassed (American Association of University Women [AAUW], 2001; Harned, 2000; Larkin & Rice, 2005), and most "teasing" and bullying of high school girls by male schoolmates appears to be sexualized (Shute, Owens, & Slee, 2008). About one-quarter of college women are likely to be victims of rape or attempted rape (Koss, Heise, & Russo, 1994). The social control model of rape proposes that the existence of sexual violence keeps women in a state of fear, in which they are ironically dependent on men for protection (e.g., Sheffield, 2007).

In many ways, then, adolescent girls and women do not control their own sexuality. The culture gives greater credence to men's sexual interests and desires than to women's. Perhaps one way girls and women try to control the threat of men's dominance is through the use of their sexuality. Though there are potential costs to this strategy, the rewards are more tangible. Girls hear about the advantages of being sexy starting in early childhood, making self-sexualization seem natural and normal (Levin & Kilbourne, 2008). Thus, there are reasons for women to engage in self-sexualization.

Patriarchal Society Promotes Gendered Roles

Strong societal forces uphold women's self-sexualization. First, according to social role theory (e.g., Eagly, Wood, & Johannesen-Schmidt, 2004), gendered social roles likely developed from some biological differences between women and men, including women's smaller body size and their ability to bear children, but the differences become magnified and perpetuated through social and interpersonal processes. Men have traditionally been in the provider role and women in the caretaking role. Thus, women need to attract men so they and their children are protected and provided for. As women and men enacted these different societal roles, they developed particular personality characteristics that suited the roles. Further, members of society have developed expectations for behavior around these gendered roles, such that we believe and encourage women as a group to express more "feminine" traits and men more "masculine." Thus, gendered roles are associated with gender stereotypes that are perpetuated through various social and cognitive processes (Eagly et al., 2004).

Although it could be argued that gendered social roles are complementary and should promote a well-functioning society, the differentiation perpetuates status inequality on the basis of gender. Male roles and traits associated with "agency" put them in leadership positions that are associated with status, whereas stereotyped female roles and traits associated with "communion" do not. Although women's increased participation in the workforce has changed their access to leadership roles, it is still the case that men are more likely to be leaders and that they make more money than women (Eagly & Carli, 2007). Thus, women continue to need to attract men to ensure economic stability. And, according to much of American culture, sexiness is what attracts men.

Gendered social roles and social processes are structured around, and help reinforce, male dominance and hence the sexualization of women for the pleasure of men. In addition, heterosexual interdependence exists between women and men that has helped to further shape social roles (Rudman & Glick, 2008). In a patriarchal society, men need to maintain dominance over women while simultaneously having sexual relations with them. In order to support these conflicting goals, our society has developed attitudes of *hostile sexism* and *benevolent sexism* (Glick & Fiske, 1996). Hostile sexism includes the ideas of *dominant paternalism* (men dominate and control women), *competitive gender differentiation* (emphasizing differences between genders and devaluing characteristics associated with women), and *hostile heterosexuality* (e.g., relationships between women and men are adversarial; women's sexuality can be used as a resource, but this is met with hostility). In complement, benevolent sexism includes the attitudes of *protective paternalism* (men protect women, who are weaker), *complementary gender differentiation* (men and women are different, but women's qualities are valued), and *heterosexual intimacy* (women and men need each other). Much research has validated the existence of these constructs. Women are less likely to agree with hostile sexist beliefs than men, but women often agree with benevolent ones (Rudman & Glick, 2008).

Because benevolent sexism and hostile sexism attitudes often co-occur in the same individual (especially among men), the greater social acceptability of the benevolent beliefs can sometimes excuse the unacceptable hostile beliefs. For example, we might judge a man a "nice guy" because he thinks "men can't live without women," even if he also believes that women who use their sexuality for influence deserved to be scorned. In societies with high levels of gender inequality, men have high levels of hostile sexism and benevolent sexism beliefs, and women have high levels of benevolent sexism beliefs as well (Eastwick, 2006). In sexist cultures, it might make sense for women to adopt benevolent sexism in order to receive protection from men. Thus, we can see from this research that women might adopt attitudes that serve their immediate individual interests, but not necessarily their long-term interests or those of their group. To the extent that women depend on men for economic resources, romantic love, and social status, it makes sense for them to value their "benefactors" and to work to attract men by engaging in self-sexualization (Glick & Fiske, 1996). Indeed, women who agree with benevolent sexist attitudes are more likely to believe that beauty and thinness are important, that beauty requires effort, that body hair is unsightly, and that appearance is more important than competence (Forbes, Collinsworth, Jobe, Braun, & Wise, 2007).

Cultural Promotion of Sexualization

So, gendered roles exist, but how much pressure do they exert on girls and women? There is much evidence that the heterosexual script, and specifically the idea that women should be sexual objects, is promoted in the mass media. In general, there are two important themes related to sexualization that can be learned from the mass media. First, women are taught that being sexually attractive to men should be of supreme importance. Second, there is a particular body type associated with sexual attractiveness, one that includes thin hips and waist, large breasts, and long legs (Levine & Murnen, 2009). The ideal woman generally has characteristics that distinguish her from men and masculinity and emphasize her sexual appeal and youth. A variety of beauty practices support the enactment of the ideal woman including the use of makeup and hair products; clothing that emphasizes the distinctive shape of women's bodies; efforts directed at creating and maintaining thinness; hair removal practices for face, legs, "bikini area," and possibly the entire pubic area; and perhaps cosmetic surgery to attain ideal breasts, thinness, or the appearance of youth. Indeed, the unrealistic nature of the ideal body virtually requires that women spend time, money, and energy on sometimes dangerous activities in order to even approximate this body type.

Along with the portrayal of the heterosexual script, the portrayal of sexual activity in general has become more prevalent in the mass media. For example, in prime-time television, the number of sex scenes doubled between 1998 and 2005 (Kunkel, Eyal, Finnerty, Biely, & Donnerstein, 2005). With an emphasis on "spontaneous, glamorous, unmarried, nonrelational sex," along with the objectification and degradation of women (Ward, 2003, p. 355), prime-time television portrays the sexualization of women as normative. Grauerholz and King (1997) found that 84% of the TV episodes they examined portrayed at least one incident of sexual harassment of women in the form of sexist comments (e.g., women called "babes"), verbal sexual comments (e.g., comments about women's body parts), and men or adolescent boys leering at girls and women. Magazines are also problematic. In magazines aimed at adolescent girls, a dominant focus is placed on the importance of women attracting men, the idea that women rather than men maintain romantic relationships, and that sexual activity is more acceptable for men than women (the sexual double standard) (Ward, 2003). Given that research suggests that 60% of middle school girls read "teen" magazines at least 2–5 times per month (Field et al., 1999), this is a widely received message. Similarly, Stankiewicz and Rosselli (2008) analyzed advertisements and found that only men's magazines were more likely to show women as sex objects than magazines aimed at adolescent girls and at women. Reichert and Carpenter (2004) found that the sexualization of women in advertisements increased significantly between 1983 and 2003. Peter and Valkenburg (2007) concluded that there is increased sexual content in the media, particularly with the advent of the Internet. Pornographic pages on the Internet increased by 1,800% between 1998 and 2004 (Paul, 2005).

In addition to the media, self-sexualization is encouraged by other practices. Clothing, hairstyles, make-up, and various practices can be used to emphasize women's sexuality. A recent emphasis has been placed on women adopting a "pornified" sexuality (see Paul, 2005, for a discussion of "pornification"). For example, beauty practices that used to be portrayed only in pornography are now appearing in popular culture, such as thong underwear and stiletto heels (Jeffries, 2005; Paul, 2005). Women, and even adolescent girls, are being encouraged to accept a view of sex that legitimizes their role as sex objects (Paul, 2005). Paul (2005, p. 110) wrote that, "Today, the pornography industry has convinced women that wearing a thong is a form of emancipation, learning to pole dance means embracing your sexuality, and taking your boyfriend for a lap dance is what every sexy and supportive girlfriend should do." Levy (2007) has also written about women's acceptance of "raunch culture," as evident in their participation in such cultural events as *Girls Gone Wild* videos. Sometimes sexualized products are even aimed at young girls. For example, there are t-shirts for young girls with sayings like, "future hottie" or "future trophy wife."

Social and cognitive theories are important to understanding the likely effects of consumer culture on girls' and women's sexualization and self-sexualization (APA Task Force Report, 2007). Social learning theories discuss the impact of rewards and punishment on behavior, as well as the influence of modeling. Cognitive perspectives add the idea that girls and women actively try to make sense of the information provided by the culture. Girls and women might internalize messages from the culture and develop stereotypes and schemas that guide their perceptions and behavior. One social-cognitive theory, *cultivation theory*, proposes that television can provide people with the norms for behaviors, ranging from what levels and types of violence are common to the normative treatment of women in heterosexual relationships (Gerbner, Gross, Morgan, & Signorelli, 1994). The more one is exposed to sexualizing, objectifying media images of women, the more likely one is to internalize these images and use them to guide one's own self-related attitudes and behaviors. Thus, self-sexualization becomes a social norm. Television viewing has been related to attitudes about thinness, breast size, and breast augmentation surgery (Harrison & Hefner, 2008). The consumption of sexualized media portrayals has been linked with an acceptance of the belief that women are sexual objects (Peter & Valkenburg, 2007; Ward, 2002; Ward & Friedman, 2006).

Objectification has received considerably more research attention than have other forms of sexualization. This is substantially because of objectification theory (Fredrickson & Roberts, 1997). Objectification theory provides a pathway linking objectification to self-objectification via consistent cultural messages. The self-objectification, which may include self-sexualization, leads to self-monitoring that, in turn, contributes to body shame. These developments occur within the context of the belief that women can thoroughly control how they look (McKinley & Hyde, 1996). There is much empirical support for objectification theory, particularly concerning the links between self-monitoring, body shame, and eating disorders (Moradi & Huang, 2008).

Evidence suggests that consumption of the media and other cultural products influences self-objectification and attitudes about the body. For example, the available data suggest a causal relationship between media exposure to the thin ideal and consequent body dissatisfaction (Levine & Murnen, 2009). In a recent meta-analysis (Grabe, Ward, & Hyde, 2008), there was a homogenous significant relationship between media and body dissatisfaction. There is also research that supports the idea that the process of self-sexualization starts at young ages. Murnen, Smolak, Mills, and Good (2003) found that first- through fifth-grade girls were aware of sexualized images of female celebrities. Girls who were more aware of the images were more likely to want to look like the thin, sexy celebrities and to have poorer body esteem. They were also more likely to think that it was important to look that way. Lindberg and her colleagues (Lindberg, Grabe, & Hyde, 2007) demonstrated that self-objectification occurs among adolescent girls and that it is already gendered by middle school. Longitudinal studies of the relationship between exposure to cultural models of sexual objectification, direct experience with being objectified by others, internalization of objectification, and self-sexualizing behavior could lead to models that incorporate important developmental processes. Of particular interest is the possibility that self-sexualization is part of the feminine gender role, a relationship that would render self-sexualization both culturally sanctioned and normative.

Peers also enforce self-sexualization. By adolescence, girls can become part of an all-female appearance subculture in which much of the talk and behavior is associated with maintaining appearance. Participation in image-oriented cultures is associated with body image dissatisfaction (Clark & Tiggemann, 2006; Jones, Vigfudsottir, & Lee, 2004). Nichter (2000) found that girls were likely to engage in ritualized "fat talk," to self-disparage their bodies, perhaps as a way to indicate their compliance with the body dictates of contemporary culture. "Fat talk" has been related to body dissatisfaction in experimental work (Stice, Maxfield, & Wells, 2003) and in correlational studies (Clarke, Murnen, & Smolak, 2010). The most common form of peer teasing focuses on appearance, and such teasing has frequently been related to body dissatisfaction (Menzel, Mayhew, Thompson, & Brannick, 2009). Sexual harassment in middle school has been associated with self-surveillance in girls (Lindberg et al., 2007).

Rewards and Costs Associated with Self-Sexualization

So far, we have argued that there are social roles that encourage women to treat themselves as sexual objects, and that many aspects of consumer culture, most notably the media, encourage this practice. There are also direct rewards that can be anticipated for attaining the societal ideal. In a meta-analytic review, Eagly and colleagues concluded that attractive women and men are assumed to be more popular and sociable (Eagly, Ashmore, Makhijani, & Longo, 1991). Gueguen (2007) found that men were more likely to approach large-breasted women compared to medium or small-breasted women in the field settings of a bar and night club. Women who are thinner and more attractive are routinely more successful in their careers in terms of job title and salary (McKinley, 1999; Smolak & Murnen, 2004).

Presenting oneself as a sex object might be a successful strategy for women to use when trying to persuade men. Matschiner and Murnen (1999) presented male and female college students with an audio-taped persuasive speech given by one of two women. In one condition, the woman presented herself as a sexual object (by expressing high agreement with some hyperfeminine (hf) attitudes). In the other condition, the woman expressed low hf. Men who heard the high hf speaker agreed with her more than did men who heard the low hf speaker, despite the fact that the high hf speaker was judged less competent. (The high hf speaker was judged to be more sexually and physically attractive than the low hf woman.) On the other hand, women participants who heard the low hf woman agreed with her more and judged her more competent than did women participants who heard the high hf speaker. Thus, to be influential to men, women might need to present themselves as compliant with their sexual objectification so as not to threaten the "status quo." This does come at a cost, though, in terms of perceptions of competence.

The results of this study are indicative of the double bind that women face in the realm of sexuality. They are supposed by be sexy, but that sexiness can reinforce their low status. Glick, Larsen, Johnson, and Branstiter (2005) found that women portrayed as sexy were not seen as competent for a high-status managerial job, compared to women portrayed in more business-like clothing. Olympic athletes shown in sexualized clothing versus athletic clothing were seen as less intelligent, capable, and strong (Gurung & Chrouser, 2007). Double binds arise from the precarious position that women face in a heterosexist society. Women need to maintain heterosexual relations with men to be socially successful (and to experience heterosexual sexual activity), so they might indicate some interest in being a sexual object, but being an object puts them under male control. If a woman is perceived as being too powerful either through expressing overt ownership of her own sexuality (she is a subject rather than an object), or by engaging in other autonomous behavior, she will likely receive sanctions from the male-dominated society to ensure she stays in "her place."

Women don't need to experience direct rewards of sexiness to believe that it is a positive attribute, according to social-cognitive perspectives. Young women who were asked to imagine their lives if they embodied the societal ideal for attractiveness thought their lives would be better in multiple ways. For example, more than half of the women associated the ideal with positive social attention, and romantic and employment success (Engeln-Maddox, 2006). Dellinger and Williams (1997) found that women associated wearing makeup with being perceived as heterosexual, healthy, and competent at work.

Given these data, it is understandable that there is confusion among women and adolescent girls about the extent to which capitalizing on "sexiness" is empowering. Some young feminists argue that female sexuality is an important source of women's empowerment that should be celebrated (Lorber, 2010). The popularity of the television show *Sex and the City*, which depicted sexuality from four women's points of view, emphasizing female sexual choice and agency, has probably had an influence on many young women. The commercial culture tries to sell products such as lingerie, sexualized clothing, and vibrators by associating them with ideas of women's sexual freedom (Attwood, 2005). However, it is questionable whether sexual cultural products are really designed for women's own pleasure, or whether they are designed to enhance women's appeal to men (Attwood, 2005; Paul, 2005; Rosalind, 2008). Further, rarely do popular images of sexy women also convey the potential degradation and violence that can be part of women's experiences as sexual objects in a male-dominated society (Rosalind, 2008).

Women who have been treated as sexual objects suffer consequences related to their empowerment. Considering just the "everyday" aspects of sexual objectification, in a cross-sectional study, it was found that grade school girls who experienced sexual harassment experienced greater body dissatisfaction (Murnen & Smolak, 2000). Links have also been found between the experience of sexist events and psychiatric symptoms (e.g., Klonoff, Landrine, & Campbell, 2000; Landrine et al., 1995; Swim, Hyers, Cohen, & Ferguson, 2001).

Women who are seen as using their sexuality for influence are possible targets of male violence, according to Glick and Fiske's (1996) model of hostile and benevolent sexism. There is likely a relationship between the objectification and degradation of women's bodies. For example, Greenwood and Isbell (2002) used the concept of ambivalent sexism to explain the popularity of "dumb blonde" jokes. Men feel ambivalence toward sexy women because, although they are attractive, they have the potential to be sexually manipulative. Telling a joke about them reduces their status, so that they are less threatening to men. Other research has shown that women and men are more likely to use degrading terms to refer to women's bodies than men's and that people who are sexually degraded are seen as less intelligent and moral (Murnen, 2000), perhaps indicating that we hold them responsible for being degraded. Negative stereotypes directed at feminists and lesbians might be related to the fact that the behavior of such women does not support a male-dominant, heterosexist society.

Thus, there are potential individual benefits if one is a "successful" sex object, including the idea that looking good is of value, especially in romantic relationships; doing "beauty work" associated with self-sexualization means fulfilling expected roles leading to acceptance by others; sexuality can sometimes be used to influence men; sexiness might attract romantic partners who can increase social status (the idea of trading looks for money); sexiness could lead to the attraction of a partner with whom to experience sexual activity; sexiness could lead to limited rewards in the work world associated with looking more "feminine"; and self-objectification could increase bonding with appearance-oriented peers. However, there are costs. Sexiness is a limited form of power, and its use could lead one to be the target of hostility and violence. It may also lead to superficial relationships that won't fulfill intimacy needs. Self-sexualization may result in less authentic connection to the body, perhaps greater body dissatisfaction and less sexual satisfaction, and may increase the likelihood of engaging in dangerous beauty practices, such as dieting or cosmetic surgery. Sexy women are perceived as less competent, which may lower work status. Finally, self-sexualization will not increase the status of women as a group. A direct comparison of benefits to costs might suggest that the potential costs of self-sexualization outweigh the benefits, but girls and women are not typically encouraged to make this direct comparison. Indeed, the cultural investment in sexualization discourages such critiques. Thus, many young women have been encouraged to engage in self-sexualization processes without "informed consent."

Girls are socialized to accept various aspects of sexualization starting at young ages, which makes the process of self-sexualization seem "normal." First, even though young girls are not culturally appropriate "sexual objects," they are exposed to sexualizing messages. Little girls may be dressed in bikinis or pretend stiletto heels (heelarious.com). Preschool-aged girls might be given toy make-up kits, jewelry, or nail polish. In addition, only about 10% of 3- to 10-year-old American girls do not own a Barbie (Dittmar, Halliwell, & Ive, 2006). Barbie's physical proportions are unrealistic, with large breasts relative to a tiny waist (Dittmar, Halliwell, & Ive, 2006). Barbie's image is sexualized and appearance-oriented. As indicated earlier, multiple media messages are aimed at girls and women. It is likely that most girls do not critically evaluate the large volume of sexualizing messages they receive from the culture, and that many of them adopt self-sexualization as a normative process.

Furthermore, normal pubertal development in girls brings increased peer harassment and self-surveillance (Lindberg et al., 2007). Sexual harassment is even more common in high school than in middle school (AAUW, 2001). Up to 90% of high school girls (and boys) report sexual harassment experiences (AAUW, 2001; Leaper & Brown, 2008). The most frequent forms of sexual harassment during high school, reported by 50–67% of the girls as occurring at least once, include unwanted romantic attention, demeaning comments about gender, teasing about appearance, and unwanted physical contact (Leaper & Brown, 2008). Girls who perceive themselves as less typically feminine and less content with the feminine gender role are more likely to perceive themselves as victims of sexism, primarily from male peers (Leaper & Brown, 2008). One possibility is that male peers who notice adolescent girls who stray from the culturally defined path attempt to bring them back in line via sexual harassment and sexist comments about academics and sports. Thus, peer enforcement of sexualization intensifies throughout childhood and adolescence, bringing the cost of noncompliance to a personal level.

The societal encouragement of women to value themselves primarily as sexual objects costs individual women and devalues the status of women in society. Engaging in the beauty practices necessary for meeting standards created by sexualization can, in and of itself, be dangerous (e.g., the risks associated with dieting and cosmetic surgery), but it also diverts energy from other potentially empowering activities. Women who are sexually objectified in our culture are seen, and treated, as if they are of lower status, which further limits their opportunities (Hesse-Biber, Leavy, Quinn, & Zoino, 2006; Smolak & Murnen, 2007). Further, various studies have shown that when women are experimentally induced to self-objectify, they perform worse on cognitive tasks (e.g., math tests) compared to those who don't self-objectify (Fredrickson, Roberts, Noll, Quinn, & Twenge, 1998; Hebl, King, & Lin, 2004; Quinn, Kallen, Twenge, & Fredrickson, 2006).

Thus, feminist theorists view sexualization as a form of oppression of women (e.g., Bordo, 1993, Brumberg, 1997). It functions to keep women in a subordinate position in society, a position that defines women's success primarily in terms of their appeal to men. In critiquing the thinness ideal, Martin (2007, p. 31) wrote, "If you spend precious time and energy worrying about your weight instead of your soul, you have been cheated. If you waste your sharp intellect on comparing and contrasting diet fads instead of the state of the world, we are all cheated."

Women might be particularly vulnerable to pressures for self-sexualization at this point in time because of the sheer prevalence of the supportive messages in the culture, the link between sexuality and power that is promoted, and current confusion about expected roles for women. Martin (2007) suggests that in a culture where girls and women have been told that they "can do anything," there have developed expectations that they should do everything perfectly—which is, of course, impossible. Women might focus attention on trying to manipulate their bodies since this might appear more manageable than performing multiple roles with perfection. Although women undoubtedly have greater access to some societal roles today than did women of previous generations, they also need to contend with greater pressures of self-sexualization that threaten their well-being.

Individual and Societal Change

In this chapter, we have argued that women's self-sexualization is a predictable phenomenon given a societal backdrop of male dominance and the culturally promoted heterosexual script. Gendered social roles and the existence of hostile and benevolent sexism function to constrain the sexual and self-expression of women in disempowering ways. Within this social setting, girls' and women's behavioral choices are limited. Perhaps the most socially acceptable role is the "nice girl" who is self-silencing, self-objectifying, and sexually passive, but she is at risk for various problems such as eating disorders, depression, and sexual dysfunction. Thus, she is not empowered. To the ambitious, outgoing teenage girl, the sex object role might seem more promising. After all, girls who fit this role are conventionally attractive, portrayed as socially successful, and have the means to attract boys, which is something girls are supposed to want to do at almost any cost. Further, sexiness is increasingly shown as a form of power, and there are a variety of consumer products available to support this role. It seems quite easy and acceptable for girls and young women to become preoccupied with time-consuming, energy-depleting beauty practices associated with self-sexualization. We have argued that there are costs to individual girls and women associated with the sex object role, and costs to the status of women as a group. For example, it is not clear what the line is between being sexualized, dehumanized, degraded, and violated. Girls and women need more empowering roles.

Obviously, many women escape societal constraints and arrive at sexual and self-definitions that are empowering. We need to learn more about these women and apply that knowledge to promote healthy development for girls. Such programs need to start by elementary school in order to inhibit the development of adherence to the social norms concerning sexualization. Girls should be given instruction and support in critiquing the social culture around them. Media literacy programs, for example, may prove valuable, as might interventions that include parents and other adults in the child's environment (Levine & Smolak, 2006). We might need to provide extra support to vulnerable girls. For example, it seems important to look at the issue of social class since lower class girls might be particularly vulnerable to the ramifications of self-sexualization. The sex object role is glorified for working class girls in the genre of "Cinderella" stories and movies like *Pretty Woman*, which promote the idea that girls with few economic resources can be "rescued" by higher status men if they are sufficiently attractive (and sexy). Such women must be able to "pass" as middle or upper class. Further, though, women of lower social class might be more vulnerable to hostility targeted at women who are sexually objectified. It is interesting to note that the term "slut" was used in a derogatory way in the 1700s in England by both upper-class women and men toward female servants who were expected to do more than clean the house (Attwood, 2007).

Empowerment may serve as a framework for such prevention efforts (Worell, 2006). Empowerment models recognize the interrelationship between social contexts and individual behavior, emphasizing that one's own identity is related to the roles one plays in social situations (O'Leary & Bhaju, 2006). Furthermore, with its focus on increasing a sense of competency and personal control within a supportive social community and with flexible gender roles, empowerment theory provides a potential road map for changing both individual outlooks and ecological contexts (Worell, 2006).

We also need to pay much more attention to the role of boys and men in promoting a sexist culture. In this chapter, we have critiqued women's roles in the "heterosexual script," but men's roles are complementary and very important to consider in the advancement of women's status. Extreme adherence to masculine gender roles that promote violence and the sexual degradation of women has been associated with perpetrating violence against women (Murnen, Wright, & Kaluzny, 2002). Further, men who spend more time in all-male groups of fraternities and athletic teams are particularly susceptible to harmful messages about women, and to objectifying and degrading women (Bleecker & Murnen, 2005; Murnen & Kohlman, 2007).

If our efforts were aimed only at individual girls and women, and individual boys and men, we would not be addressing the heart of the problem. We also need to critically examine the entire societal structure that maintains gender inequality. Specifically with respect to the sex object role, we need more critique of personal and corporate power that is served by this role and why this structure is even willing to damage women's health. The consumer culture greatly benefits from women feeling sufficiently dissatisfied with their bodies that they will buy products and services to try to attain an impossible ideal. The feminist ecological model of eating disorders prevention (Levine & Smolak, 2006), as exemplified by Piran's (1999) work with a national ballet school, may provide some guidelines for changing the cultural, as well as individual, context. Piran's model of embodiment, which has been empirically supported, may also be helpful (Piran & Cormier, 2005). This model includes socially based violations of body ownership, as well as gender prejudice, as causes of an individual's mistreatment and exploitation of her own body. It is imperative to extend the use of these models from prevention of eating disorders (Levine & Smolak, 2006) to sexualization.

Perhaps our best hope for increasing critique of sexualization and gender roles, and working on multiple fronts to increase status opportunities for women, comes from feminism. Rubin, Nemeroff, and Russo (2004) conducted a qualitative study with feminist (or womanist) college women who agreed that feminists were more likely to celebrate bodily diversity among women and that a feminist perspective should lead to a conscious awareness of cultural messages, as well as to the development of strategies to resist cultural pressure. They believed that feminism promoted ways to reclaim the body from the objectifying gaze through "emancipatory resistance," which might occur through athletics, dance, "taking up space," "moving with confidence," and redefining beauty. However, despite an awareness of what a feminist perspective could offer women to help protect against the development of body image dissatisfaction in an objectifying culture, the women felt that they were still susceptible to cultural messages about thinness. Rubin and colleagues (2004, p. 28) described rejecting beauty ideals as a "radical act" due to the enormous pressure on young women from appearance norms. Such resistance training needs to begin early, before self-sexualization starts to becomes an automatic reaction that seems "natural." Murnen and Smolak (2009) found that, across 26 studies, possessing feminist attitudes was associated with greater body satisfaction and less internalization of the thin media ideal. Feminism challenges patriarchal and heterosexist norms that threaten gender equality.

References

American Association of University Women (AAUW). (2001). *Hostile hallways: Bullying, teasing, and sexual harassment in schools.* Washington. DC: AAUW Educational Foundation.

APA Task Force on the Sexualization of Girls. (2007). *Report of the APA task force on the sexualization of girls.* Washington, DC: American Psychological Association. Retrieved from www.apa.org/pi/wpo/sexualization.html

Attwood, F. (2005). Fashion and passion: Marketing sex to women. *Sexualities, 8,* 392–406.

Attwood, F. (2007). Sluts and riot grrrls: Female identity and sexual agency. *Journal of Gender Studies, 16,* 233–247.

Bleecker, T., & Murnen, S. K. (2005). Fraternity membership, the display of sexually degrading sexual images of women, and rape myth acceptance. *Sex Roles, 53,* 487–493.

Bordo, S. (1993). *Unbearable weight: Feminism, western culture, and the body.* Berkeley, CA: University of California Press.

Brumberg, J. J. (1997). *The body project: An intimate history of American girls.* New York: Random House.

Clark, L., & Tiggemann, M. (2006). Appearance culture in nine to 12-year old girls: Media and peer influences on body dissatisfaction. *Social Development, 15,* 628–643.

Clarke, P. M., Murnen, S. K., & Smolak, L. (2010). Development and psychometric evaluation of a quantitative measure of "fat talk." *Body Image,7,* 1–7

Dellinger, K., & Williams, C. L. (1997). Makeup at work: Negotiating appearance rules in the workplace. *Gender & Society, 11,* 151–177.

Dittmar, H., Halliwell, E., & Ive, S. (2006). Does Barbie make girls want to be thin? The effect of experimental exposure to images of dolls on the body image of 5-to-8-year-old girls. *Developmental Psychology, 42,* 283–292.

Eagly, A. H., Ashmore, R. D., Makhijani, M. G., & Longo, L. C. (1991). What is beautiful is good, but…: A meta-analytic review of research on the physical attractiveness stereotype. *Psychological Bulletin, 110,* 109–128.

Eagly, A. H., & Carli, L. L. (2007). *Through the labyrinth: The truth about how women become leaders.* Boston: Harvard Business School Press.

Eagly, A. H., Wood, W., & Johannesen-Schmidt, M. C. (2004). Social role theory of sex differences and similarities: Implications for the partner preferences of women and men. In A. H. Eagly, A. E. Beall, & R. J. Sternberg (Eds.), *The psychology of gender* (2nd ed., pp. 269–295). New York: Guilford.

Eastwick, P. W., Eagly, A. H., Glick, P., Johannesen-Schmidt, M. C., Fiske, S. T., Blum, A. M. B., et al. (2006). Is traditional gender ideology associated with sex-typed mate preferences? A test in nine nations. *Sex Roles, 54,* 603–614.

Engeln-Maddox, R. (2006). Buying a beauty standard or dreaming of a new life? Expectations associated with media ideals. *Psychology of Women Quarterly, 30,* 258–266.

Field, A., Camargo, C., Taylor, C., Berkey, C., Frazier, L., Gillman, M., et al. (1999). Overweight, weight concerns, and bulimic behaviors among girls and boys. *Journal of the American Academy of Child and Adolescent Psychiatry, 38,* 754–760

Forbes, G. B., Collinsworth, L. L., Jobe, R. L., Braun, K. D., & Wise, L. M. (2007). Sexism, hostility toward women, and endorsement of beauty ideals and practices: Are beauty ideals associated with oppressive beliefs? *Sex Roles, 56,* 265–273.

Fredrickson, B. L., & Roberts, T. A. (1997). Objectification theory: Toward understanding women's lived experiences and mental health risks. *Psychology of Women Quarterly, 21,* 173–206.

Fredrickson, B. L., Roberts, T. A., Noll, S. M., Quinn, D. M., & Twenge, J. M. (1998). That swimsuit becomes you: Sex differences in self-objectification, restrained eating, and math performance. *Journal of Personality and Social Psychology, 75,* 269–284.

Gerbner, G., Gross, L., Morgan, M., & Signorelli, N. (1994). Growing up with television: The cultivation perspective. In J. Bryant, & D. Zillmann (Eds.), *Media effects: Advances in theory and research* (pp. 17–41). Hillsdale, NJ: Erlbaum.

Glick, P., & Fiske, S. T. (1996). The Ambivalent Sexism Inventory: Differentiating hostile and benevolent sexism. *Journal of Personality and Social Psychology, 70,* 491–512.

Glick, P., Larsen, S., Johnson, C., & Branstiter, H. (2005). Evaluations of sexy women in low- and high-status jobs. *Psychology of Women Quarterly, 29,* 389–395.

Grabe, S., Ward, L. M., & Hyde, J. S. (2008). The role of the media in body image concerns among women: A meta-analysis of experimental and correlational studies. *Psychological Bulletin, 134,* 460–476.

Grauerholz, E., & King, A. (1997). Prime time sexual harassment. *Violence Against Women, 3,* 129–148.

Greenwood, D., & Isbell, L. M. (2002). Ambivalent sexism and the dumb blonde: Men's and women's reactions to sexist jokes. *Psychology of Women Quarterly, 26,* 341–350.

Gueguen, N. (2007). Women's bust size and men's courtship solicitation. *Body Image, 4,* 386–390.

Gurung, R. A. R., & Chrouser, C. J. (2007). Predicting objectification: Do provocative clothing and observer characteristics matter? *Sex Roles, 57,* 91–99.

Harned, M. (2000). Harassed bodies: An examination of the relationships among women's experiences of sexual harassment, body image, and eating disturbances. *Psychology of Women Quarterly, 24,* 336–348.

Harrison, K., & Hefner, V. (2008). Body image and eating disorders. In S. L. Calvert, & B. J. Wilson (Eds.), *Handbook of child development and the media* (pp. 645–689). Malden, MA: Blackwell.

Hebl, M., King, E., & Lin, J. (2004). The swimsuit becomes us all: Ethnicity, gender, and vulnerability to self-objectification. *Personality and Social Psychology Bulletin, 30,* 1322–1331.

Heelarious.com. (2008). Accessed March 9, 2009.

Hesse-Biber, S., Leavy, P., Quinn, C. E., & Zoino, J. (2006). The mass marketing of disordered eating and eating disorders: The social psychology of women, thinness, and culture. *Women's Studies International Forum, 29,* 208–224.

Hyde, J. S. (2005). The gender similarities hypothesis. *American Psychologist, 60,* 581–592.

Jeffries, S. (2005). *Beauty and misogyny: Harmful cultural practices in the West.* New York: Routledge.

Jones, D. C., Vigfudsottir, T. H., & Lee, Y. (2004). Body image and the appearance culture among adolescent girls and boys: An examination of friend conversations, peer criticism, appearance magazines, and the internalization of appearance ideals. *Journal of Adolescent Research, 29,* 323–339.

Kim, J. L., Sorsoli, C. L., Collins, K., Zylbergold, B. A., Schooler, D., & Tolman, D. (2007). From sex to sexuality: Exposing the heterosexual script on prime-time network television. *Journal of Sex Research, 44,* 145–157.

Klonoff, E. A., Landrine, H., & Campbell, R. (2000). Sexist events may account for well-known gender differences in psychiatric symptoms. *Psychology of Women Quarterly, 24,* 93–99.

Koss, M. P., Heise, L., & Russo, N. F. (1994). The global health burden of rape. *Psychology of Women Quarterly, 18,* 509–537.

Kunkel, D., Eyal, K., Finnerty, K., Biely, E., & Donnerstein, E. (2005). *Sex on TV 5: A biennial report to the Kaiser Family Foundation.* Menlo Park, CA: Kaiser Family Foundation.

Landrine, H., Klonoff, E. A., Gibbs, J., Manning, V., et al. (1995). Physical and psychiatric correlates of gender discrimination: An application of the Schedule of Sexist Events. *Psychology of Women Quarterly, 19,* 473–492.

Larkin, J., & Rice, C. (2005). Beyond "health eating" and "healthy weights": Harassment and the health curriculum in middle schools. *Body Image, 2,* 219–232.

Leaper, C., & Brown, C. (2008). Perceived experiences with sexism among adolescent girls. *Child Development, 79,* 685–704.

Levin, D., & Kilbourne, J. (2008). *So sexy, so soon: The new sexualized childhood and what parents can do to protect their kids.* New York: Ballantine.

Levine, M. P., & Murnen, S. K. (2009). "Everybody knows that mass media are/are not (pick one) a cause of eating disorders": A critical review of evidence for a causal link between media, negative body image, and disordered eating in females. *Journal of Social & Clinical Psychology, 28,* 9–42.

Levine, M. P., & Smolak, L. (2006). *The prevention of eating problems and eating disorders: Theory, research and practice.* Mahwah, NJ: Lawrence Erlbaum Associates.

Levy, A. (2005). *Female chauvinist pigs: Women and the rise of raunch culture.* New York: Free Press.

Lindberg, S., Grabe, S., & Hyde, J. S. (2007). A measure of objectified body consciousness for preadolescent and adolescent youth. *Psychology of Women Quarterly, 30,* 65–76.

Lorber, J. (2010). *Gender inequality: Feminist theory and politics* (4th ed.). New York: Oxford University Press.

Mahalik, J., Locke, B., Ludlow, L., Diemer, M., Scott, R., Gottfried, M., et al. (2003). Development of the Conformity to Masculine Norms Inventory. *Psychology of Men & Masculinity, 4,* 3–25.

Mahalik, J. R., Mooray, E. B., Coonerty-Femiano, A., Ludlow, L. H., Slattery, S. M., & Smiler, A. (2005). Development of the conformity to feminine norms inventory. *Sex Roles, 52,* 417–435.

Martin, C. E. (2007). *Perfect girls, starving daughters: The frightening new normalcy of hating your body.* New York: Free Press.

Matschiner, M., & Murnen, S. K. (1999). Hyperfemininity and influence. *Psychology of Women Quarterly, 23*, 631–642.

McKinley, N. M (1999). Women and objectified body consciousness: Mothers' and daughters' body experience in cultural, developmental, and familial contexts. *Developmental Psychology, 35*, 760–769.

McKinley, N. M., & Hyde, J. S. (1996). The Objectified Body Consciousness Scale: Self-objectification, body shame, and disordered eating. *Psychology of Women Quarterly, 22*, 623–636.

Menzel, J. E., Mayhew, L. L., Thompson, J. K., & Brannick, M. T. (2009, May). *Teasing, body dissatisfaction, and restrictive eating: A meta-analysis.* Paper for presentation to the Academy of Eating Disorders Conference, Cancun, Mexico.

Moradi, B., & Huang, Y. (2008). Objectification theory and psychology of women: A decade of advances and future directions. *Psychology of Women Quarterly, 32*, 377–398.

Murnen, S. K. (2000). Gender and the use of sexually degrading language. *Psychology of Women Quarterly, 24*, 319–327.

Murnen, S. K., & Byrne, D. (1991). Hyperfemininity: Measurement and initial validation of the construct. *Journal of Sex Research, 28*, 479–489.

Murnen, S. K., & Kohlman, M. H. (2007). Athletic participation, fraternity membership, and sexual aggression among college men: A meta-analytic review. *Sex Roles, 57*, 145–157.

Murnen, S. K., & Smolak, L. (2000). The experience of sexual harassment among grade-school students: Early socialization of female subordination? *Sex Roles, 43*, 1–17.

Murnen, S. K., & Smolak, L. (2009). Are feminist women protected from body image problems? A meta-analytic review of relevant research. *Sex Roles, 60*, 186–197

Murnen, S. K., Smolak, L., Mills, J. A., & Good, L. (2003). Thin, sexy women and strong, muscular men: Grade-school children's responses to objectified images of women and men. *Sex Roles, 49*, 427–437.

Murnen, S. K., Wright, C., & Kaluzny, G. (2002). If "boys will be boys," then girls will be victims? A meta-analytic review of the research that relates masculine ideology to sexual aggression. *Sex Roles, 46*, 359–375

Nichter, M. (2000). *Fat talk: What girls and their parents say about dieting.* Cambridge, MA: Harvard University Press.

O'Leary, V., & Bhaju, J. (2006). Resilience and empowerment. In J. Worell, & C. Goodheart (Eds.), *Handbook of girls' and women's psychological health* (pp. 157–165). Oxford, UK: Oxford University Press.

Paul, P. (2005). *Pornified: How pornography is transforming our lives, our relationships, and our families.* New York: Times Books.

Peter, J., & Valkenburg, P. M. (2007). Adolescents' exposure to a sexualized media environment and their notions of women as sex objects. *Sex Roles, 56*, 381–395.

Piran, N. (1999). Eating disorders: A trial of prevention in a high risk school setting. *Journal of Primary Prevention, 20*, 75–90.

Piran, N., & Cormier, H. C. (2005). The social construction of women and disordered eating patterns. *Journal of Counseling Psychology, 52*, 549–558.

Quinn, D. M., Kallen, R. W., Twenge, J. M., & Fredrickson, B. L. (2006). The disruptive effect of self-objectification on performance. *Psychology of Women Quarterly, 30*, 59–64.

Reichert, T., & Carpenter, C. (2004). An update on sex in magazine advertising: 1983 to 2003. *Journalism & Mass Communication Quarterly, 81*, 823–837.

Rosalind, G. (2008). Empowerment/sexism: Figuring female sexual agency in contemporary advertising. *Feminism and Psychology, 18*, 35–60.

Rubin, L. R., Nemeroff, C. J., & Russo, N. F. (2004). Exploring feminist women's body consciousness. *Psychology of Women Quarterly, 28*, 27–37.

Rudman, L. A., & Glick, P. (2008). *The social psychology of gender: How power and intimacy shape gender relations.* New York: Guilford Press.

Sanchez, D. T., Kiefer, A. K., & Ybarra, O. (2006). Sexual submissiveness in women: Costs for sexual autonomy and arousal. *Personality and Social Psychology Bulletin, 32*, 512–524.

Sheffield, C. J. (2007). Sexual terrorism. In L. L. O'Toole, J. R. Shiffman, & M. L. K Edwards (Eds.), *Gender violence: Interdisciplinary perspectives* (2nd ed., pp. 111–130). New York: New York University Press.

Shute, R., Owens, L., & Slee, P. (2008). Everyday victimization of adolescent girls by boys: Sexual harassment, bullying or aggression? *Sex Roles, 58*, 477–489.

Smolak, L., & Murnen, S. K. (2004). A feminist approach to eating disorders. In J. K. Thompson (Ed.), *Handbook of eating disorders and obesity* (pp. 590–605). Hoboken, NJ: John Wiley.

Smolak, L., & Murnen, S. K. (2007). Feminism and body image. In V. Swami, & A. Furnham (Eds.), *The body beautiful* (pp. 236–258). London: Palgrave Macmillan.

Stankiewicz, J. M., & Rosselli, F. (2008). Women as sex objects and victims in print advertisements. *Sex Roles, 58*, 579–589.

Stice, E., Maxfield, J., & Wells, T. (2003). Adverse effects of social pressure to be thin on young women: An experimental investigation of the effects of "fat talk." *International Journal of Eating Disorders, 34*, 108–117.

Swim, J. K., Hyers, L. L., Cohen, L. L., & Ferguson, M. J. (2001). Everyday sexism: Evidence for its incidence, nature, and psychological impact from three daily diary studies. *Journal of Social Issues, 57*, 31–53.

Ward, L. M. (2002). Does television exposure affect emerging adults' attitudes and assumptions about sexual relationships? Correlational and experimental confirmation. *Journal of Youth and Adolescence, 31*, 1–15.

Ward, L. M. (2003). Understanding the role of entertainment media in the sexual socialization of American youth: A review of empirical research. *Developmental Review, 23*, 347–388.

Ward, L. M., & Friedman, K. (2006). Using TV as a guide: Associations between television viewing and adolescents' sexual attitudes and behavior. *Journal of Research on Adolescence, 16*, 133–156.

Worell, J. (2006). Pathways to healthy development: Sources of strength and empowerment. In J. Worell, & C. Goodheart (Eds.), *Handbook of girls' and women's psychological health* (pp. 25–35). Oxford, UK: Oxford University Press.

RESISTANCE, ACTIVISM, AND ALTERNATIVES

PART FIVE

RESISTANCE, ACTIVISM AND
ALTERNATIVES

13

"Not Always a Clear Path"

Making Space for Peers, Adults, and Complexity in Adolescent Girls' Sexual Development

LAINA Y. BAY-CHENG, JENNIFER A. LIVINGSTON, AND

NICOLE M. FAVA

The "madonna/whore" dichotomy has been decried for decades for its narrow and rigid depiction of female sexuality: that a woman is either chaste and good or promiscuous and bad. Despite the fact that changes in gender relations and sexual values challenge the sexist and moralist foundation of these categories, they still exist. Girls continue to contend with dueling messages of sexuality, albeit in updated forms. The moralist (i.e., madonna) sexuality education provided by schools and families has been expanded to idealize not only virtue and purity but also unflagging responsibility and achievement (especially in academic and professional realms). Meanwhile, the sexualized discourse that permeates American popular culture has rebranded the "whore" as a pseudo-liberated, self-determining woman who makes no apologies for her sexual desires or her desirability. The oft-critiqued double bind experienced by girls is perhaps better described as a complicated knot.

The "hyper-responsibility" promoted through sexuality education has been critiqued for relying on fear and misinformation while concealing social inequality (Burns & Torre, 2004; Fields, 2008; Fine & McClelland, 2006), and the current volume clearly exposes the troubling consequences of sexualization. Although these approaches to girls' sexuality may seem diametrically opposed in some ways, and each riddled with their own idiosyncratic problems, they also share common flaws. Both hyper-responsibility and sexualization stem from the cultural value of self-interest and position young women as passive targets of others' visions of an ideal sexuality, be it chaste or promiscuous. In this chapter, we question the real-world applicability of either of these clear-cut prescriptions for young women's sexuality. Drawing on what we have learned through focus group research, we argue that for young women to cultivate positive, healthy sexualities, they require opportunities to move beyond the limits of simplistic representations of female sexuality and to engage in candid discussions of its complexity and ambiguity.

Moralism and Hyper-responsibility

Ideas of female adolescent sexuality—whether presented in sexuality education classrooms or in the popular media—are dominated by the themes of vulnerability and risk. Sexually transmitted infections, unwanted pregnancies, and sexual coercion dominate discussions by researchers, teachers, parents, and the public at large. This is particularly true when conversations are about or aimed at adolescents, who are presumed to be especially at-risk as a result of a volatile combination of raging hormones and cognitive immaturity (Lesko, 1996).

It is almost indisputable that adolescents are disproportionately vulnerable to negative consequences of partnered heterosexual activity, such as infection (Weinstock, Berman, & Cates, 2004) and unintended pregnancy (Finer & Henshaw, 2006), and there is compelling evidence that developmental factors may lead them to be more likely than adults to take risks (Steinberg, 2007). Nevertheless, Americans' preoccupation with adolescent sexual risk often veers away from these public health concerns (and the social norms and conditions that perpetuate them) and extends into moral territory, much of which is grounded in gender norms. For instance, even sexual behavior that is consensual and "safe" (insofar as it involves measures to prevent sexually transmitted infections [STIs] and pregnancy) is often presented as potentially perilous since it might damage a girl's social reputation, a relationship can end in betrayal and heartbreak (which is presumed to be exacerbated if there has been sexual activity), and one might come to regret not saving one's virginity for marriage, or at least for a partner deemed "the one." In fact, cautionary tales about the emotional, social, and moral dangers of adolescent sexual activity are mandated components of federally funded, abstinence-only sexuality education programs, although sexuality education has historically relied on such moralistic, fear-based messages (Fields, 2008; Fine & McClelland, 2006; Moran, 2000).

Although moralism remains a cornerstone of sexuality education, abstinence and safe sex are also often presented as pragmatic matters of self-interest. Appealing to personal ambition, schools and parents urge adolescents to postpone sexual activity lest it distract or detract from one's other pursuits and objectives. The scare tactics employed in secular sexuality education are not primarily concerned with virtue or sin, but instead focus on what it takes to succeed (e.g., grades, extracurricular activities) and how sexuality and relationships can hinder one's ability to compete. Burns and Torre (2004) described the effect of this fear-based emphasis on hyper-responsibility as promoting a sense of "anxious achievement" in which girls, especially those without race and class privilege, are perpetually "reminded of the fragility of their success" (p. 130). Therefore, girls are encouraged to resist sexual temptations in order to maintain and maximize their chances for future academic, professional, and financial success.

We certainly do not dispute the importance of sexual responsibility (i.e., engaging in consensual behaviors and taking precautions to safeguard the well-being of all partners) and accurate, comprehensive sexuality education. Nevertheless, we are wary of a simplistic discussion of personal responsibility that ignores social inequalities (such as those based on gender, class, and race) and how these complicate individual choice and behavior. The abilities to refuse unwanted or unprotected sex, to access reliable contraception and health care, and to advocate for one's sexual interests do not just arise from within an individual; these are enabled or constrained by an array of other interpersonal and social factors. Such complexity is obscured by blanket directives about how girls should conduct themselves sexually and in relationships. Furthermore, responsibility is often idealized as the total avoidance of risk: to be responsible is to absent oneself from settings and interactions that carry any potential danger. This protectionist and perfectionist notion is not only unrealistic, but also denies the possibility that some degree of risk-taking and experimentation is itself positive, growth-promoting, and, in fact, a normal, and perhaps even unavoidable, aspect of adolescent development (Erikson, 1968; Fortenberry, 2003; Graber, Brooks-Gunn, & Galen, 1998; Steinberg, 2007; Tolman & McClelland, 2011).

In keeping with the perspective that some degree of experimentation can lead to positive developmental outcomes, safe (i.e., protected and consensual) sexual activity allows adolescents to gain an understanding of their own sexuality and of how to negotiate sexual relationships (Hensel, Fortenberry, O'Sullivan, & Orr, 2011; Horne & Zimmer-Gembeck, 2005; Rostosky, Dekhtyar, Cupp, & Anderman, 2008). Using cross-sectional data, Horne and Zimmer-Gembeck (2005) found that girls who had engaged in sexual exploration (e.g., self-masturbation, noncoital orgasm, and coitus) achieved several positive gains, including but not limited to more positive views of their sexuality and themselves, an ability to share their opinions with their intimate partners, and less acceptance of societal double standards. In addition, the initiation of coitus prior to age 16 was associated with positive attitudinal outcomes.

These results are bolstered by the findings from Harden and colleagues' (2008) quasi-experimental study of the impact of coital debut and subsequent delinquency. Using a sample of same-sex twins from the National Longitudinal Study of Adolescent Health that allowed them to control for genetic influence and shared environment, Harden et al. found that earlier age of sexual debut did not lead to higher levels of delinquency in early adulthood; instead, they found that within a twin pair, the twin who had initiated coitus earlier demonstrated lower levels of delinquency. In reporting their findings, Harden et al. acknowledge that the bulk of research focused on adolescent sexual activity has found coitus to be associated with negative physical and psychological outcomes. They use the discrepancy between these findings and their own to advocate for more rigorous and nuanced analyses of adolescent sexual behavior. Similarly, we do not discount evidence that adolescent sexual activity can carry serious consequences, especially in the absence of freely given consent, mutual feelings of sexual interest and desire, and protection against infection or pregnancy (Basile et al., 2006; Howard & Wang, 2005; Kilpatrick et al., 2003). However, we feel it is also important to consider findings that challenge the common equation of responsibility with abstinence—and abstinence alone.

Sexualization and Pseudo-Empowerment

In Fine's (1988) analysis of school-based sexuality education, she critiqued its reliance on moralism and fear, as well as the absence of a discourse of desire. As Harris (2005) points out, however, female sexual desire and pleasure can no longer be regarded as "missing" in popular discourse. The rampant availability and growing acceptability of sexually explicit media content and consumer goods are sometimes purported to be evidence of women's sexual liberation. But, as Levy (2006) argues in her critique of "raunch culture," we must not mistake female sexualization for female sexuality. Instead, the performance of sexualized pseudo-empowerment ought to be read as just that: a performance of sexuality, scripted for the pleasure of others, rather than an expression of sexuality, enacted for the pleasure of oneself or in mutual satisfaction with a partner. Moreover, sexualization indentures girls and women to consumerism as they seek to outfit themselves with the costumes and props necessary to play their assigned role (Harris, 2005; Levy, 2006). Far from liberating girls and women from gendered sexual norms, sexualization entrenches them even more deeply as sexual objects rather than as sexual agents. Studies have demonstrated the wide-ranging, detrimental impact of sexualization on girls' health and well-being, including greater depressive symptomatology, body dissatisfaction and eating disorders, and lower self-esteem and academic performance (American Psychological Association, Task Force on the Sexualization of Girls [APA], 2007).

Comments by a participant in a recent qualitative analysis of unwanted sex (i.e., sexual encounters to which one consents but does not want; Bay-Cheng & Eliseo-Arras, 2008) exposed the downside of illusory pseudo-empowerment.

Over the course of an interview, an affluent, white, heterosexual young woman at an elite private university casually described multiple experiences of consenting to unwanted sexual encounters, seeming to regard them as relatively inconsequential. Near the end of the interview, however, she offered the interviewer a different, rawer insight into her experience: "I would come home [after an unwanted sexual experience], actually...I didn't mention this [earlier in the interview], but there were some times I'd come home and I started crying. I was just really upset with what I did." We interpreted the participant's reluctance in acknowledging how troubling her unwanted sexual experiences had been, as well as similar feelings expressed by other participants, as evidence of just how much girls want to appear (to themselves and to others) to be in charge and in control, even when what occurs is something they did not choose or consent to. Sexualization is appealing precisely because it offers girls the cover and façade of individual empowerment: that they are invulnerable, self-determining, and unapologetically self-interested. Although this role, one that is typically reserved for boys and men, has cultural cache and the illusion of power, the evidence presented in the original APA Task Force Report (APA, 2007) and this volume's chapters make it clear how deceptive and ultimately detrimental the pseudo-empowerment of sexualization can be.

Complexity and Ambiguity

Although it is easy to identify a gaping ideological divide between sexuality education's idealization of hyper-responsible "alpha girls" (to borrow Kindlon's [2006] phrase), who are too achievement-oriented to risk their futures on sex, and popular culture's consumerist pretense of young women as carefree sexual players, both tap into dominant cultural values of self-determination and meritocracy. Indeed, at first glance, these ideologies may seem at odds with one another, and yet, both rely on the rhetoric of "girl power" and on notions of girls and women beating boys and men at their own game, whether judged in terms of academic success (e.g., "At Colleges, Women are Leaving Men in the Dust"; Lewin, 2006) or sexual wantonness (Levy, 2006). In the study of unwanted sex cited earlier (Bay-Cheng & Eliseo-Arras, 2008), as well as in a recent set of focus group analyses (Bay-Cheng, Livingston, & Fava, 2011), we have observed young women struggling to cover their vulnerability and distress in an effort to uphold the coinciding, post-feminist expectations of both unfettered achievement and carefree sexuality. In a critical reflection on feminist scholarship regarding adolescent female sexual subjectivity, Lamb (2010) pointed out the potential limitations of and paradoxes within it. She argued that not only within moralistic and sexualized discourses, but also within some feminist discourse of female sexual subjectivity, girls themselves are targeted as sites in need of improvement (whether in terms of moral willpower, sexualized allure, or sexual agency). Feminist critiques of the social construction of adolescent female sexuality and surrounding conditions of inequality have been invaluable to the advancement of scholarship, policy, and practice in the field. Nevertheless, Lamb offers an important warning against the unwitting promotion of yet another unattainable sexual ideal toward which girls are supposed to strive, this one of unfailing agency and authenticity.

All fixed categories, whether the original madonna/whore dichotomy or their modern day equivalents, share the same fundamental flaw: they are equally rigid, narrow, and static and, therefore, equally unrealistic. As noted earlier, sexual activity is not necessarily antithetical to responsibility or positive development, as is often asserted in moralist modes of sexuality education. In addition, studies of the existence and basis of unwanted sex have exposed the multidimensionality of sexual wanting (e.g., someone might want to have a sexual experience for one reason and simultaneously not want to for another; Peterson & Muehlenhard, 2007) and the implausibility of models that presume sexual desire, wanting, and consent to align neatly. Instead, several permutations are possible: a woman might consent to a sexual encounter in the absence of sexual arousal because she wants it for some reasons (though maybe not for others); she might also not consent in spite of desiring and wanting to do so. Sexual interactions are influenced by countless personal (e.g., one's physical, emotional, and cognitive functioning), relational (e.g., with a romantic partner, peers, and parents), and societal factors (e.g., norms and values). Studies of adolescent female sexual experiences shed light on the complexity and ambiguity of sexual interactions, including the coexistence of danger, pleasure, uncertainty, and gratification (Holland, Ramazanoglu, Sharpe, & Thomson, 2004; Muehlenhard & Peterson, 2005; Phillips, 2000; Tolman & Higgins, 1996). Furthermore, Diamond's (2008) research on the fluidity of women's sexual desire disrupts the notion that sexual attraction is fixed and divided simply into the categories of heterosexual or homosexual.

Other calculations and considerations also enter into sexual and relational decision making. In focus groups conducted by Banister and Jakubec (2004), adolescent girls openly discussed the dilemma of breaking up with a boyfriend, noting that ending a relationship might free one from an abusive or emotionally taxing relationship but may also result in being ostracized by friends and a loss in social status. Other research suggests that, for young women with limited access to resources and opportunities, sexuality can be viewed as a strategy for gaining access to resources (Baumeister & Vohs, 2004); as an affordable means of gaining a sense of achievement and validation (Martin, 1996; Travis, Meginnis, & Bardari, 2000); as a refuge from poverty, violence, and neglect in their communities and homes (Bay-Cheng et al., 2011; Brooks-Gunn & Paikoff, 1997); or sometimes as "gravy" to be set aside until more basic needs are met (Burns & Torre, 2004). In light of the damage that can be done by sexualization and the vast complexity of sexuality and relationships, it is critical that simplistic ideals and false dichotomies be eroded.

The multidimensionality and dynamism of sexuality and sexual relationships defy pat categorization or simple models of rational decision making. Dominant approaches to the topic with adolescents, however, persist in pretending otherwise. Whether allied with an abstinence-only or comprehensive agenda, sexuality education is predominantly aimed at the dissemination of knowledge (about biological processes, infection transmission, and prevention tactics) rather than in the provocation of discussion and debate (Allen, 2004; Fields, 2008). Although the transmission of comprehensive, accurate information regarding sexual health is a necessary component of developing healthy sexuality, on its own it is insufficient. Even if conducted through interactive exercises and modules, sexuality education relies on the top-down transfer of facts and instructions from adult experts to youth novices. Similarly, while sexualized depictions of girls and women may be criticized and worried over, there are far fewer opportunities to examine and discuss the appeal and semblance of power conveyed by these characterizations (see Murnen & Smolak, 2013; Chapter 12, this volume). Superficial critiques of sexualization also run the risk of placing blame on girls and women (e.g., for their dress or behavior) and subsequently reinforcing a sexual double standard (Bay-Cheng & Lewis, 2006). Whatever good intentions and best efforts may underlie these attempts at sexuality education, directive, one-size-fits-all prescriptions are disconnected from the complexity of sexuality and interpersonal relationships for all people, young and old.

Although it may seem counterintuitive, we propose supporting girls' sexual health and well-being by making room for their confusion, ambivalence, and contradictions. We view the airing and consideration of these as necessary for the development of critical insight into one's own feelings and behaviors, as well as into the surrounding social world (e.g., gender norms, sexualized media). Alarm regarding the sexual threats posed to girls may be well-placed, but attempts to simply impart knowledge and directives for how to avoid these, without accompanying discussion and contextualization, are often ineffective (see Kirby, 2001, for a review of the effectiveness of various sexuality education models). Likewise, failure to acknowledge adolescents' burgeoning feelings of sexual interest and desire presents an intellectualized and decontextualized view of sexual behavior that is inconsistent with real-life experience. Aside from the well-established gap between knowledge and behavior, simplistic and universal directions for avoiding sexual missteps—however these might be defined—neglect the complexity and ambiguity of gender, sexuality, interpersonal relationships, and the diverse, intersecting conditions of young women's lives. Positive, healthy sexuality is not something that can be instilled in or delivered to girls; it is something that they cultivate and produce for themselves over the course of education, experience, contemplation, and conversation.

In her contribution to this volume, Lamb calls for a more relational perspective on healthy adolescent female sexuality, one that prioritizes mutuality and negotiation between sexual partners. To this, we would like to add the value of expanding conversations and exchanges about sexuality beyond the sexual dyad to include peers and adults. In a special issue of *Feminism & Psychology* dedicated to Fine's (1988) original observation of the "missing discourse of desire," Harris (2005) revisited the need for "safe spaces" in which girls "engage in unregulated dialogue and debate with one another" (p. 42) about their personal experiences, as well as about broader social forces related to sexuality. Such safe spaces should not be sanitized or censored such that the only permissible voice is one of unwavering self-assurance and entitlement; rather, they must be able to accommodate, and treat as legitimate, the ambivalence and uncertainty that are often either left out of discussions about sexuality or used to mark girls as incompetent. Girls must feel confident that their candor will not be minimized, dismissed, or used against them.

We base our recommendation for the creation of such safe spaces on a series of recent focus groups with adolescent girls. Although the groups were originally conceived as a preliminary step in a larger research program led by the second author regarding sexual risk and substance use, they also served an unintentional but critical purpose: the opportunity for the participants to express and exchange their views and experiences. Specifically, we were struck by instances in which the participants disputed the simplistic information and advice they were given by adults regarding sexuality and by their occasional willingness to admit their own ambivalence and uncertainty about how to navigate sexual relationships. In addition, participants described wishing that they had adults with whom they could engage in conversations about sexuality without fear of negative consequence (e.g., judgment or punishment). These adolescents were struggling to construct their own understanding of sexuality and were frustrated by the inadequacy of the resources available to them. We view these conversations and comments as evidence of how safe spaces might be developed through peer communication among adolescent girls about the complexity of their sexual and relational lives; and through evocative, rather than directive, relationships between women and girls.

Study Overview

A total of seven adolescent focus groups were conducted with 43 adolescent girls between the ages of 14 and 17 years. Participants were on average 15 years old (*SD* = 1.19), predominantly European American (68%), and living with two parents (57%). The median household income was between $40,000 and $54,900, consistent with the median income for the county from which the sample was recruited, and 40% of participants' mothers had obtained a college degree. The sample was recruited through newspaper advertisements in Erie County, New York. Eligibility requirements consisted of age (14–17 years old) and residence with a mother. Parental consent and adolescent assent were obtained before focus group participation. Focus groups were organized based on the girls' ages (14–15; 16–17). Each group consisted of 4–11 participants (*Mode* = 5). Discussions lasted about 1.5 hours, were audio recorded and then transcribed. Participants were compensated $25 for their time. All groups were led by the second author, a European American woman, with a background in educational psychology, whose work has focused on adolescent substance use and the causes and prevention of sexual aggression perpetrated against young women and adolescent girls. A more detailed discussion of the procedures of this study is available in Bay-Cheng et al. (2011).

Several steps were taken in an endeavor to establish rapport with participants and foster an open, nonjudgmental atmosphere for the group (see Krueger & Casey, 2000). The ground rules were presented at the outset of the discussion and included: (a) treating all members of the group with respect; (b) acknowledging that there will be a diversity of opinions expressed throughout the discussion, and that each person's opinion is valid; (c) having only one person speak at a time; (d) treating everything discussed in the group as confidential, not to be shared outside of the group; (e) stating that everyone's participation is encouraged, though not required; (f) no one should reveal private, sensitive information about themselves or their experiences; and importantly, (g) assuring all that there is no need to come to a group consensus on any topic. To further promote participation by all group members, the facilitator employed several of the moderation strategies recommended by Krueger and Casey (2000), including use of innocuous round-table ice breakers to open the discussion. These techniques were reasonably effective; in all of the sessions, every group member contributed to the group discussion at some point.

The aim of the interviews was to gain insight into the ways in which adolescent girls reconcile the conflicting messages they receive about sex: that its risks are ubiquitous, but that girls are expected to present, through their dress, attitude, and behavior, in highly sexualized ways. Some of the key questions that were asked of all the groups included: What concerns do girls have about having sex? About not having sex? What have you been told about sex from your school? How useful was this information? What information do girls your age wish they had, that they are not getting? (see Bay-Cheng et al. [2011] for a complete list of focus group questions). These questions were raised to stimulate conversations about dating, sexual behavior, and sexual risks between the girls in the focus groups and to elicit their personal perspectives. Sexual risk was not formally defined by the interviewer; rather, participants were asked to describe what concerns girls had about being sexually active. The phrasing of the initial questions did not specify heterosexual relationships as a point of interest. Although this technically left open the opportunity for participants to consider same-gender relationships and risks, the groups' conversations focused exclusively on heterosexual interactions. As a result, any conclusions drawn from these data refer only to heterosexual interactions and risks.

Results and Discussion

Our proposal that safe spaces be developed through peer communication and evocative relationships is based on inductive analyses of the focus group transcripts. The first principle, focused on the importance of peer communication, emerged in previous analyses, in which we noted instances of participants challenging each other and dominant scripts (Bay-Cheng et al., 2011). The second, regarding the participants' desire for evocative relationships with adults, especially women, was articulated in response to a particular set of questions in the interview protocol. In both of the following sections, we enlist these focus group data to illustrate and substantiate our recommendations.

Peer Communication

Over the course of the focus group conversations, participants repeatedly referred to the risks of sexuality while also arguing that these risks were avoidable given the right constellation of personal qualities and values (Bay-Cheng et al., 2011). Participants criticized girls who suffered negative sexual consequences (e.g., pregnancy, infection, coercion) as inept in some regard and simultaneously distanced themselves from risk by proclaiming their own maturity, goal-directedness, and responsibility. The common attribution of negative experiences to character flaws and poor judgment allowed the girls to assert their own superiority and invulnerability. In doing so, participants cast themselves as hyper-responsible: too clear-headed, self-directed, and high-achieving to put themselves or their futures on the line, particularly for the sake of a boy. As one participant stated:

> Yeah, like, there are so many things I want to do, like, scholarship applications, college applications, and I want to do this musical composition contest. So, now I'm going to be working on that and school musicals. It's just like I wouldn't have time to spend, time to dedicate to, like, a boyfriend.

Participants also invoked many common refrains and value positions regarding adolescent sexuality: "I think, while you're still a teenager, you're still too young [to engage in coitus]. In my opinion"; "I think you should save yourself for marriage"; and "it [coitus] shouldn't be after, like, two weeks [as a couple]. It should be, like, a year, two years, three years. You should trust him enough." Girls also mentioned strategies they could employ to deter unwanted sexual advances. These included, "say 'no,'" have friends "watch your back," and "try screaming really loudly, so someone that's maybe walking by or hears it goes to see what's going on, or use self-defense."

In each of the groups, however, there were also instances in which individual girls or the conversation belied the self-assurance and clarity inherent in these statements. For instance, contrary to several participants' insistence that they were unwilling to subordinate their own interests to those of their male partners, there were times when participants acknowledged feeling drawn to do so. In one group, girls discussed how to respond to sexual pressure from a boy. Although the conversation began with two participants taking strong positions about what they would do, this initial certainty soon dissolved as participants weighed how contextual factors (e.g., the boyfriend's approach and the seriousness of the relationship) could complicate what the "right" response would be:

Interviewer: How comfortable are girls responding to that pressure [to have sex]?

Participant 1: I would pour a drink on him or stop him, or something. Like, "Are you crazy?!"

Interviewer: But, what if it's a boyfriend?

Participant 1: Break up with him.

Participant 2: Depends on how they bring it up....

Participant 3: Or maybe I might talk to him.

Participant 1: Like, if they're like, "We have to do this." Then it's like, "No."

Participant 2: It depends on how serious you are.

Participant 1: ... If it's like, "I want to talk about this." Then it's like ...

Participant 2: Yeah. If you've been going out for, like, a year, I don't think...I don't know.

Participant 3: ... Yeah.

In this same group, participants also suggested including content in school-based sexuality education on "[h]ow to say, 'No' [to an unwanted sexual interaction] in a way that, like, if you actually really do like the guy, like, not so that he would break up with you." A participant in another group also described the challenge in balancing one's interest (or lack thereof) in a sexual interaction with one's interest in preserving or developing a relationship with a boy:

> You can be really into a guy, and if he doesn't like you, or if he likes you but he just wants to have sex with you, and you say "No," then he's gonna be upset or something. Then it's like, now you're like, "No, I like you," and now you're you know, you want to do it now just because he's not gonna like you, so. I don't know, it's kinda hard.

These excerpts exemplify the competing interests and desires that comprise sexuality and relationships. Although it is concerning that anyone, regardless of age or gender, feels compelled to consent to unwanted sex in an effort to preserve a relationship, it is also important to recognize that this is a commonplace occurrence: studies indicate that more than half of college women have consented to unwanted sex (Crown & Roberts, 2007; O'Sullivan & Allgeier, 1998). Moreover, as the participants in an earlier example suggested, the benefits and costs of sexual and relational compromises can vary depending on contextual factors (Impett, Gable, & Peplau, 2005; O'Sullivan & Allgeier, 1998).

Despite how complicated and context-dependent relational negotiations are, the advice issued by adult authorities (e.g., parents and schools) rarely accommodates this complexity. At different points, participants objected to the directives and certainties often imparted by adults and each other. For example, although the dominant, explicitly articulated stance across groups was that abstinence until marriage was ideal, that adolescent pregnancy could be disastrous, and that girls who were assertive enough could withstand sexual coercion, these absolutes were also contested at different points as unrealistic. Participants offered a more nuanced view of when and in what contexts sex should occur, with one girl disputing the notion of the "right age" to start having sex: "There's a lot of ages that's too young, but I don't know what the right age is. Like, I can't say because people got different life stories, so." In another group, one participant countered others' automatic disapproval of sex outside the context of a romantic relationship:

> Um. I agree with them on the context of a one night stand, that, that's never acceptable, like, if you just met somebody that night and had sex with them. That's never acceptable. But, like, there's a difference between knowing somebody and just meeting them that night. Sex is not always completely, like, one hundred percent wrong at all times. That's what I'm trying to say.

With regard to pregnancy, a participant ventured to suggest that it might not be unequivocally negative by telling others about a 15-year-old mother she knew: "She's happy she has a baby. So, it depends on who the girl is." And, as a final example of how girls occasionally took issue with the simplistic and unrealistic messages they received, one participant pointedly dispelled the blanket utility of just saying "no," a common refrain in the girls' sexuality education:

> But, like, I mean, if you say "no" a guy's not just gonna be like…I mean, if that were the case, that a guy would believe "no" then there wouldn't be those rapes that you hear about. There wouldn't be all that stuff. Obviously "no" doesn't mean "no" to guys.

These admissions of ambiguity and complexity provoked further discussions of just how vexing sexuality could be. One participant described the Catch-22 position of girls trying to avoid rumors that might ensue if they consent to sex (e.g., being seen as promiscuous) or if they do not (e.g., being seen as a prude): "So, it's like stuck between a rock and a hard place about what to do. There's not always, like, a clear path." Such acknowledgments represented meaningful deviations from the script of invulnerability (given the right qualities) that otherwise dominated group discourse. As McClelland and Fine (2008) observed in their own focus group research, after a period of what they referred to as "discursive foreplay" (p. 239), conversations within a group gradually and intermittently opened up to diverse topics, experiences, and perspectives. The airing of difference and complexity is an important step toward dissolving shame and validating experience, although it may also be a rare opportunity for adolescent girls who are typically regarded as targets of information, not sources of insight. We do not dispute that adults have an important role to play in helping younger generations navigate and think through the complexities of sexuality and relationships; however, participants in our focus groups and data from other sources suggest that a revision of conventional modes of adult–youth interaction is in order.

Evocative Relationships

During the interviews, several questions were posed to each focus group about what sort of sexuality education they had received from their families and schools and what information girls their age wish they had but are not getting. In response to these questions, participants described schools' reliance on medical facts (e.g., "I got the whole baby thing, and I got why not to have sex, like, all the diseases and what are they, and then basically our teacher showed us how to use a condom. So, I mean, that's about it."), simple directives (e.g., "They just say, 'Use protection.'"), and scare tactics (e.g., "Really more about the bad of it, kind of like to get you to stay abstinent. They try, like, to scare you not to have sex."). They also expressed feeling uncomfortable and constrained when confiding in teachers:

> I mean, sometimes I think it's helpful that you talk to your health teacher, but sometimes it's uncomfortable. You don't want to talk to

your teachers about stuff like that. I mean, that's their job to teach you the consequences and stuff about it, but sometimes it's uncomfortable. 'Cause you want to really, like, get information, you want to really know, and you want to really tell them or really ask questions, and then it's just uncomfortable.

In addition, participants doubted that parents could be relied on to reserve judgment or provide full information. One participant noted that parents "try to shelter people, and that's the worst thing to do, not to tell you. It would be better for them to just tell you what's going to happen or how to be safe if you do it, instead of just not telling you at all." Another participant stated, "It's like your mom's like, 'Don't have sex 'til you're married. It's better that way.'" Many participants described parents taking such positions, but these seemed to lack merit for the girls because parents did not provide explanations or engage in discussion beyond such declarations. This left the impression that most parents were motivated by their own agenda (i.e., to discourage sexual activity) and therefore could not be counted on for open exchange. As one participant commented, parents "have one, just, narrow mind on that subject, 'cause they don't want their little daughters, you know, their little babies, having sex and stuff." Participants also felt that parents were out of touch with or did not take seriously the challenges of girls' lives:

Adults think that being young now is easy and, like, we shouldn't be stressed out, and we're not facing this serious…Like, my dad thinks being young is easy. I'm applying for college. I'm fighting off, like, all these different influences and, like, being young now is a lot different than just being young ten years ago. You're exposed to a lot of different pressure. And, like, academically, physically, and a lot of girls are developing faster. Like, I know that I did. And, like, when I was twelve I had, like, seventeen year old guys coming up to me, like, "You want to get in my car?"

This participant continued by describing which people and places she found informative and validating:

That's how I learned how to fend off, like, 'cause my cousin was right behind me, like, "No, we don't want to get in your car!" It's a lot if you have that support network. Like, you need a variety of different tools when you have to educate someone about how…And, like, open dialogue like this [the focus group] is perfect. Like, if you just have girls and you sit them down and be like, "Let's talk about what it feels like to be a girl."

Other participants also valued conversations and support from same-aged or slightly older individuals, "because they're more likely to listen. You're like, 'Oh. Hey. You live now. You're my age. You know what's going on.'" Cousins, older siblings, and aunts were among those named as people adolescent girls could count on for guidance and practical assistance:

> Then I have those few aunts that say, "You can come to me if you need help or anything. If you ever go to a party and you just want to get out of there, I can come pick you up. I won't say anything." 'Cause, like, they have that, they're not your parents, but they're still your family. They're still looking out for you, but they're not gonna be as strict. So, like, you can talk to them and stuff, and they're not just gonna go run out to your parents and stuff. So, I think you just have to have that level of trust, or that relationship, with some other family member that you can just go to them if you need to, if there's no one else to go to, so you don't feel completely alone. I wouldn't think I'd ever be able to go to my mom or my parents about this stuff, definitely not, but with an aunt I could.

We identify in these excerpts girls' wishes not just for information but also for conversation and exchange with adults who are knowledgeable without being dismissive or judgmental. Their frustrations and suggestions call for a move away from protectionist, condescending modes of interaction between adults and youth in which the latter are presumed to be deficient (Fields, 2008) and expected to be passive. It is worth noting the irony that conventional, "adultist" dynamics in sexuality education—whether in schools or families—cast girls in precisely the same role that is argued to jeopardize their sexual well-being in the first place (Gavey, 2005; Slater, Guthrie, & Boyd, 2001): that of passive recipient. In contrast, feminist literature on mentorship and cross-generational ties proposes the value of "relational hardiness zones" in which adult women forge authentic, supportive relationships with adolescent girls (Brown, 2003; Debold, Brown, Weseen, & Brookins, 1999; for specific guidance on how to foster such relationships, see the website for the "Hardy Girls Healthy Women" initiative, http://hghw.org/index.php). Sullivan (1996) urged adult women to cultivate *evocative*, rather than directive or didactic, relationships with adolescent girls. Such relationships are not predicated solely on the transmission of knowledge from an adult to an adolescent. Instead, they operate from the premise that youth already possess the capacity for knowledge, wisdom, resilience, and critical thinking; the relationship serves as a platform for that potential to be realized. Bannister and Leadbeater (2007) also pointed out that such evocative relationships also present adolescent girls with models of and practice in relationships built on mutual respect and regard, qualities that they might then be better able to replicate in their romantic and sexual relationships.

An emphasis on the capacity of individuals—young and old—for careful, critical thinking about complex issues does not presuppose that those same individuals have the right answers, or any answers at all. Admissions of confusion and ignorance, especially if combined with the perspective and input of a supportive other, can stimulate an evolving process of critical reflection on one's self, relationships, and surrounding social conditions. In contrast, relationships founded on the reception and recitation of correct answers can inhibit critical thinking and discussion as girls simply parrot back what they have been told. Whether they do so out of disengagement or a desire to please, the result is the same: a missed opportunity to exercise the skills needed to negotiate the lifelong complexity and ambiguity of sexual and romantic relationships.

The cultivation of evocative relationships with girls is not simply a new tactic for engaging and winning over youth; rather, it represents a significant shift in our orientation toward adolescents and adult authority. The dominant characterization of adolescence and adolescent sexuality (at least in the United States; see Schalet [2011] for a cultural comparison) as inherently dangerous, irresponsible, and impulsive is often invoked as justification for adults' surveillance of and attempts at restricting youth sexuality (Lesko, 1996). Whether perceived as menacing or vulnerable—a depiction that often hinges on race, class, and sexual orientation (Fields, 2008; Tolman, 1996)—adolescent girls are commonly seen as "[l]acking the capacity psychologically or physically to manage the pressure, expectations, and attention that are heaped upon their sexually developing bodies" (McClelland & Fine, 2008, p. 236). Evocative relationships between adolescent girls and adults contest the fundamental presumptions of adolescent deficiency and adult superiority.

Inherent in these recommendations for both freer peer communication among young women and the development of evocative relationships between adult and adolescent women is a call for adults to hold back from imposing our authority or views. We do not mean to take a naïve stance regarding the value of adults' life experiences and accumulated wisdom, nor are we encouraging adults to abdicate our ethical obligation to bring that wisdom to bear in supporting youth. Instead, we suggest that adults make available our own experiences and also allow young women opportunities to explore, express, and experiment for themselves, with the hope that, in doing so, they will strengthen their own skills, strategies, and insights. All of us, when learning new skills, need opportunities to try out and exercise them for ourselves. Infants do not learn to transition from sitting to crawling by having a caregiver position their bodies for them each time they indicate the urge to move. Watching an infant struggle to manipulate her body to reach a desired object can be difficult: it takes so long, can be so frustrating (for her and for onlookers), and might result in a few falls and bumps. But it is only through these efforts, as inefficient and clumsy as they may be, that skills are mastered and autonomy can be achieved. Just as a caregiver must resist the urge to help too much (and thereby thwart a child's development and ability to manage frustration), adults must hold their tongues—and most especially their judgment—and relinquish some control when it comes to youths' negotiation of sexuality. In a study of youths' use of electronic bulletin boards to discuss sexuality, Bay-Cheng (2005) found that, given time and opportunity, adolescents demonstrated the ability to debate complicated issues, to respect differing values and views, and to correct each other's misconceptions or misinformation about sexual health and responsibility. Although an adult moderator might have stepped in sooner, doing so would have not only forestalled adolescent discussants' self-expression but also deprived them of the opportunity to practice skills of critical thinking and dialogue.

However, we also do not mean to understate the prevalence of sexual risks or the severity of their fallout, particularly for young women. Reducing the rates of infection, unwanted pregnancy, and coercion are rightfully identified as critical objectives for safeguarding the health and well-being of young women. We understand that it may seem unconscionable to abide youth sexual experimentation when the stakes are so great. Yet, we also maintain that some degree of sexual and relational experimentation and engagement among youth is to be both expected and accepted as normal and necessary. Therefore, we recommend that well-meaning adults channel our protectionist urges not into restricting adolescent girls' sexuality but into reducing the magnitude of the dangers associated with it. We propose that adults accomplish this by combating social (e.g., sexism, racism, homophobia) and economic inequalities and by advocating for more comprehensive and accessible services. To return to the analogy of the infant child, if crawling is unsafe because the floor is dirty or littered with broken glass, the appropriate response is not to confine and restrict the child from crawling, but to clean up the mess. In his review of findings regarding adolescent neurological development, Steinberg (2007) argues that since risk-taking may be a normal, expected part of adolescent development, adults should focus on providing youth with the safest possible contexts and safety nets for their exploration of potentially risky domains (e.g., providing access to condoms and contraception). Similarly, we propose that young women may be best served by adults who are available for counsel and who can help enable youth dialogues, but who also work to promote social conditions that allow youth to take up and hone the skills required for lifelong sexual and relational well-being.

Conclusion

Judging from its proliferation in our popular and news media, there can be little doubt of the cultural significance and centrality of adolescent sexuality. Unfortunately, whether erring on the side of hyper-responsibility, as most modes of sexuality education are wont to do, or pseudo-empowerment, as sexualization pretends to be, our discourse of adolescent female sexuality is sorely lacking in nuance, realism, and the voices of adolescent girls themselves. As an alternative to these simplistic and top-down (i.e., adult-down) renditions of adolescent female sexuality, we recommend the cultivation of safe spaces in which adolescent girls are free to engage in open, candid discussion and debate with one another and with adults to construct their own individual views of sexuality and form a basis for making sexual decisions. This proposal is not a prescription for ensuring that adolescent girls perfect their sexual decision-making skills and avert all related risks. Rather than approach adolescent girls as objects to be shaped and directed, we recommend that adults rework our understanding of adolescent girls and our power in relation to them such that we honor their subjectivity and rights: to their own perspectives and opinions; to experimentation and exploration, which are the keys to innovation and mastery (Horne & Zimmer-Gembeck, 2005; Rostosky et al., 2008); and to ambivalence and confusion. In addition to a shift in our view of adolescents and adult authority, we advocate for a redefinition of positive and healthy sexuality among adolescent girls. Rather than an achieved state with specific features and criteria (e.g., the absence of sexual risk-taking), it can be viewed as a dynamic and subjective capacity to consider, examine, and weigh all of the factors and angles of sexuality and related life domains, and as one that fluctuates in concert with one's changing relational, developmental, social, and material life circumstances. Given how complex and changeable sexuality can be (and as many adults personally know it to be), it is unreasonable, unrealistic, and disingenuous to define positive, healthy sexuality as easy, simple, or flawless. Positive, healthy sexuality is also not a matter of young women parroting platitudes and living out the vision of sexuality that others deliver. Instead, we call for a dedication of efforts to the creation of spaces in which girls are safe to express confusion, ambivalence, and disagreement (including with adults) without fear of being judged or typecast, whether as a madonna or a whore.

Acknowledgments

This research was supported by grant K01 AA15033 from the National Institute of Alcohol Abuse and Alcoholism, awarded to Jennifer A. Livingston. We wish to thank Janelle Baker, Florence Leong, Margalit Post, and Maria Testa for their assistance with recruitment, interviewing, and transcribing. Portions of this chapter were previously presented at the American Psychological Association Annual Conventions in Boston (August, 2008) and Toronto (August, 2009).

References

Allen, L. (2004). Beyond the birds and the bees: Constituting a discourse of erotics in sexuality education. *Gender and Education, 16,* 151–167.

American Psychological Association (APA) Task Force on the Sexualization of Girls. (2007). *Report of the APA task force on the sexualization of girls.* Washington, DC: American Psychological Association.

Banister, E., & Jakubec, S. (2004). "I'm stuck as far as relationships go": Dilemmas of voice in girls' dating relationships. *Child & Youth Services, 26,* 33–52.

Bannister, E., & Leadbeater, B. J. R. (2007). To stay or to leave? How do mentoring groups support healthy dating relationships in high-risk girls? In B. J. R. Leadbeater, & N. Way (Eds.), *Urban girls revisited: Building strengths* (pp. 121–141). New York: NYU Press.

Basile, K. C., Black, M. C., Simon, T. R., Arias, I., Brener, N. D., & Saltzman, L.E. (2006). The association between self-reported lifetime history of forced sexual intercourse and recent health-risk behaviors: Findings from the 2003 National Youth Risk Behavior Survey. *Journal of Adolescent Health, 39*(5), 752.e1–752.e7.

Baumeister, R. F., & Vohs, K. D. (2004). Sexual economics: Sex as female resource for social exchange in heterosexual interactions. *Personality and Social Psychology Review, 8,* 339–363.

Bay-Cheng, L. Y. (2005). Left to their own devices: Disciplining youth discourse on sexuality education electronic bulletin boards. *Sexuality Research and Social Policy, 2,* 37–50.

Bay-Cheng, L. Y., & Eliseo-Arras, R. K. (2008). The making of unwanted sex: Gendered and neoliberal norms in college women's unwanted sexual experiences. *Journal of Sex Research, 45,* 386–397.

Bay-Cheng, L. Y., & Lewis, A. E. (2006). Our "ideal girl": Prescriptions of female adolescent sexuality in a feminist mentorship program. *Affilia, 21,* 71–83.

Bay-Cheng, L. Y., Livingston, J. A., & Fava, N. M. (2011). Adolescent girls' sexual risk assessment and management. *Youth & Society, 43,* 1167–1193.

Brooks-Gunn, J., & Paikoff, R. (1997). Sexuality and developmental transitions during adolescence. In J. Schulenberg, J. L. Maggs, & K. Hurrelmann (Eds.), *Health risks and developmental transitions during adolescence* (pp. 190–219). New York: Cambridge University Press.

Brown, L. M. (2003). *Girlfighting: Betrayal and rejection among girls.* New York: NYU Press.

Burns, A., & Torre, M. E. (2004). Shifting desires: Discourses of accountability in abstinence-only education in the United States. In A. Harris (Ed.), *All about the girl: Culture, power, and identity* (pp. 127–137). New York: Routledge.

Crown, L., & Roberts, L. J. (2007). Against their will: Young women's nonagentic sexual experiences. *Journal of Social and Personal Relationships, 24,* 385–405.

Debold, E., Brown, L. M., Weseen, S., & Brookins, G. K. (1999). Cultivating relational hardiness zones for adolescent girls: A reconceptualization of resilience in relationships with caring adults. In N. G. Johnson, M. C. Roberts, & J. Worell (Eds.), *Beyond appearance: A new look at adolescent girls* (pp. 181–204). Washington, DC: American Psychological Association.

Diamond, L. M. (2008). *Sexual fluidity: Understanding women's love and desire.* Cambridge, MA: Harvard University Press.

Erikson, E. H. (1968). *Identity: Youth and crisis.* New York: Norton.

Fields, J. (2008). *Risky lessons: Sex education and social inequality*. New Brunswick, NJ: Rutgers University Press.

Fine, M. (1988). Sexuality, schooling, and adolescent females: The missing discourse of desire. *Harvard Educational Review, 58*, 29–53.

Fine, M., & McClelland, S. I. (2006). Sexuality education and the discourse of desire: Still missing after all these years. *Harvard Educational Review, 76*, 297–338.

Finer, L. B., & Henshaw, S. K. (2006). Disparities in rates of unintended pregnancy in the United States, 1994 and 2001. *Perspectives on Sexual and Reproductive Health, 38*, 90–96.

Fortenberry, J. D. (2003). Adolescent sex and the rhetoric of risk. In D. Romer (Ed.), *Reducing adolescent risk: Toward an integrated approach* (pp. 293–300). Thousand Oaks, CA: Sage.

Gavey, N. (2005). *Just sex? The cultural scaffolding of rape*. New York: Routledge.

Graber, J. A., Brooks-Gunn, J., & Galen, B. R. (1998). Betwixt and between: Sexuality in the context of adolescent transitions. In R. Jessor (Ed.), *New perspectives on adolescent risk behavior* (pp. 270–316). Cambridge, UK: Cambridge University Press.

Harden, K. P., Mendle, J., Hill, J. E., Turkheimer, E., & Emery, R. E. (2008). Rethinking timing of first sex and delinquency. *Journal of Youth and Adolescence, 37*, 373–385.

Harris, A. (2005). Discourses of desire as governmentality: Young women, sexuality and the significance of safe spaces. *Feminism & Psychology, 15*, 39–43.

Hensel, D. J., Fortenberry, J. D., O'Sullivan, L. F., & Orr, D. P. (2011). The developmental association of sexual self-concept with sexual behavior among adolescent women. *Journal of Adolescence, 34*, 675–684.

Holland, J., Ramazanoglu, C., Sharpe, S., & Thomson, R. (2004). *The male in the head: Young people, heterosexuality, and power*. London: Tufnell Press.

Horne, S., & Zimmer-Gembeck, M. J. (2005). Female sexual subjectivity and well-being: Comparing late adolescents with different sexual experiences. *Sexuality Research and Social Policy, 2*, 25–40.

Howard, D. E., & Wang, M. Q. (2005). Psychosocial correlates of U.S. adolescents who report a history of forced sexual intercourse. *Journal of Adolescent Health, 36*, 372–379.

Impett, E., A., Gable, S. L., & Peplau, L. A. (2005). Giving up and giving in: The costs and benefits of daily sacrifice in intimate relationships. *Journal of Personality and Social Psychology, 89*, 327–344.

Kilpatrick, D. G., Ruggiero, K. J., Acierno, R., Saunders, B. E., Resnick, H. S., & Best, C. L. (2003). Violence and risk of PTSD, major depression, substance abuse/dependence, and comorbidity: Results from the National Survey of Adolescents. *Journal of Consulting and Clinical Psychology, 71*, 692–700.

Kindlon, D. (2006). *Alpha girls: Understanding the new American girl and how she is changing the world*. New York: Rodale.

Kirby, D. (2001). *Emerging answers: Research findings on programs to reduce teen pregnancy*. Washington, DC: National Campaign to Prevent Teen Pregnancy.

Krueger, R., & Casey, M. A. (2000). *Focus groups: A practical guide for applied research*. Thousand Oaks, CA: Sage.

Lamb, S. (2010). Feminist ideals for a healthy female adolescent sexuality: A critique. *Sex Roles, 62*, 294-306.

Lesko, N. (1996). Denaturalizing adolescence: The politics of contemporary representations. *Youth and Society, 28*, 139–161.

Levy, A. (2006). *Female chauvinist pigs: Women and the rise of raunch culture*. New York: Free Press.

Lewin, T. (2006, July 9). At colleges, women are leaving men in the dust. *New York Times*. Retrieved March 27, 2009, from http://www.nytimes.com/2006/07/09/education/09college.html

Martin, K. A. (1996). *Puberty, sexuality, and the self*. New York: Routledge.

McClelland S. I., & Fine, M. (2008). Writing on cellophane: Studying teen women's sexual desires, inventing methodological release points. In K. Gallagher (Ed.), *The methodological dilemma: Critical and creative approaches to qualitative research* (pp. 232–260). London: Routledge.

Moran, J. P. (2000). *Teaching sex: The shaping of adolescence in the 20th century.* Cambridge, MA: Harvard University Press.

Muehlenhard, C. L., & Peterson, Z. D. (2005). Wanting and not wanting sex: The missing discourse of ambivalence. *Feminism and Psychology, 15,* 15–20.

Murnen, S. K., & Smolak, L. (2013). "I'd rather be a famous fashion model than a famous scientist": The rewards and costs of internalizing sexualization. In E. L. Zurbriggen & T.- A. Roberts (Eds.), *The sexualization of girls and girlhood: Causes, consequences, and resistance* (Chapter 12). New York: Oxford University Press.

O'Sullivan, L. F., & Allgeier, E. R. (1998). Feigning sexual desire: Consenting to unwanted sexual activity in heterosexual dating relationships. *Journal of Sex Research, 35,* 234–243.

Peterson, Z. D., & Muehlenhard, C. L. (2007). Conceptualizing the "wantedness" of women's consensual and nonconsensual sexual experiences: Implications for how women label their experiences with rape. *Journal of Sex Research, 44,* 72–88.

Phillips, L. M. (2000). *Flirting with danger: Young women's reflections on sexuality and domination.* New York: NYU Press.

Rostosky, S. S., Dekhtyar, O., Cupp, P. K., & Anderman, E. M. (2008). Sexual self-concept and sexual self-efficacy in adolescents: A possible clue to promoting sexual health? *Journal of Sex Research, 45,* 277–286.

Schalet, A. T. (2011). *Not under my roof: Parents, teens, and the culture of sex.* Chicago: University of Chicago Press.

Slater, J. M., Guthrie, B. J., & Boyd, C. J. (2001). A feminist theoretical approach to understanding health of adolescent females. *Journal of Adolescent Health, 28,* 443–449.

Steinberg, L. (2007). Risk taking in adolescence: New perspectives from brain and behavioral science. *Current Directions in Psychological Science, 16,* 55–59.

Sullivan, A. M. (1996). From mentor to muse: Recasting the role of women in relationship with urban adolescent girls. In B. J. R. Leadbeater, & N. Way (Eds.), *Urban girls: Resisting stereotypes, creating identities* (pp. 226–249). New York: NYU Press.

Tolman, D. L. (1996). Adolescent girls' sexuality: Debunking the myth of The Urban Girl. In B. Leadbeater, & N. Way (Eds.), *Urban girls: Resisting stereotypes, creating identities* (pp. 255–271). New York: NYU Press.

Tolman, D. L., & Higgins, T. E. (1996). How being a good girl can be bad for girls. In N. B. Maglin, & D. Perry (Eds.), *Women, sex, and power in the nineties* (pp. 205–225). New Brunswick, NJ: Rutgers University Press.

Tolman, D. L., & McClelland, S. I. (2011). Normative sexuality development in adolescence: A decade in review, 2000–2009. *Journal of Research on Adolescence, 21,* 242–255.

Travis, C. B., Meginnis, K. L., & Bardari, K. M. (2000). Beauty, sexuality, and identity: The social control of women. In C. B. Travis, & J. W. White (Eds.), *Sexuality, society, and feminism* (pp. 237–272). Washington, DC: American Psychological Association.

Weinstock, H., Berman, S., & Cates, Jr., W. (2004). Sexually transmitted diseases among American youth: Incidence and prevalence estimates, 2000. *Perspectives on Sexual and Reproductive Health, 36,* 6–10.

14

Toward a Healthy Sexuality for Girls and Young Women

A Critique of Desire

SHARON LAMB

The charge of the American Psychological Association (APA) Task Force on the Sexualization of Girls (TFSG) was to define sexualization, determine how present it is in the lives of girls, and to examine the evidence that suggests that it may be harmful (APA, 2007). Thus, the TGSG began with a hunch that sexualization and the kind of sexuality presented through sexualization in society, by the media, and in marketing are harmful to girls. This focus also begged the question of healthy sexuality, because defining unhealthy sexuality necessarily has implications for the definition of healthy sexuality. Within the report, the authors made a number of suggestions with regard to healthy sexuality, in particular for adolescent and preadolescent girls. These suggestions were based on psychological research and clinical practice, in addition to feminist theory that has advocated for a sex education that acknowledged female desire. The recommendations were made as antidotes to the rampant sexualization of women that young and adolescent girls are exposed to and which must affect their developing sexuality, broadly defined.

Defining healthy sexuality for adolescent girls in particular was and still is an important goal of such projects like that of the TFSG, given that becoming a "sexual person" remains a task of adolescence in U.S. culture (Sigelman & Rider, 2009). For young girls, it is clear that sexualization is harmful because premature exposure to sexual material is inappropriate and because young girls are presumed to be particularly vulnerable, according to current theories (APA, 2007; Brown, 2003; Duits & van Zoonen, 2007; Levin & Kilbourne, 2008). Adolescent girls, however, are appropriately interested in sexual material and are introduced to such material via their peer culture, media, and other cultural sources in ways that may be both helpful and problematic but that also acknowledge that they are developing sexual attitudes, feelings, and behaviors. The way that adolescents become sexual in this culture is informed by the options available in the world around them (APA, 2007). The TFSG report emphasized that these options are limited, narrowly defining sexual as looking sexy and physically attractive according to a narrow, unrealistic standard.

This chapter looks at how healthy sexuality is currently defined and discussed, where these notions came from, and what additional or alternative views of healthy sexuality might be developed. To do so, I examine first the version of healthy sexuality that is suggested by comprehensive sex education (CSE) advocates, in opposition to the abstinence-only-until-marriage (AOUM) advocates. Then I go on to examine what feminist theorists, myself among them, have proposed as a healthy sexuality and how these ideas of sexuality developed. I then raise questions about these popular ideas of what a healthy sexuality is and provide an alternative.

Healthy Sexuality in Comprehensive Sex Education

Sex education in the United States has been under siege. While the media explodes with television news shows about adolescent sexuality and a wide variety of sexual material in television programs, websites, and movies about adolescents, the debate about what kind of sex education is most appropriate for adolescents continues. An examination of this debate shows what two camps, the AOUM camp and the CSE camp believe to be healthy sexuality and why. For over a decade now, CSE advocates like the Congressional Committee on Government Reform (Committee, 2004) have shown that AOUM curricula contain false, misleading, or distorted information, as well as stereotypes with regard to male and female behavior, and have been making arguments based on a particular notion of healthy sexuality. Their arguments focus on the rights of adolescents to accurate health information; their definition of sexual health relies on the notion that freedom, autonomy, and access to public health and public health information are at its foundation.

Recently, we have seen changes with regard to U.S. sex education. President Barack Obama, in his May 2009 budget, called for an end of funding for AOUM programs that did not have evidence to support their effectiveness. In his budget, he recommended no longer funding programs that ignore or denigrate the effectiveness of contraceptives and safe-sex behaviors. He also recommended increasing funding for comprehensive adolescent pregnancy prevention programs (Guttmacher Institute, 2009) and has begun to fund Personal Responsibility and Education programs (PREP) while continuing to fund abstinence only education (Guttmacher Institute, 2010).

This welcome news came after almost 20 years of support for abstinence-only programming that was first endorsed by President Clinton, a Democrat; that endorsement continued and was strengthened under George W. Bush (a Republican). By the late 1990's, 86% of schools required that abstinence be promoted as either the only or preferred means of contraception (Kendall, 2008b; Landry, Kaeser, & Richards, 1999). This is because in 1996 Clinton signed a bill (Section 510 of the Personal Responsibility and Work Opportunity Reconciliation Act of 1996) that gave $50 million a year in federal grants to states for AOUM education (Dailard, 2005). Since then, more than a billion dollars have gone to AOUM education (Kendall, 2008b; SIECUS, 2007). AOUM programming was even required in international initiatives (Kendall, 2008a). And, in 2001, another bill, the Children and Families Community-Based Abstinence-Education (CBAE) Program, only increased funding because it bypassed state governments and gave directly to organizations (e.g., faith-based or pregnancy crisis services). The catch was that this funding was only provided to organizations that followed the eight tenets of AOUM education, one of which required that no information regarding contraception was to be provided to adolescents and that abstinence was to be promoted as the only safe way to avoid pregnancy and disease.

The CBAE bill was passed in spite of a report released that same year by the Surgeon General, David Satcher, that argued that scientific evidence showed that CSE is effective and that parents want their adolescent children to receive this type of sex education. This report cited the goals of sex education as including "the ability to understand and weigh the risks, responsibilities, outcomes and impacts of sexual actions and to practice abstinence when appropriate," and "freedom from sexual abuse and discrimination and the ability of individuals to integrate their sexuality into their lives, derive pleasure from it, and to reproduce if they so choose" (Satcher, 2001). An interesting thread that ran through this report brought attention to the fact that sexual violence as a public health issue is often not a part of the current discussion with regard to sex education. The report said that 22% of all women have been victims of forced sexual acts and that 104,000 children are victims of sexual abuse each year. The report also importantly indicated that sexual orientation could not be altered through force of will.

Those who have been battling for CSE in the years following do not always follow Satcher's lead to include in their definition of healthy sexuality a sexuality free from abuse; instead, they focus on two issues. The first issue is that adolescents have a right to receive information about contraception in order to support their physical health. That is, for these advocates, a healthy sexuality means physically healthy. The research they use to support this view shows the ineffectiveness of AOUM curricula in preventing disease and pregnancy (e.g., Kirby, 2007). The second focus of CSE advocates is human rights. This perspective encompasses the right to health information but also the right to be free from discrimination (for example, for gay, bisexual, lesbian, transsexual, or queer [GBLTQ] youths) and the right to make one's own decisions about sex (the right to autonomy). An adolescent boy or girl, has, in their view, the right to say either "yes" or "no" to sex, and has the right to information that will help him or her make that decision wisely and carry out any decision safely.

Earlier AOUM curricula (e.g., *Sex Respect*; Mast, 1990) described non-heterosexual practices as unhealthy and then later changed the curriculum to simply describe a healthy sexuality as one that is grounded in a monogamous, marital relationship, because only in such a relationship could one be sure to avoid disease (Lamb, 2010a). These curricula also spoke to mental health, describing the anguish and worry premarital sex would, in their opinion, bring to adolescents who engaged in such behavior. They have been roundly criticized for distorting information about the safety of contraception (Kirby, 2007; Manlove, Romano-Papillo, & Ikramullah, 2004).

The CSE curricula describe a healthy sexuality as one in which the adolescents are autonomous in decision making (that is, they are uninfluenced by each other and make the decision to engage in sex without pressure or persuasion), where they have all the information they need with regard to having safe sex, and that this information is accurate. They also describe relationships as egalitarian. Some address non-heterosexual sex (e.g., by using names such as Lee and Lee in hypothetical scenarios) (Taverner & Montfort, 2005) and some even mention desire, although none discuss desire as part of a *healthy* sexuality (Lamb, 2010a).

One reason that CSE advocates focus on adolescents' rights to obtain accurate information about and access to contraception (as the foundation of a healthy sexuality) is not only because they are addressing what is missing in AOUM curricula, but also because this focus leads to measurable outcomes. An effective program can be measured in terms of self-reports of unprotected sex, unwanted pregnancies, and disease. In the end, therefore, CSE advocates present a view of healthy sexuality that is synonymous with physical health, pregnancy prevention, and autonomous decision making (Lamb, 2010a).

Feminist Versions of Healthy Sexuality

While sex educators were debating, feminists were envisioning what a healthy sexuality might look like in terms of sex education, and the idea of "desire" (or "pleasure," which is often used synonymously with desire) became the lynchpin or trope for feminist work in this area. Beginning with Fine's important piece, "The Missing Discourse of Desire," published in 1988, one argument made by feminist critics (including Fine) is that sex education was too risk-focused, with sexuality constituted as always problematic and dangerous for girls (Fine, 1988). Other feminist theorists also describe these risk-focused curricula as picturing girls as potential victims (Allen, 2007a,b; Bay-Cheng, 2003; Fine, 1988; Tolman, 1994) not only of the sexual harassment and violence that affect the majority of girls in schools (American Association of University Women [AAUW], 2001) but also of boys' uncontrollable sexuality and pressure to have sex (Fine, 1988; Whatley, 1991). A risk model, they argue, disproportionately affects girls and women (Fine & McClelland, 2006) and interferes with girls' rights to a curriculum that might focus on desire rather than risk (Fine, 1988; Kendall, 2008b). A curriculum that focuses on girls' greater risk also places greater responsibility on girls for birth control (Ashcraft, 2006; Bay-Cheng, 2003; Fine, 1988; Lamb, 1997; Tolman, 2002). Although it may be true that girls are at greater risk of sexual abuse, rape, and pregnancy, the discourse around sexuality does not have to focus on these factors. This discourse, so theorists have argued, makes it appear as if uncontrollable male sexuality is natural and that girls are supposed to manage or watch out for it (Ashcraft, 2006, Fine, 1988; Hollway, 1989; Lamb, 1997, Whatley, 1991). Feminist theorists bemoan the absence of a way of talking about sex that captures agency, initiation, and subjectivity (Bay-Cheng, 2003; Fine, 1988; Tolman, 2002).

Following Fine's article, many feminists have explored problems in sex education with regard to silence around pleasure and desire (Bay-Cheng, 2003; Harrison, Hillier, & Walsh, 1996; Horne, 2005; Horne & Zimmer-Gembeck, 2005; Kehily 2002; Rasmussen, 2004; Lamb, 1997; Tolman, 2000, 2002; Welsh, Rostosky, & Kawaguchi, 2000). Through these arguments, a feminist version of healthy sexuality has been formed, and it highlights that girls learn to be subjects, not objects, through recognizing feelings of desire and experiencing pleasure.

The writing on the subject of girls' sexual subjectivity has been evocative and inspiring, describing a kind of preciousness around girls' sexuality "delicious and treacherous" (Fine & McClelland, 2006, p. 305). And desire is represented as the foundation of all health: "developing sexual subjectivity is at the heart of the adolescent developmental task of becoming a 'self-motivated sexual actor'" (Tolman, 2002, p. 20; see also Fine & McClelland's 2006 idea of "thick desire"). Martin (1994, as cited in Welles, 2005) wrote that for adolescent girls, "sexual subjectivity (the ability to feel confident in and in control of one's body and sexuality) shapes their ability to be agentic (the ability to act, accomplish, and feel efficacious in other parts of one's life) and vice versa." Sometimes sexuality seems to be overvalued as a goal of female development: "When sexual desire is truncated, all desire is compromised—including girls' power to love themselves and to know what they really want" (Debold, Wilson, & Malave, 1993, p. 211). Unlike boys' sexuality, which generally has been ignored by researchers and is presumed uncomplicated, girls' sexuality is presented by feminist writers as a suppressed story that needs airing and development: "To take possession of sexuality in the wake of the anti-erotic sexist socialization that remains the majority experience, most teenagers need an erotic education" (Thompson, 1990, p. 358).

This description of what healthy female sexuality should look like suggests a number of capacities that seem idealized and unconcerned that teenage girls are developing, not yet fully formed, sexual beings (Russell, 2005). Healthy sexuality requires that a teenage girl be knowledgeable about her own desires; use full reasoning ability in making choices; remain uninfluenced by television, books, or movies; pursue her own pleasure as much as her partner's; and always stay a subject not an object for someone else's pleasure. She is never passive, always responsible, knows both how to consent and how to refuse sex, and, even more importantly, always unambivalently knows if she wants to consent or refuse (see Muehlenhard & Peterson, 2005, for their discussion on the missing discourse on ambivalence). Where do these fervent wishes for girls come from? Why would feminist theorists heap these expectations on adolescent girls?

Healthy Sexuality as Subjectivity, Desire, and Pleasure

Desire and pleasure may be signs of subjectivity. And feminists who hope for a healthy sexuality for adolescent girls based on desire and pleasure believe that those girls who experience desire and are interested in pleasure already feel like subjects not objects. Girls who are subjects, not objects, can better resist objectification, can stand up to victimization, and can make more fully autonomous sexual choices (Fine, 1988; Tolman, 2002). These three hopes—that girls are subjects, that they resist victimization, and that they make autonomous choices—are the foundation of the desire model of adolescent girl sexuality.

Desire as an Antidote to Objectification

A healthy sexuality for adolescent girls that emphasizes subjectivity would seem to be an antidote to the objectification all around them. We know from the TFSG report that objectification is harmful (APA, 2007) and that exposure to and endorsement of sexually objectifying images (often described merely as "narrow beauty ideals," although such ideals are often objectifying) can affect self-esteem and body image, and can lead to depression and eating disorders or to self-objectification, which in turn leads to depressive symptoms, cognitive impairment, and lower self-esteem (APA, 2007; Durkin & Paxton, 2002; Fredrickson, Roberts, Noll, Quinn, & Twenge, 1998; Hawkins, Richards, Granley, & Stein, 2004; Tolman, Impett, Tracy, & Michael, 2006). Research has shown that having an objectified image of oneself or of women in general affects how one sees one's body and oneself as a sexual person (e.g., Impett, Schooler, & Tolman, 2006; Ward, Merriwether, & Caruthers, 2006).

Objectification of girls and, for that matter, of anyone can be seen as harmful for other reasons that do not lend themselves to empirical studies. There may be moral reasons, such as that one should never treat another person as a means to an end (Kant, 1785/1998; Nussbaum, 2000), or that rampant objectification appears to have some connection to the second sex status of women globally (Nussbaum, 2000). Theorists continue to describe women as subjected to scrutiny, defined by their bodies and appearances, and constituted as bodies for consumption (Bartky, 1990; Fredrickson & Roberts, 1997; Gill, 2006; McKinley & Hyde, 1996). Through objectification, they are denied their autonomy and subjectivity and are treated as objects, fungible and violable, denying that they are ends themselves, not means for another's use (Nussbaum, 2000).

Thus, given the longstanding concern about objectification and what it means for women and girls, it is understandable that a new model of sexuality would require a vision of subjectivity and desire, and an emphasis on girls experiencing the pleasure rather than giving someone else pleasure through their bodies or performances. It is also understandable why sexual subjectivity has been taken up by third-wave theorists as an alternative to objectification and has come to mean a position that defies any strictures, feminist or oppressive, that seek to control and define what girls can or can't wear, look like, or what girls need to wear or do to feel sexual (e.g., Edut, 2003).

Desire as an Antidote to Abuse and Victimization

It also seems clear to feminists that a healthy sexuality that emphasizes subjectivity (desire, pleasure, etc.) will help an adolescent girl to resist victimization and not see herself primarily as a potential victim. In the 1980s, as a feminist voice brought to light the widespread experience of victimization of girls and women through sexual abuse, rape, and harassment, women became aware of the effects of such violence on our psyches and bodies. Sexual violence, like no other act, makes a woman into an object for another's use. This was described in the second wave by Susan Brownmiller (2000), who, in 1975, described rape as a "victorious conquest over her being" (1975, p. 197, as reprinted in Baxandall & Gordon, 2000). The acknowledgment of the pervasiveness and harm of sexual violence was very powerful and came in some ways to define women's sexuality (Gavey, 2005; Lamb, 1999). More recently, empirical and theoretical work in psychology has shown that abuse and victimization harm girls in numerous ways, but in particular in terms of their developing sexuality. The sexually abused girl may grow up taking on the perpetrator's perspective, viewing herself as good for nothing but sex (Herman, 1992). The refusal of perpetrators to respect boundaries may also result in difficulties asserting boundaries or in impaired self-protection (Classen, Palesh, & Aggarwal, 2005; Quina, Morokoff, Harlow, & Zurbriggen, 2004).

Desire as an Antidote to Lack of Autonomy

Subjectivity, in the form of desire and pleasure—that is, desiring and seeking pleasure—also works as an antidote to passivity that historically has been at the center of women's sexual lives. Both legal and popular writings confirmed a sexuality for women that suggested their sexuality was in service to men, passive in relation to men's active stance (e.g., Bartky, 1990; Gavey, 2005).

Proponents of the desire, pleasure, and subjectivity view of healthy sex for adolescent girls infer in their writing that it is equally as important for a woman or girl to have sex and to have pleasure as it is for a man or a boy, and that ideals of femininity work against girls' experiencing desire and developing a healthy sexuality (Tolman, 1999). Horne wrote that within a discourse of traditional femininity, "sexual subjectivity is suppressed... and self-silencing is likely elevated" (p. 57, Horne, 2005) and includes "sexual exploration" in her definition of a healthy sexuality. The concept of "desire" also is used to undo the double standard, in which a man is applauded for his lust and a woman is shamed and called a slut (Tolman, 2002).

The notion of female passivity as opposed to male agency permeates much of our understanding of gender differences and has been associated with greater freedoms and privileges for men, particularly if they are white, middle-class men who not only are imagined as more agentic but more in control of this agency. Mohanty (1991) wrote of the binary positioning of masculine and feminine sexualities in a way in which the feminine was always the less powerful, less sexual, and had more to lose. As this applies to the world of adolescent sexuality, adolescent boys, particularly, heterosexual adolescent boys, masculinity theorists point out, have been pictured as agents, choosers, actors, ready to go, unconfused about their wants and needs, out for pleasure, demanding, and entitled (Kimmel, 2005; Kindlon & Thompson, 1999, Pleck, 1981). Until recently, adolescent girls' sexuality has been pictured as more hesitant and fragile. Girls who do show some sexual agency risk being described as sluts (Attwood, 2007; Brown, 2003; Lamb, 2002; Tanenbaum, 2000).

Thompson (1990) described a group of adolescent girls who were not sexually passive. She called them "pleasure narrators" and said they took "sexual subjectivity for granted" (p. 351). Tolman (2002) also described a group of "desiring girls" she interviewed. She noted that these girls were not likely to let sex "just happen," and they took more responsibility for contraception. This position was not without risk, as Tolman points out, as some girls were brave and lived life as agentic and pleasure-seeking adolescent girls in the open while others could hardly find "breathing room" for their desires and sacrificed authenticity (p. 164).

Third-wave theorists also appear to be trying to undo binaries such as the passive versus active in heterosexual relations (Baumgardner & Richards, 2003; Edut, 2003). Images of chastity, of girls needing to be pursued, of being a container for other people's fluids or passion, as there to serve or please, are exchanged for images of lust, orgasm, pleasure, and "self-pleasuring" (Gill, 2007) in an era in which there has been a widening of sexual attitudes, in general, among the young, as well as a greater acceptance of gay partners, more sexual partners, and earlier sex (Jackson & Scott, 2004). If girls have grown up with a message that sex is for boys and their bodies are for other people's use, pleasure and self-pleasure is certainly an antidote.

In spite of third-wave efforts to undo the binary, the idea of female passivity and the idea that sex is for men live on in women's magazines, "girl talk," and romance narratives (Carpenter, 1998; Duffy & Gotcher, 1996; Garner & Sterk, 1998; Kim & Ward, 2004; Tolman, 2000; Walkerdine, 1990). Thus, a healthy sexuality for adolescent girls also must counteract notions of female passivity that girls may receive. A focus on desire would seem to do so.

Critique of Desire Model of Adolescent Female Sexuality

Desire, autonomy, and pleasure are all important goals for female sexuality but there are problems with a model that places these at its center. The expectations for a healthy female adolescent sexuality seem exaggerated and unrealistic, especially when considering that adolescent girls are newly developing their sexual attitudes, feelings, and behaviors (Lamb, 2010b). The desire model pictures an adolescent girl always clear about whom she desires and when and where, quite knowledgeable about sexual feelings, and in particular sexual feelings at the site of her genitals (Tolman, 2002). In this model, she exercises subjectivity by making sexual choices uninfluenced by romance narratives and beauty ideals, uninfluenced by TV, books, or movies, or at least the "wrong kind" of TV, books, or movies. She pursues her own pleasure and thinks of pleasure as the purpose of sex. If she wants to be admired or look sexy, she's suspect. And, if she borrows conventions of sexy appearance that are part of the culture at large, she may be pictured as a dupe of culture. Her sexual desire must also be connected to political issues. Desire, now called "a stew of desires" (p. 326) in Fine and McClelland (2006), means desire for economic and social equalities and reproductive freedom. Not only is she responsible for her own subjectivity but she also is desiring of all freedoms for other girls and women. Not that these aren't noble goals, but when did the blossoming of sexuality get so exhausting?

Another problem with this model as it may play out in girls' lives is that a girl must be a "supergirl" (Girls, Inc., 2006) to live up to this ideal. In the West, these kinds of ideals often serve as part of an overarching goal of self-improvement in that sexual fulfillment becomes a central life goal (Jackson & Scott, 2004) and is treated (if women's and teen girl magazines are indicators of their concerns) as something to be constantly improved upon (Jackson & Scott, 2004). This attitude toward sex isn't questioned by, and indeed is taken up into, girls' empowerment groups (Bay-Cheng, 2003). It's taught as a form of girl power, sometimes with little discussion of how the relationship of girl power and sexuality can be problematic (Bay-Cheng, 2003, 2012). Sex and relationships are thus projects, and the adolescent girl is brought into the culture of adult sexuality with yet another project to work on, not just her body, not only her self, but now also her subjectivity, her pleasure.

A second issue with the desire model is the conflation of sexual freedom with sexual pleasure. Desire isn't only a stand-in for autonomy. To be desirous does not only mean having one's own thoughts and feelings and ideas and plans about sex (being an autonomous sexual person) but links the idea of autonomy with sexual longing. In so doing, it suggests that pleasure (for oneself) is the endpoint of sex. It is understandable why desire might serve as a way to talk about autonomy. And autonomy in sexual decision making is an important goal of adolescent girls, to the extent that autonomy can be achieved. Sexual autonomy for adolescent girls means freedom, freedom to make their own choices with regard to who they have sex with, how "far" they will go, and when they can refuse. Autonomy thus seems the cornerstone of good sex education in the service of pregnancy and victimization prevention. But while the ability to feel and seek pleasure may be *correlated* (Horne & Zimmer-Gembeck, 2005; Impett et al., 2006; Tolman et al., 2006) with sexual autonomy, it may be important to keep these notions separate. There can indeed be autonomy without desire and without the pursuit of pleasure.

In emphasizing pleasure as the endpoint or purpose of sex, a third problem arises—girls seem to be positioned as teenage boys, or at least, as the cultural stereotype of adolescent boys (Kimmel, 2008). It's as if theorists are informing girls that the only way to resist objectification and victimization, the only way to find one's desire, is to be more like the stereotypical boy and focus on one's own pleasure. Besides reifying a dichotomy, this suggests that boys' sexuality and the discourse about it in U.S. culture are not problematic. Boys and men in U.S. culture are depicted as always active, as knowing what they want and able to ask for it, as interested in sex for sex's sake, as able to feel and experience sexual pleasure unambivalently (Giordano, Longmore, & Manning, 2006). If this "boys' sex" is set out as the better way to be sexual, then a duality is reified and the passive role (usually associated with the girl), or, the role of the one admired and sexually desired (a form of objectification) (Hollway, 1989), is always a "one down" position rather than one role among a myriad of roles one can take within a complex and changing sexual relationship. In this dichotomy, any desire to be physically admired or longed for becomes an enactment of one's self-objectification or passivity. It makes active pursuit and pleasure-seeking the only correct position from which to have sex.

And then, if pleasure is the endpoint of sex, whether or not sex is pleasurable may come to mean "good" sex for the adolescent girl when "good" can and should refer to all sorts of ethical and expressive aspects of sex (Stoltenberg, 1990). If pleasure is the gold standard of whether an act of sexuality is good or not, then unethical forms of sex will fall under the category of good sex (e.g., it is wrong and doesn't make sense to weigh a rapist's pleasure against a victim's harm). Moreover, some experiences of objectification can be sexually pleasurable (Nussbaum, 1995). Those adolescents that the media seem most worried about today, those who call their lap dancing and breast flashing empowered (Levy, 2005), may be feeling a lot of pleasure. Some research suggests that objectifying performances aren't connected to physical pleasure (England & Thomas, 2006; Lamb, 2006); however, if these experiences *are* pleasurable, would that then make these forms of self-objectification right or good in an ethical or personal sense for adolescent girls? Although the current privileging of pleasure for girls and women is an important response to the centuries-long oppression of women that reflected that their own pleasure didn't count, the reverse of this is a problematic position. And although sexual pleasure is a right (WHO, 2004), it is important to be wary of views that describe all pleasures as good and as signifying of freedom, naturalness, or innocence, rather than learned and bound up with power (Kellner, 1995; Stoltenberg, 1990).

There is yet another problem in making pleasure the gold standard by which "good" sex is defined and that is, as Harris, Aapola, and Gonick (2000) point out, it supports a view that women and girls are their bodies, that satisfaction with one's body "becomes integral to a sense of happiness with one's self" (p. 380). And this is a position that has been harmful to girls over time, producing excessive worry and concern over body image, as well as leading to eating disorders. As with beauty, weight, and fitness, once again girls are asked to competently understand their bodies, now managing their orgasms, ensuring pleasure for themselves. Experiencing one's body positively and autonomously thus becomes an act of self-management, requiring expert advice.

Another problem with the desire model of adolescent sexuality is the way it may play out differently for racial and ethnic minority girls (Gill, 2012; Lamb, 2010b). Pleasure, subjectivity, voice, and desire, words that can evoke a delicateness and specialness about adolescent girls' sexuality, unwittingly also can evoke conceptions of a white heterosexual femininity that needs to be protected (as in Stillman's [2007] "missing white girl syndrome"). Historically, this description of sexuality that was fragile and precious was part of a discourse that served to "other" black women as hypersexual and present white women in opposition to uncontrollable and bestial male sexuality (Collins, 1990/2000; Tolman, 1996; Wilson, 1986; Wyatt, 1997). Thus, rather than counteracting objectification, passivity, and the culture's lack of interest in their sexual pleasure, black girls must also counteract stereotypes of being booty-shaking, "p-popping" girls on MTV, oversexed when not invisible as sexual beings (Sharpley-Whiting, 2007). Tolman (2002) wrote of the vulnerabilities in seeking pleasure for black girls, given that they are more associated with society's fears of adolescent sexuality. In an effort to not reproduce stereotypes, researchers hold out very different examples of black girls when depicting them as models of sexual agency. Instead of using "pleasure seekers," they emphasize agentic black girls as those who show their ability to say no and hold back (Weekes, 2002). Weekes points out that researchers in the past described black girls as taking a "no-nonsense" approach to male attention and/or sexual harassment (Lees, 1986; Griffin, 1985; Griffiths, 1995). Such constructions of black girls as refusing to be objects of male desire position them as invulnerable or "superstrong," but as "superstrong" is associated with masculinity, it may leave them with little to work with in constructing their own versions of female sexuality (Weekes, 2002).

And what of immigrant adolescents, some eager to join modern media culture while still practicing the religion and tradition of their families? If we recognize that true multiculturalism means respecting differences and seeing individuals as having complex identities (Blum, 2009; Song, 2007), then we must consider religious views in any definition of healthy sexuality. A definition of a healthy sexuality must not subsume all girls under one form and must take seriously girls who grow up in religious communities for whom religion provides sexual values. This is not to say that psychologists must endorse oppressive practices (Okin, 1999), for certain cultural and religious practices may be equally as oppressive as Western oppressive forces that come from media and marketing of girls' sexuality; but any claim to healthy or an "authentic sexuality" can't be found by asking a girl to look deep within herself for what she truly desires, because the bedrock of identity is not emotion divorced from context. A sexuality that she both wants and chooses needs to represent the complexity of her identity by taking into consideration her cultural history, religion, familial history, and how girls' bodies are acknowledged within these. It seems a very Western notion to separate girls' sexuality from the contexts in which she lives in order to help her to find a place from which she can resist oppressive media. It seems as if the assumption that all religious claims on sexuality will be oppressive is also problematic.

A final problem with the desire model of adolescent girl sexuality stems from the way this discourse has been taken up by young women, some of whom understand desire and empowerment as the freedom to become sexual objects for men (Bay-Cheng, 2012; Gill, 2007, 2008, 2012). Bailey (1997) writes that third-wave feminists define themselves as resisting limiting and oppressive aspects of second-wave feminism, regarding sexuality and personal aesthetics, although their depiction of second-wave politics is hotly contested (Bailey, 1997; Baxandall & Gordon, 2000; Chidgey, 2008; Henry, 2004). Third-wave theorists view the third-wave girl as "a new, robust young woman with agency and a strong sense of self" (Aapola, Gonick, & Harris, 2005, p. 39; Kelly, 2005), welcoming multiple sexual encounters, partners, sexualities, and ways of being, as well as the choice to empower themselves by ironically taking on stereotypically feminine roles and performing them. In these performances, empowerment is synonymous with the idea of sexual autonomy, as these young women choose to enact whatever sexuality they might like to enact, mocking traditional feminism by showing that they remain in control even when mimicking what might have been seen earlier as an oppressive sexuality (e.g., performing a striptease). I want to separate out third-wave feminists who were trying to undo gender and sexual categories from what Levy has titled "female chauvinist pigs" who may be their legacy. The former were trying to find a sexual way of being that was neither male nor female, and that would feel empowering to diverse groups of women. Nevertheless, they were the harbingers for a modern-day version of female sexuality sold as empowerment but that is more closely associated with pornography (Dines, 2010; Gill, 2008; Levy, 2005; Paul, 2005; Sarracino & Scott, 2008). Indeed, many of the images today of a young woman in charge of her sexuality come from the world of pornography and reproduce very old exploitative scenes of male voyeurism and women's victimization and/or oppression (Levy, 2005). This porn image of sexuality is marketed to increasingly younger girls as an adolescent sexuality they can aspire to (Lamb, 2006; Lamb & Brown, 2006). In this version of sexuality, an adolescent girl can feel empowered by *choosing* to lap dance, striptease, or perform other acts traditionally associated with pornography, and, in doing so, she can still consider herself to be an autonomous agent who is having fun. Her choice and experience of fun make her voyeurs not exploiters, but admirers, although these "admirers" somehow seem to still have the power to redefine the "striptease" (Lamb, 2010b,c; see Lamb & Peterson [2012] and commentaries by Bay-Cheng [2012], Gavey [2012], Gill [2012], and Tolman [2012], for a discussion of this point).

Is There an Authentic Sexuality?

A final problem with the desire model of sexuality is the way feminist theorists sometimes describe an "authentic sexuality" that is meant to be the alternative to a sexuality defined by looking sexy (a sexuality that has at its heart the appearance of sexiness and which requires purchases of make-up, fashion, and, increasingly, plastic surgery). Some theorists have tried to describe sexual authenticity as the gold standard of sexual health (Chalker, 1994; Daniluk, 1993; Lamb, 2002; Lorde, 1984; Thompson, 1990, 1995; Tolman, 1991, 1994, 2002; Welles, 2005) using the term "embodied" and discussing being "fully present" (Welles, 2005, p. 1) for sex in opposition to being dissociated (not fully aware). For example, Impett et al. (2006) describe sexual self-efficacy as an embodied, responsible girl in touch with her own feelings. The emphasis on "embodiment" derives in part from philosopher Iris Marion Young's (1980) writing on embodiment for girls who play sports. A girl, she argues, typically throws a softball as if there is a crowd watching, and, because of this, can't throw very well because she is both in her body and looking at it from the outside, simultaneously judging it and protective of it against a male gaze. Using this framework, self-sexualization is a performance, and a duality is set up between within (what a girl feels) and without (who is watching).

The theories that focus on authenticity see desiring as a liberatory act, and the adolescent girl is pictured as naturally desirous in a world that sees desire and subjectivity as unnatural for girls. As Fine writes, desire "insists: it carves underground irrigation systems of radical possibility" (2005, p. 55). Coming from a liberal individualist perspective, the adolescent girl is free, actually freed of something (the media, the oppressive expectations of others, her own insecurities) in order to make individual, healthy choices. And choice is tied to freedom (as in Horne's [2005] inclusion of "sexual exploration" as an aspect of healthy sexuality).

Thus, the girl who resists a prepackaged, often pornographic, sexuality based on looking sexy is both "natural" and autonomous. She chooses an inner sexuality after recognizing ideological forces that seek to shape her from the outside. The natural girl who looks within is set up in opposition to the "packaged" one. The choosing girl is set up in opposition to girls-as-dupes (of patriarchy, of the marketplace).

Both of these images can serve as a way to critique the girl who, say, does a striptease at a party. The stripping girl is not "natural" because she does the striptease to perform for onlookers. If she might argue that it is embodied in that she feels pleasure in her body and enjoys performing, one could argue that this pleasure is not original or "natural," but is rather pleasure that's derived from what a male-privileged society deems pleasurable for girls or women (that a woman should feel pleasure pleasing a man). And her choice to perform the striptease does not appear to be a fully free choice as it is heavily influenced by the rewards her peer group gives her for that performance. And that peer group is also heavily influenced by male privilege. Thus, she expresses sexuality through a striptease because she's ruled by a system that doesn't support other forms of female agentic behavior and limits her to performing her sexuality for boys and men (Bussey & Bandura, 1999; Fredrickson & Roberts, 1997). This is an appealing argument.

And if this girl insists that she is not stripping for rewards from others and says she doesn't care about other people watching but does so because it makes her feel powerful and sexy, then she is said to have developed a false kind of subjectivity. This perspective was described in a general way by the philosopher Althusser (1971), who explained the process in which an individual might believe he or she is acting autonomously while the discourse of the day has, in a sense, recruited her to represent this discourse and the ideology behind it. That is, individuals identify with certain value positions that are supported ideologically by systems in power, but belie they are the authors of their meaning. Applied to the adolescent girl who claims empowerment, she believes she is autonomous, choosing to be the kind of object that has been defined as sexy by marketers and a highly media-influenced audience, just as she believes her choice to wear name brand clothing over generic brands is a free one. She becomes a part of, even a representative of, the commercial discourse that defines her subjectivity within a framework of choice, equality, and freedom (McRobbie, 2007).

This elevation of choice is what makes the CSE curricula problematic for girls, even if it does serve to enforce autonomy along with sexual health. The curricula's insistence on adolescents' choice (as opposed to the limits on their choice presented by the AOUM curricula) naïvely hopes that, if given all the information possible, adolescents will be less influenced by social forces that impinge on their autonomy. Freedom may not be as free for adolescent girls as it seems.

The discourse of autonomy, "choice" for adolescent girls, is also a marketing discourse. Marketers rely on the belief that people, in this case adolescent girls, can self-create, construct their own identities (Gill, 2008). Consumers are set up as hyperagents, making choices from an array of alternatives in a free market. As Becker (2005) points out in her critique of the self-empowerment movement, feminism has long incorporated male discourses of autonomy, individual rights, and agency that have influenced what we've seen as cures for women's ills. Gill (2003) has called this discourse of endless choices "subjectification" that has replaced objectification. A girl who is said to be developing a more authentic sexuality is asked to know herself, know her body, and know her desires, not unlike the discourse Becker (2005) writes about regarding the self-empowerment movement.

If a girl looks within to find an "authentic" sexuality, it may be that she will come up with yet another but different packaged version of adolescent sexuality. For example, the discourse of romance can and has been set in opposition to the discourse of the slut, and narratives of the "slut," which often end in the realization that all a girl ever wanted was to be loved (Freitas, 2008). In "chick lit," for example, a common theme is for wild girls to become "re-virginized" when they meet Mr. Right, seeing how shallow pursuit of pleasure was before

(Gill, 2006). And, with a nod to the new vampire series (Meyer, 2005), written by a woman who hoped to describe the tortures of abstinence as well as desire within adolescent love, exchanging the power porn sexually active female for the old-fashioned girl who longs but can't have merely reiterates an oppressive gender dichotomy. Recreating oneself as a sexual agent along pornographic lines cannot be replaced with another myth of the good girl who just wants to be loved, calling the latter authentic because it is a traditional feminine position, the former inauthentic because it is for boys or it imitates a male sexuality.

Thus, proposing to girls that they find an authentic sexuality, one unmarketed, that they feel from within in an embodied way, may be wrong-minded. There may be no authentic sexuality to be found. Conversely, as Duits and van Zoonen (2007) point out, construing adolescent girls as always ruled by patriarchy or the marketplace or dominant ideologies, contributes to the culture's ability to dismiss girls and women as politically relevant actors. One way to address this problem has been to look for moments of resistance in which girls seem to be acting against a mainstream version of what it might mean to be sexy. In what might seem a hall of mirrors of discourses, there may still be choices to be made (Lamb & Peterson, 2011; Peterson & Lamb, 2012). Gill (2006) wisely asks, "why is acknowledging cultural influences deemed so shameful? Conversely, why are autonomous choices so fetishized?" (p. 73). And Gavey (2012) points out that certain regressive acts can sometimes be used toward progressive ends. That is to say, we do not have to throw out what is good in the liberal ideal of individual choosing (Nussbaum, 2000) if we are careful not to call girls' sexuality authentic but instead name for them, and more importantly with them, where they are restricted, where they are presented with alternatives, and why certain alternatives are placed in their paths whereas others need to be discovered in less public places. And we may not have to propose individual and individualized sexuality as an answer when—and this is true for adults, too—sexuality mostly exists in relationship to other people.

New Ways of Defining a Healthy Sexuality for Adolescent Girls

Descriptions of the embodied, agentive, subjective, authentic, desiring sexuality that is the ideal set out for adolescent girls lacks one important element—the other person. Authentic sexuality is often depicted as something an adolescent girl must discover in herself and not in relation to another person. Perhaps this is because girls and women have traditionally been directed outward in their sexual expression, toward pleasing a man. For girls, that other person, within a heterosexual model of sexual relationships, presents a danger to their autonomy and agency, and girls are typically presented as "Ophelias" in need of protection from boys (Marshall, 2007). Isn't it problematic that adolescent girls are said to discover their most authentic, embodied sexuality, alone, in the privacy of their bedrooms? What theorists have really neglected to do with regard to adolescent female sexuality is carve out a way to be sexual in relation to others.

A different alternative to the directive of looking within for an embodied or authentic sexuality, discovering a suppressed or nascent desire and then making healthy choices, is a model of mutuality. Love tied to sexuality is another model that some sex education curricula advocate but not one I propose here because it doesn't have the ethical meaning that mutuality does. Also, it has been shown that adolescent girls do self-denying, self-destructive things in the name of love, so the sex-in-love model hasn't worked very well for them to date (Holland, Ramazanoglu, Sharpe, & Thomson, 1998; Lamb, 2006; Thompson, 1990, 1995; Tolman, 2000). The idea of mutuality begins with the notion that sex occurs between people and is something more than a contract that autonomous individuals enter into, if only for a night. In moments of joining, collaboration, uniting, or transcending, individuals can be both embodied and, in the moment, with someone else. Mutuality does imply an ethic of fairness and equality, good values within the liberal tradition, but it also implies that sex happens in relation to and with someone else, and that for sex to be good, in both and all meanings of the word, moving beyond an individual focus, to think about and feel with and through another may be an alternative model. As we think about compassion, caring, and empathy as moral goals for all human interactions, we can think about pleasure for oneself and for someone else as being deeply connected.

A notion of mutuality can incorporate pleasure and desire in terms of mutual pleasure and mutual desire and doesn't have to be reduced to one person's pleasure deriving from only giving pleasure to another (Lamb, 2011a). Still, the ideal of mutuality may be difficult to achieve in heterosexual relationships, given cultural inequities. This model of mutuality is not a reiteration of a self-sacrificing femininity that privileges male pleasure but can be consistent with subjectivity and choice—that is, girls can choose to give as well as to receive, to seek pleasure for themselves and for others, to love or to play, and do this all within an ethic of caring that mutuality employs. Stoltenberg wrote of this when he described, for want of a better phrase, an " erotic potential between humans such that mutuality, reciprocity, fairness, deep communion and choice-making and decision-making are merged with robust physical pleasure, intense sensation, and brimming-over expressiveness" (Stoltenberg, 1990, p. 112). Is this too idealistic? Perhaps the "brimming-over expressiveness" may be beyond the typical self-conscious adolescent, but otherwise, I think not.

How would we teach this model to girls—and to boys as well? I argue that sex education as it is taught to adolescents today, in terms of making autonomous choices for a healthy sexuality, needs to be supplemented by ethics and relationship sex education (Lamb, 2010a). Today's adolescents need to understand the liberties at stake and the harms at risk in our culture with regard to topics such as pornography and prostitution, so that they might be good sexual citizens. And they ought to be asked to think about relationships in terms of fairness and compassion and apply principles of justice and caring to all relationships, in particular, sexual relationships. Although the sexual rights of adolescents are important, they ought to be asked to consider what kinds of sexual relationships adolescents and adults should have—which will be most gratifying, least harmful, most fair, least disturbing. This may mean sex educators will need to put aside notions of empowerment; but, consistent with a health perspective, an ethics perspective of mutuality may be able to ask adolescents to think about their own health, physical, and psychological needs, alongside of what is healthy for others.

The desire model of sexuality for adolescent girls is a romanticized model that once served a political purpose. Although adults—feminist researchers included—may have ambivalent feelings about how adolescent girls can express a healthy sexuality, we need a model that goes beyond the problematic messages consistent with desire, as well as one that goes beyond a discussion of sexual rights. In a new era of sex education, we can build on the sexual rights focus, the right to information, to contraception, and ask educators to address a broader view of "healthy" sexuality, to provide discussion of values, as well as practices cognizant of multicultural differences. We can ask sex educators to explore with adolescents the ideologies present that teach adolescents in subtle ways what is expected in sexual relationships and to think about what ethical sex might look like in the face of desire and longing (Lamb, 2010b). To the extent that cultural critique and sexual ethics are embedded in a sex education curriculum, girls may be free to examine what it might mean to construct a healthy sexuality. Using mutuality as a guide, they will at least be able to explore this alongside someone else.

References

Aapola, S., Gonick, M., & Harris, A. (2005). *Young femininity: Girlhood, power, and social change.* London: Palgrave.

Allen, L. (2007a). Doing "it" differently: Relinquishing the disease and pregnancy prevention focus in sexuality education. *British Journal of Sociology of Education, 28,* 575–588.

Allen, L. (2007b). "Pleasurable pedagogy": Young people's ideas about teaching "pleasure" in sexuality education. *21st Century Society, 2,* 249–264.

Althusser, L. (1971). Ideology and ideological state apparatuses. In L. Althusser (Ed.), *Lenin and philosophy and other essays* (127–188). New York: Monthly Review Press.

American Association of University Women (AAUW). (2001). *Hostile hallways: Bullying, teasing, and sexual harassment in school.* Retrieved on March 18, 2009, from http://www.aauw.org/research/upload/hostilehallways.pdf

APA Task Force on the Sexualization of Girls. (2007). *Report of the APA task force on the sexualization of girls.* Washington, DC: American Psychological Association. Retrieved on April 12, 2008, from www.apa.org/pi/wpo/sexualization.htm

Ashcraft, C. (2006). "Girl, you better go get you a condom": Popular culture and teen sexuality as resources for critical multicultural curriculum. *Teachers College Record, 108,* 2145–2186.

Attwood, F. (2007). Sluts and riot grrrls: Female identity and sexual agency. *Journal of Gender Studies, 16,* 233–247.

Bailey, C. (1997). Making waves and drawing lines: The politics of defining the vicissitudes of feminism. *Hypatia, 12,* 17–28.

Bartky, S. L. (1990). *Femininity and domination: Studies in the phenomenology of oppression.* New York: Routledge.

Baumgardner, J., & Richards, A. (2003). The number one question about feminism. *Feminist Studies, 29,* 448–452.

Baxandall, R., & Gordon, L. (Eds.). (2000). *Dear sisters: Dispatches from the women's liberation movement.* New York: Basic Books.

Bay-Cheng, L. (2003). The trouble of teen sex: The construction of adolescent sexuality through school-based sexuality education. *Sex Education, 3,* 61–74.

Bay-Cheng, L. (2011). Recovering empowerment: De-personalizing and re-politicizing adolescent female sexuality. *Sex Roles, 66*(11–12), 713–717.

Becker, D. (2005). *The myth of empowerment.* New York: New York University Press.

Blum, L. (2009, July). *Modood's defense of multiculturalism.* Paper presented at the Association for Moral Education 35th Annual Conference, Utrecht, The Netherlands.

Brown, L. M. (2003). *Girlfighting: Betrayal and rejection among girls.* New York: NYU Press.

Brownmiller, S. (2000). The mass psychology of rape. In R. Baxandall & L. Gordon (Eds.), *Dear sisters: Dispatches from the women's liberation movement* (pp. 196–197). New York: Basic Books.

Bussey, K., & Bandura, A. (1999). Social cognitive theory of gender development and differentiation. *Psychological Review, 106,* 676–713.

Carpenter, L. (1998). From girls into women: Scripts for sexuality and romance in *Seventeen* magazine, 1974–1994. *The Journal of Sex Research, 35,* 158–168.

Chalker, R. (1994). Updating the model of female sexuality. *SIECUS Report, 22,* 1–6.

Chidgey, R. (March, 2008). *The Fword: Contemporary UK Feminism* (blog). Retrieved June 12, 2012, from http://www.thefword.org.uk/reviews/2008/12/cunning_stunts

Classen, C., Palesh, O., & Aggarwal, R. (2005). Sexual revictimization: A review of the empirical literature. *Trauma, Violence, and Abuse, 6,* 103–129.

Collins, P. H. (1990/2000). *Black feminist thought: Consciousness and the politics of empowerment. Revised 10th anniversary edition.* New York: Routledge.

Committee on Government Reform—Minority Staff. (2004). *The content of federally funded abstinence-only education programs.* Washington, DC: United States House of Representatives.

Dailard, C. (2005). Administration tightens rules for abstinence education grants. *The Guttmacher Report on Public Policy, 8.* Retrieved January 24, 2009, from http://www.guttmacher.org/pubs/tgr/08/4/gr080413.html

Daniluk, J. C. (1993). The meaning and experience of adolescent sexuality. *Psychology of Women Quarterly, 17,* 53–70.

Debold, E., Wilson, M., & Malave, I. (1993). *Mother daughter revolution: From good girls to great women.* New York: Random House.

Dines, G. (2010). *Pornland: How pornography has hijacked our sexuality*. Boston: Beacon Press.

Duffy, M., & Gotcher, J. M. (1996). Crucial advice on how to get the guy: The rhetorical vision of power and seduction in the teen magazine YM. *Journal of Communication Inquiry, 20*, 32–48.

Duits, L., & van Zoonen, L. (2007). Who's afraid of female agency?: A rejoinder to Gill. *European Journal of Women's Studies, 14*, 161–170.

Durkin, S. J., & Paxton, S. J. (2002). Predictors of vulnerability to reduced body image satisfaction and psychological well-being in response to exposure to idealized female media images in adolescent girls. *Journal of Psychosomatic Research, 53*, 995–1005.

Edut, O. (2003). *Body outlaws: Rewriting the rules of beauty and body image*. Berkeley, CA: Seal Press.

England, P., & Thomas, R. J. (2006). The decline of the date and the rise of the college hook up. In A. S. Skolnick & Skolnick, J. (Eds.). *Families in transition* (14th ed.). Boston: Allyn & Bacon.

Fine, M. (1988). Sexuality, schooling, and adolescent females: The missing discourse of desire. *Harvard Educational Review, 58*, 29–53.

Fine, M. (2005). Desire: The morning (and 15 years) after. *Feminism & Psychology, 15*, 54–50.

Fine, M., & McClelland, S. (2006). Sexuality education and desire: Still missing after all these years. *Harvard Education Review, 76*, 297–338.

Fredrickson, B. F., & Roberts, T. -A. (1997). Objectification theory: Toward understanding women's lived experience and mental health risks. *Psychology of Women Quarterly, 21*, 173–206.

Fredrickson, B. L., Roberts, T., Noll, S. M., Quinn, D. M., & Twenge, J. M. (1998). That swimsuit becomes you: Sex differences in self-objectification, restrained eating and math performance. *Journal of Personality and Social Psychology, 75*, 269–284.

Freitas, D. (2008). *Sex and the soul: Juggling sexuality, spirituality, romance, and religion on America's college campuses*. New York: Oxford University Press.

Garner, A., & Sterk, H. M. (1998). Narrative analysis of sexual etiquette in teen magazines. *Journal of Communication, 48*, 59–79.

Gavey, N. (2005). *Just sex?: The cultural scaffolding of rape*. London: Routledge.

Gavey, N. (2011). Beyond "empowerment"? Sexuality in a sexist world. *Sex Roles,66*(11–12), 718–724.

Gill, R. C. (2003). From sexual objectification to sexual subjectification: The resexualisation of women's bodies in the media. *Feminist Media Studies, 3*, 99–106.

Gill, R. C. (2006). *Gender and the media*. Cambridge, UK: Polity Press.

Gill, R. C. (2007). Critical respect: The difficulties and dilemmas of agency and "choice" for feminism: A reply to Duits and van Zoonen. *European Journal of Women's Studies Journal, 14*, 69–80.

Gill, R. (2008). Empowerment/sexism: Figuring female sexual agency in contemporary advertising. *Feminism and Psychology, 18*, 35–60.

Gill, R. (2012). Media, empowerment and the 'sexualization of culture' debates. *Sex Roles, 66*(11–12), 758–763.

Giordano, P., Longmore, M., & Manning, W. (2006). Gender and the meanings of adolescent romantic relationships: A focus on boys. *American Sociological Review, 71*, 260–287.

Girls, Inc. (2006). *The supergirl dilemma: Girls grapple with the mounting pressure of expectations*. New York: Author.

Griffin, C. (1985). *Typical girls: Young women from school to the job market*. London: Routledge & Kegan Paul.

Griffiths, V. (1995). *Adolescent girls and their friends: A feminist ethnography*. Aldershot, UK: Avebury.

Guttmacher Institute. (2009, May 8). *President Obama's 2010 budget: A decidedly mixed bag*. Retrieved July 20, 2009 from http://www.guttmacher.org/media/inthenews/2009/05/08/index.html

Guttmacher Institute (2010, Spring) Sex education: Another big step forward – and a step back. Retrieved June 12, 2012, from http://www.guttmacher.org/pubs/gpr/13/2/gpr130227.html.

Harris, A., Aapola, S., & Gonick, M. (2000). Doing it differently: Young women managing heterosexuality in Australia, Finland and Canada. *Journal of Youth Studies,* 3, 373–388.

Harrison, L., Hillier, L., & Walsh, J. (1996). Teaching for a positive sexuality: Sounds good, but what about fear, embarrassment, risk and the "forbidden" discourse of desire? In L. Lasky & C. Beavis (Eds.), *Schooling and sexualities: Teaching for a positive sexuality* (pp. 69–82). Geelong, AU: Deakin University Press.

Hawkins, N., Richards, P., Granley, H. M., & Stein, D. M. (2004). The impact of exposure to the thin-ideal media image on women. *Eating Disorders,* 12, 35–50.

Henry, A. (2004). *Not my mother's sister: Generational conflict and third-wave feminism.* Bloomington, IN: Indiana University Press.

Herman, J. L. (1992). *Trauma and recovery: The aftermath of violence—from domestic abuse to political terror.* New York: Basic Books.

Holland, J., Ramazanoglu, C., Sharpe, S., & Thomson, R. (1998). *The male in the head: Young people, heterosexuality, and power.* London: Tufnell Press.

Hollway, W. (1989). Theorising heterosexuality: A response. *Feminism & Psychology,* 3, 412–417.

Horne, S. (2005). *Female sexual health: The definition and development of sexual subjectivity, and linkages with sexual agency, sexual experience and well being in late adolescents and emerging adults.* Doctoral dissertation, School of Health, Griffiths University. Retrieved July 23, 2009 from http://www4.gu.edu.au:8080/adt-root/uploads/approved/adt-QGU20060726.165349/public/02Main.pdf

Horne, S., & Zimmer-Gembeck, M. J. (2005). Female sexual subjectivity and well-being: Comparing late adolescents with different sexual experiences. *Sexuality Research & Social Policy,* 2, 25–40.

Impett, E. A., Schooler, D., & Tolman, D. L. (2006). To be seen and not heard: Femininity ideology and adolescent girls' sexual health. *Archives of Sexual Behavior,* 21, 628–646.

Jackson, S., & Scott, S. (2004). Sexual antimonies in late modernity. *Sexualities,* 7, 233–247.

Kant, I. (1785/1998). *Groundwork of the metaphysics of morals* (M. J. Gregor, Trans.). New York: Cambridge University Press. (Original work published 1785.)

Kehily, M. J. (2002). Sexing the subject: Teachers, pedagogies and sex education. *Sex Education,* 2, 215–231.

Kellner, D. (1995). *Media culture: Cultural studies, identity and politics between the modern and the postmodern.* New York: Routledge.

Kelly, E. (2005). A new generation of feminism? Reflections on the 3rd wave. *New Political Science,* 27(2), 233–243.

Kendall, N. (2008a). Introduction to special issue: The state(s) of sexuality education in America. *Sexuality Research & Social Policy,* 5, 1–11.

Kendall, N. (2008b). Sexuality education in an abstinence-only era: A comparative case study of two U.S. states. *Sexuality Research & Social Policy,* 5, 23–44.

Kim, J. L., & Ward, L. M. (2004). Pleasure reading: Associations between young women's sexual attitudes and their reading of contemporary women's magazines. *Psychology of Women Quarterly,* 28, 48–58.

Kimmel, M. S. (2005). *The gender of desire: Essays on male sexuality.* Albany, NY: State University of New York Press.

Kimmel, M. S. (2008). *Guyland: The perilous world where guys become men.* New York: Harper.

Kindlon, D., & Thompson, M. (1999). *Raising Cain: Protecting the emotional life of boys.* New York: Ballantine.

Kirby, D. (2007). *Emerging answers 2007: Research finding on programs to reduce teen pregnancy and sexually transmitted diseases.* Washington, DC: The National Campaign to Prevent Teen and Unplanned Pregnancy.

Lamb, S. (1997). Sex education as moral education. *Journal of Moral Education, 27*(4), 301–316.

Lamb, S. (1999). Constructing the victim: Popular images and lasting labels. In S. Lamb (Ed.), *New versions of victims: Feminists struggle with the concept* (pp. 108–138). New York: New York University Press.

Lamb, S. (2002). *The secret lives of girls: What good girls really do—sex play, aggression, and their guilt.* New York: Free Press.

Lamb, S. (2006). *Sex, therapy, and kids: Addressing their concerns through talk and play.* New York: W.W. Norton.

Lamb, S. (2010a). Towards a sexual ethics curriculum: Bringing philosophy and society to bear on individual development. *Harvard Educational Review, 80*(1), 81–105.

Lamb, S. (2010b) Feminist ideals of healthy female adolescent sexuality: A critique. *Sex Roles, 62*(5/6), 294–306.

Lamb, S. (2010c). Porn as a pathway to empowerment? A response to Peterson's commentary. *Sex Roles, 62*(5/6), 314–317.

Lamb, S. (2011). The place of mutuality and care in democratic sexuality education: Incorporating the other person. In D. Carlson & D. Roseboro (Eds.), *The sexuality curriculum and youth culture: Youth culture, popular culture, and democratic sexuality education* (pp. 29–43). New York: Peter Lang.

Lamb, S., & Brown, L. M. (2006). *Packaging girlhood: Rescuing our daughters from marketers' schemes.* New York: St. Martin's Press.

Lamb, S., & Peterson, Z. (2012). Adolescent girls' sexual empowerment: Two feminists explore the concept. *Sex Roles, 66*(11–12),703–712.

Landry, D., Kaeser, L., & Richards, C. (1999). Abstinence promotion and the provision of information about contraception in public school sexuality education policies. *Family Planning Perspectives, 31,* 280–286.

Lees, S. (1986). *Losing out: Sexuality and adolescent girls.* London: Hutchinson.

Levin, D., & Kilbourne, J. (2008). *So sexy so soon: The new sexualized childhood and what parents can do to protect their kids.* New York: Ballantine.

Levy, A. (2005). *Female chauvinist pigs: Women and the rise of raunch culture.* New York: Free Press.

Lorde, A. (1984). Uses of the erotic: The erotic as power. In *Sister outsider: Essays and speeches* (p. 55). Freedom, CA: Crossing Press.

Luker, K. (2006). *When sex goes to school: Warring views on sex—and sex education—since the sixties.* New York: Norton.

Manlove, J. M., Romano-Papillo, A., & Ikramullah, E. (2004). *Not yet: Programs to delay first sex among teens.* Washington, DC: National Campaign to Prevent Teen Pregnancy.

Marshall, E. (2007). Schooling Ophelia: Hysteria, memory, and adolescent femininity. *Gender and Education, 19,* 707–728.

Martin, K. (1994). Puberty, sexuality, and the self: Gender differences at adolescence (Doctoral Dissertation, University of California, Berkeley, 1994). *University of California Dissertation Services.*

Mast, C. (1990). *Sex respect: The option of true sexual freedom.* Bradley, IL: Respect Incorporated.

McKinley, N. M., & Hyde, J. S. (1996). The objectified body consciousness scale. *Psychology of Women Quarterly, 20,* 181–215.

McRobbie, A. (2007). Top girls: Young women and the post-feminist contract. *Cultural Studies, 21,* 718–737.

Meyer, S. (2005). *Twilight (Book 1),* New York: Little, Brown, & Co.

Mohanty, C. T. (1991). Under western eyes: Feminist scholarship and colonial discourses. In C. T. Mohanty, A. Russo, & L. Torres (Eds.), *Third world women and the politics of feminism* (pp. 51–80). Bloomington: Indiana University Press.

Muelhlenhard, C., & Peterson, Z. D. (2005). Wanting and not wanting sex: The missing discourse of ambivalence. *Feminism & Psychology, 15,* 15–20.

Nussbaum, M. (1995). Objectification. *Philosophy and Public Affairs, 24,* 249–291.

Nussbaum, M. C. (2000). *Women and human development: The capabilities approach.* Cambridge/ New York: Cambridge University Press.

Okin, S. (1999). Is multiculturalism bad for women? In S. Okin, et al (Eds.), *Is multiculturalism bad for women?* Princeton, NJ: Princeton University Press.

Paul, P. (2005). *Pornified: How pornography is changing our lives.* New York: Times Books.

Peterson, Z., & Lamb, S. (2012). The political context for personal empowerment: Continuing the conversation. *Sex Roles, 66*(11–12), 758–763.

Pleck, J. H. (1981). *The myth of masculinity.* Cambridge, MA: MIT Press.

Quina, K., Morokoff, P. J., Harlow, L. L., & Zurbriggen, E. L. (2004). Cognitive and attitudinal paths from childhood trauma to adult HIV risk. In L. J. Koenig, A. O'Leary, L. S. Doll, & W. Pequegnat (Eds.), *From child sexual abuse to adult sexual risk: Trauma revictimization and intervention* (pp. 135–157). Washington, DC: American Psychological Association.

Rasmussen, M. L. (2004). Wounded identities, sex and pleasure: "Doing it" at school. Not! *Discourse: Studies in the Cultural Politics of Education, 25,* 445–458.

Russell, S. T. (2005). Introduction to positive perspectives on adolescent sexuality: Part 2. *Sexuality Research and Social Policy: Journal of NSRC, 2*(4), 1–3.

Sarracino, C., & Scott, K. (2008). *Porn culture in America.* Boston: Beacon Press.

Satcher, D. (2001). *The Surgeon General's call to action to promote sexual health and responsible sexual behavior.* Retrieved June 12, 2012 from http://www.ncbi.nlm.nih.gov/books/ NBK44216/Sharpley-Whiting, T. (2007). *Pimps up, ho's down: Hip hop's hold on young Black women.* New York: NYU Press.

SIECUS—Sexuality Information and Education Council of the United States. (2007). *Public policy office state profile: Wyoming.* New York: Author.

Sigelman, C. K., & Rider, E. A. (2009). *Life-span human development.* Belmont, CA: Wadsworth Publishing.

Song, S. (2007). *Justice, gender, and the politics of multiculturalism.* New York: Cambridge University Press.

Stillman, S. (2007). "The missing white girl syndrome": Disappeared women and media activism. *Gender & Development, 15,* 491–502.

Stoltenberg, J. (1990). *Refusing to be a man: Essays on sex and justice.* New York: Meridien.

Tanenbaum, L. (2000). *Slut: Growing up female with a bad reputation.* New York: Harper Collins.

Taverner, B., & Montfort, S. (2005). *Making sense of abstinence: Lessons for comprehensive sex education.* Morristown, NJ: Planned Parenthood of Greater Northern New Jersey.

Thompson, S. (1990). Putting a big thing into a little hole: Teenage girls' accounts of sexual initiation. *Journal of Sex Research, 27*(3), 341–361.

Thompson, S. (1995). *Going all the way: Teenage girls' tales of sex, romance, and pregnancy.* New York: Hill and Wang Winter.

Tolman, D. L. (1991). Adolescent girls, women and sexuality: Discerning dilemmas of desire, *Women & Therapy, 11,* 55–69.

Tolman, D. (1994). Doing desire: Adolescent girls' struggle for/with sexuality. *Gender & Society, 8,* 324–342.

Tolman, D. (1996). Adolescent girls' sexuality: Debunking the myth of the urban girl. In B. J. Leadbeater & N. Way (Eds.), *Urban girls: Resisting stereotypes, creating identities* (pp. 255–257). New York: New York University Press.

Tolman, D. (1999). Femininity as a barrier to positive sexual health for girls. *Journal of the American Medical Women's Association, 54*(3), 133–138.

Tolman, D. L. (2000). Object lessons: Romance, violence and female adolescent sexual desire. *Journal of Sex Education and Therapy, 25*(1), 70–79.

Tolman, D. L. (2002). *Dilemmas of desire: Teenage girls talk about sexuality.* Cambridge, MA: Harvard University Press.

Tolman, D. L. (2012). Female adolescents, sexual empowerment, and desire: A missing discourse of gender inequity. *Sex Roles, 66*(11–12), 758–763.

Tolman, D. L., Impett, E. A., Tracy, A. J., & Michael, A. (2006). Looking good, sounding good: Feminist ideology and adolescent girls' mental health. *Psychology of Women Quarterly, 30,* 85–95.

Walkerdine, V. (1990). *Schoolgirl fictions.* London: Verso.

Ward, L. M., Merriwether, A., & Caruthers, A. (2006). Breasts are for men: Media use, masculinity ideology, and men's beliefs about women's bodies. *Sex Roles, 55,* 703–714.

Weekes, D. (2002). Get your freak on: How black girls sexualise identity. *Sex Education in England and Scotland, 2,* 251–262.

Welles, C. E. (2005). Breaking the silence surrounding female adolescent sexual desire. *Women & Therapy, 81,* 31–45.

Welsh, D. P., Rostosky, S. S., & Kawaguchi, M. C. (2000). A normative perspective of adolescent girls' developing sexuality. In J. W. White (Ed.), *Sexuality, society, and feminism* (pp. 111–140). Washington, DC: American Psychological Association.

Whatley, M. (1991). Raging hormones and powerful cars: The construction of men's sexuality in school sexuality education and popular adolescent films. In H. Giroux (Ed.), *Postmodernism, feminism, and cultural politics* (pp. 119–143). New York: SUNY Press.

WHO. (2004). Sexual health—A new focus for WHO. *Progress in Reproductive Sexual Health, 67,* 1–8.

Wilson, P. (1986). Black culture and sexuality. *Journal of Social Work and Human Sexuality, 4*(3), 29–47.

Wyatt, G. E. (1997). *Stolen women: Reclaiming our sexuality, taking back our lives.* New York: John Wiley & Sons.

Young, I. M. (1980). Throwing like a girl: A phenomenology of feminine body comportment motility and spatiality. *Human Studies, 3,* 137–156.

15

Fighting Sexualization

What Parents, Teachers, Communities, and
Young People Can Do

EILEEN L. ZURBRIGGEN AND TOMI-ANN ROBERTS

There is ample evidence that the sexualization of girls can have negative consequences for girls themselves, as well as having broader impacts (American
Psychological Association [APA], 2007). Thus, it is important to work on
multiple fronts to decrease the prevalence of sexualization and to mitigate
its negative effects. Many plausible strategies have been suggested by scholars (e.g., APA, 2007). Most of the chapters in this volume have either directly
addressed these questions or provided hints of promising pathways to follow.
In this chapter, we review some of these pathways and strategies.

In doing so, we follow the organization of the three spheres of sexualization
outlined in Chapter 1: cultural, interpersonal, and intrapsychic. It is easy to
fixate on the need to demand changes in the types of media representations
that saturate girls' lives. Although this is a worthy effort, other changes are
equally important—changes in the ways that parents, teachers, and peers interact with girls, as well as changes in the ways that girls think about themselves.
For each form of sexualization, we address both how we might minimize the
prevalence of that type of sexualization, as well as provide options for mitigat-
ing the negative effects, when exposure can't be completely eliminated.

Cultural Sexualization

In considering the sexualization of girls, cultural sexualization, particularly that
provided by the mass media, has received the most attention. This is not surprising, given the large number of sexualized images of girls and young women
that saturate the media landscape. In virtually every media genre that has been
examined, including video games, music videos, magazines, advertisements,

and cartoons and animation, numerous examples of highly sexualized images of women can be found (APA, 2007). The message to girls is clear: popularity and social standing are based on looking like a sex object. Moreover, concern about the media is high because its reach is so extensive and its influence so great. Thus, an adequate response to the sexualization of girls must provide ample attention to cultural sexualization, particularly by the media.

In crafting a response, we believe that a three-pronged approach is warranted. First, all of us need to work to radically change the media landscape that girls (and boys) are exposed to now. The prevalence of sexually objectifying images should be reduced and the frequency of positive, alternative images increased. Second, schools can provide media literacy programs that include attention to sexualization. Finally, by viewing media with children, parents and other interested adults can help them learn to interpret and critique these images.

Change the Media Landscape

Manufacturers and media producers could take an important step by making the decision to stop presenting sexualizing images of girls and to instead replace them with images of girls as children, active and engaged with their world, doing the things that children do. Not only would this be the right thing to do, morally, we believe it would also be economically advantageous. Parents are eager for alternatives that they can feel good about buying for their children. In so many conversations that we have had with parents, they have bemoaned the lack of options. It appears that a large market is waiting to be tapped.

More specifically, Farley and other authors in this volume have made a call for an end to the mainstreaming of prostitution-like behavior. For the vast majority of women engaged in prostitution, it has devastating consequences, emotionally, physically, psychologically, and financially. Normalizing prostitution makes these consequences invisible and, as argued by Purcell and Zurbriggen (2013; Chapter 8, this volume), contributes to a misogynistic and sexist culture that harms girls and women. Especially, we believe that marketing prostitution to adolescent and pre-teen girls as a glamorous and viable occupation (for example, by having strippers speak at school Career Days, or by teaching adolescents pole-dancing routines) does a deep disservice to girls.

Certain forms of sexualizing media may deserve special attention. Farley (2013; Chapter 9, this volume) and Tolman (2013; Chapter 5, this volume) mentioned video games, such as Grand Theft Auto, in which women are sexualized, but also killed and discarded. Emerging research suggests that interactive media such as "first-person shooter" games may be especially powerful agents of socialization in regards to violence and aggression (Dill & Dill, 1998). Interactive video games that teach boys to aggress sexually against women (even against "ho's" who are painted as deserving of such treatment) are likely to be equally powerful teachers (Dill & Thill, 2007). Our boys deserve better than this. They deserve a childhood in which they learn to relate to girls and women with respect, friendship, and joy, rather than fear, hatred, and dominance.

Music videos have also been seen as providing especially egregious examples of the sexual objectification of young women. These portrayals of women may be more frequent in rap and hip-hop (Jones, 1997), genres in which the majority of artists are black. In their systematic analysis of music videos played on the Black Entertainment Television (BET) network, Ward et al. (2013; Chapter 3, this volume) found extremely high levels of sexual objectification of women. Moreover, there was little diversity in women's activities and roles. The most frequent occupation for women was stripper. This is a clear example of the third element of sexualization—when someone is depicted as having value only for their sexuality. The fact that levels of sexualization may be especially high in videos that depict black women raises questions about the special risks that may be present for girls of color. If they see black women represented exclusively as sexual objects, their ability to envision diverse possibilities for their own futures may be hampered. In addition, it is important to note that hip-hop and rap music are very popular with white teenage male audiences. By teaching (white) boys that women of color are sexual objects, this perpetuates racist notions of the animalistic sexuality of black women. These are especially hurtful stereotypes that we need to work to eliminate, rather than perpetuate.

Another media format that may be especially important is sports media. Daniels and LaVoi (2013; Chapter 4, this volume) provided data showing how promising athletic participation is for girls. Moreover, their data suggest that when girls get to see female athletes (both girls and women) engaged in their sports, they are changed in important ways. Girls worry less about their appearance and start to internalize a more action-oriented identity (i.e., one that does not have self-objectification as its foundation). What a shame it is that this genre, one that could be a powerful force supporting girls, instead falls back on the same sexualizing standards that are common in other genres.

It can be easy to feel that we are at the mercy of multinational corporations that, to a large extent, control the choices available to us for entertainment and apparel, and who bombard us with advertisements on an hourly basis. However, there are ways both large and small in which parents, teachers, communities, and children can make a meaningful difference in this area.

Although it may seem implausible, individual efforts can have a noticeable impact. For example, Linnea W. Smith, waging a one-woman letter-writing campaign, was able to convince Hyundai Motors to pull its advertisements from the swimsuit edition of *Sports Illustrated* because of its sexualized and objectifying portrayals of women (Horovitz, 1993).

Working collectively is often an even better strategy. The Campaign for a Commercial-Free Childhood is an example of an organization that works to promote activism against inappropriate marketing to children, with grassroots letter-writing campaigns and an annual Consuming Kids Summit. The sexualization of childhood is one of their issues of interest, and they were instrumental in helping convince Hasbro to cancel a planned line of Pussycat Dolls, modeled on the sexualized musical group and marketed to girls as young as 6 (Goldiner, 2006).

Another activist organization dedicated to resisting the sexualization of girls is SPARK (Sexualization Protest: Action, Resistance, Knowledge; www.sparksummit.com). Founded in 2010, SPARK engages teen girls as part of the solution and has organized protests against marketing pink and "girly" Legos to girls, unrealistically photoshopped images in *Seventeen* magazine, and sexualized Halloween costumes.

Media Literacy

Several studies have suggested that media literacy programs can help prevent girls from internalizing a thin ideal (Irving, DuPen, & Berel, 1998) and can protect against body image problems (Levine & Murnen, 2009). For this reason, Tiggemann and other authors in this volume have called for the development—and wide implementation—of media literacy programs that include information about the sexualization of girls and women. Based on the effectiveness of media literacy programs addressing television violence (Vooijs & van der Voort, 1993) and alcohol use (Austin & Johnson, 1997), we believe that programs addressing sexualization are also likely to be effective. Because Tiggemann's work suggests that girls begin to internalize sexualizing messages at a very young age, media literacy programs should be designed for children as young as 6 or 7.

Co-Viewing

In addition to school-based media literacy programs, parents can help teach their children to become critical media consumers by watching or listening with them and initiating discussions. By commenting on the content presented by the media, and introducing your own thoughts and values, you can actually alter the influence of the media on your children. For example, in one study, children exposed to media portraying stereotypical gender roles were less accepting of nontraditional gender roles for men as compared with children exposed to the same media along with comments that contradicted the stereotypical roles (Nathanson, Wilson, McGee, & Sebastian, 2002). Although studies on the effects co-viewing sexualized materials have not yet been conducted, similar results would be expected.

Interpersonal Sexualization

The mass media sexualizes girls, but so do some peers and adults that are part of girls' lives. Working against these interpersonal sources of sexualization is equally as important as working against cultural forms of sexualization. We can work against interpersonal sexualization on a variety of levels, from changing national policies, to working within our communities, to changing the ways that we talk with girls and think about ourselves.

Comprehensive Sexuality Education

Several authors argued for the important role that comprehensive sexuality education can play in combating sexualization. By adding information about sexualization to sexuality curricula, sexualization by peers can be reduced and the effects of sexualization can be mitigated. Although girls tend not to sexually harass other girls, Petersen & Hyde (2013; Chapter 6, this volume), Thompson (2013; Chapter 7, this volume) reminds us that girls do sexually objectify each other. Thus, it will be important to help both boys and girls learn about the ways in which they may be sexualizing girls.

Thompson also points out that sexual minority girls have a double layer of sexual objectification. Because of this, sexuality education programs should address issues of compulsory heterosexuality and the objectification of sexual minority girls. To be maximally effective, they must also take into account, and respect, girls' ethnic, cultural, and religious backgrounds (Lamb, 2013; Chapter 14, this volume).

What else does the research presented in this book suggest about best practices for sexuality education programs? Bay-Cheng et al. (2013; Chapter 13, this volume) provided important data that indicate the importance of fostering "relational hardiness zones"—spaces where girls can talk with each other, not just spaces where adults provide information to girls. Sexuality education programs would be ideal locations for such communication. Girls in their focus groups also had specific requests for sexuality education courses. For example, they want advice about how to say no to unwanted sex with a boy that they like without jeopardizing the chance for a relationship with him.

Thompson's work suggests that agency is key, and that programs that foster sexual agency for girls will have positive effects. She advocates a space in which girls can get help understanding their feelings, fears, hopes, and desires. Without disagreeing, Lamb advocates for the role of mutuality as the underpinning of healthy sexuality. This leads to her recommendation that sexuality education include a focus on ethics and relationships. Empowerment and desire are fine as far as they go, but the ethics of mutuality, and the values that are inherent in that approach, are even more important.

Girls Groups

A key finding from Bay-Cheng et al.'s (2013; Chapter 13, this volume) focus groups is the essential role played by peer communication. If such communication is not possible in sexuality education courses (or if such courses are not provided), then other spaces for open communication should be created. In addition to allowing girls a place for exploration and discovery, such spaces can foster the kind of supportive friendships that both Bay-Cheng et al. and Petersen and Hyde (2013; Chapter 6, this volume) argued were important forces in buffering the negative effects of peer sexualization.

Bullying/Harassment Policies

Sexual harassment is one form of interpersonal sexualization (Petersen & Hyde, 2013; Chapter 6, this volume). Although research indicates that teachers are opposed to peer sexual harassment (Stone & Couch, 2004), students report that teachers do not intervene enough in preventing sexual harassment (American Association of University Women [AAUW], 2001). We need to do more to prevent sexualization by peers, and we need to listen to girls (and boys) to determine whether we have been successful in our prevention and intervention efforts. Good intentions are not enough—if students don't think we've changed the school climate in a meaningful way, then we haven't succeeded.

Based on the effective programs on bullying developed by Olweus (1993), a "whole-school" approach to preventing sexual harassment has the most promise of success. Such a program will involve all parties (teachers, principals, perpetrators, victims, bystanders, parents) and include significant follow-up. Examples of such programs include the Expect Respect program and the Equal Rights Advocates.

In developing sexual harassment prevention programs, we must remain aware of differences related to social identity. Ethnic and sexual minority girls (and boys) may be especially vulnerable to sexual harassment. In addition, sexual harassment is often racialized when it is directed toward ethnic minorities. These factors should be incorporated into all prevention efforts.

Prostitution

Farley (2013; Chapter 9, this volume) made a variety of suggestions geared toward eliminating the prostitution of girls, including providing safe spaces and transitional living for girls escaping prostitution and providing information and training for social service workers. The data she reviewed suggest also that efforts to prevent sexual abuse within the family and to combat homelessness among youth will help to eliminate the prostitution of youth. As a side benefit, it seems likely that reducing or eliminating prostitution will lead to a reduction in the "pornification" of everyday culture (Paul, 2005), which will have advantages for all girls.

Intrapsychic Sexualization

The third sphere of sexualization is intrapsychic sexualization, which happens when girls internalize the sexualizing messages that they receive from other people and from the broader cultural milieu. It is important to remember that girls are not passive vessels, but often are actively choosing to present themselves as sexual objects for the gaze of other people, especially boys that they want to attract or girls that they want to impress. Murnen and Smolak (2013; Chapter 12, this volume) remind us that, at some level, these choices make sense. There are many rewards for self-sexualizing, including popularity, status, power, and increased chances for romantic relationships and sexual exploration. Moreover, it often feels good to fulfill the roles we are expected to fulfill, and doing so can garner acceptance and (in the adult world) substantive rewards, such as career success and higher salaries. It would be a mistake to dismiss girls' choices as having only costs, and no benefits.

Self-sexualization has even more complexities that should be considered, as Stubbs and Johnston-Robledo (2013; Chapter 11, this volume) discussed. Mothers in their focus groups could clearly point to examples when their daughters self-sexualized (e.g., wearing clothes that the mothers thought were too sexy). They drew connections between cultural sexualization and the choices that their daughters were making (connections supported by ample research, as described by Tiggemann and others throughout this volume). They recognized that their daughters respond to and learn from what they see in the media (oftentimes, media designed for and marketed to older girls). But they note, as well, that the girls' actions and self-perceptions change from situation to situation; for example, engaging in child-like make-believe games at home, but then putting on a more sexualized persona in a dance class.

A final point worthy of note is that self-objectification is important in girls and adolescents, as well as in adult women (Tiggemann, 2013, Chapter 10, this volume). The internalization of cultural sexualization messages starts early, and there seem to be strong effects for young girls. Therefore, our efforts at helping girls to navigate these messages need to start early as well. The research reported in this volume suggests that a variety of approaches hold particular promise.

Athletics

Work described in Daniels and LaVoi (2013; Chapter 4, this volume) suggests that sports participation can help girls think differently about themselves. Sports participation is generally associated with increased self-esteem and body satisfaction. Although research has not yet been conducted to determine the exact mechanisms whereby this happens, a likely candidate is (decreased) self-objectification. The prediction is that sports participation helps girls think more about what their bodies can *do* than about how they *look*. The picture is complicated by the fact that some sports (for example, a sport like figure skating, in which judging is based partly on body appearance, or a sport like distance running, where very low body weight can improve performance) might be associated with disordered eating and body dissatisfaction, rather than having the positive effects that most sports and fitness activities seem to lead to (Daniels & LaVoi, 2013; Chapter 4, this volume; Tiggemann, 2013; Chapter 10, this volume; Tolman, 2013; Chapter 5, this volume). With a few possible exceptions, though, athletics seem to be a protective factor, and one that can be recommended to parents and girls. Given the positive impact of athletic participation, it is crucial for communities and schools to provide more access to athletic activities to all girls. Such participation will not only combat childhood obesity, but also help protect girls against the onslaught of sexualizing messages to which they are subjected. Currently, ethnic minority girls, and girls who are poor or live in urban or rural (as opposed to suburban) areas have less access to athletics (Daniels & LaVoi, 2013; Chapter 4, this volume). As a matter of public policy, ensuring equal access to all would be a positive step forward. Maximum impact will be achieved if such programs provide a "task-involving climate" (Neumark-Sztainer, Story, Hannan, Tharp, & Rex, 2003) where the focus is on skill-building, on nurturing and developing the potential of each girl, and on having fun, rather than winning at any cost.

Communication with Girls and "Informed Consent"

In their chapter discussing the costs and benefits to girls of self-sexualizing, Murnen and Smolak (2013; Chapter 12, this volume) implied that we owe girls the right to make informed decisions about whether, how much, and when to engage in this practice. In effect, it is up to adults to help provide a kind of "informed consent" procedure for girls, but then allow them the freedom to make their own decisions. Girls seem to be more aware of the benefits of self-sexualization than the costs, and adults can provide information about the latter, as well as help in weighing and balancing them against each other.

Such discussion can be part of broader, wide-ranging communications with girls about sexuality. Although communication between parents and children is important, Stubbs and Johnston-Robledo noted that it can easily be disrupted by cultural messages. Thus, is it important for parents to give these communications high priority, even if they feel uncomfortable at times. What might such communication look like? Some research (for example, Stubbs and Johnston-Robledo's work on menstruation; see Chapter 11, this volume) suggests that mothers and fathers may need more information and knowledge to do a good job of talking with their daughters, especially in a climate of rampant sexualization of girls. Providing that knowledge could help increase parents' comfort and effectiveness in talking with their children.

At the same time, the focus group work of Bay-Cheng et al. (2013; Chapter 13, this volume) supports the idea that parents should allow room for their daughters to express confusion and ambivalence, and that discussions should not be a lecture in which the parent presents factual information and force-feeds values. Rather, girls will benefit best from "evocative" relationships in which they both listen and speak, learn and teach. Although it might be uncomfortable for parents to have this kind of discussion with their daughters, it seems to be what girls need. Exploration is an essential part of all development, including sexual development. We can (and should) try to make the environment a reasonably safe one, but then we must give adolescents room to explore.

A final suggestion for parents is to be open to having other trusted family members talk with children about sex and sexualization. Bay-Cheng et al.'s focus group participants mentioned that they counted on cousins, older siblings, and aunts for accurate information and nonjudgmental discussions.

Conclusion

The research and commentary in this volume support the conclusion that the sexualization of girls is a widespread problem with serious consequences. Although many factors contribute to the problem, a patriarchal and sexist culture lies at the root. Fortunately, there are many tools and strategies that we can use to fight back. Ultimately, our goal should be to provide every girl and boy with an environment that allows for healthy development in all areas, including sexuality. The contributions in this volume are a step toward reaching that goal.

References

American Association of University Women. (AAUW). (2001). *Hostile hallways: Bullying, teasing, and sexual harassment in school.* New York: Harris/Scholastic Research.

American Psychological Association (APA). (2007). *Report of the APA task force on the sexualization of girls.* Washington, DC: Author.

Austin, E. W., & Johnson, K. K. (1997). Effects of general and alcohol-specific media literacy training on children's decision making about alcohol. *Journal of Health Communication, 2*, 17–42.

Bay-Cheng, L. Y., Livingston, J. A., & Fava, N. M. (2013). "Not always a clear path": Making space for peers, adults, and complexity in adolescent girls' sexual development. In E. L. Zurbriggen & T.- A. Roberts (Eds.), *The sexualization of girls and girlhood: Causes, consequences, and resistance* (Chapter 13). New York: Oxford University Press.

Daniels, E. A., & LaVoi, N. M. (2013). Athletics as solution and problem: Sport participation for girls and the sexualization of female athletes. In E. L. Zurbriggen & T.- A. Roberts (Eds.), *The sexualization of girls and girlhood: Causes, consequences, and resistance* (Chapter 4). New York: Oxford University Press.

Dill, K. E., & Dill, J. C. (1998). Video game violence: A review of the empirical literature. *Aggression and Violent Behavior, 3*, 407–428.

Dill, K. E., & Thill, K. P. (2007). Video game characters and the socialization of gender roles: Young people's perceptions mirror sexist media depictions. *Sex Roles, 57*, 851–864.

Farley, M. (2013). Prostitution: An extreme form of girls' sexualization. In E. L. Zurbriggen & T.- A. Roberts (Eds.), *The sexualization of girls and girlhood: Causes, consequences, and resistance* (Chapter 9). New York: Oxford University Press.

Goldiner, D. (2006, May 25). Hasbro axes dirty dancer toys for girls. *The New York Daily News*, p. 8. Retrieved May 26, 2006, from www.nydailynews.com

Horovitz, B. (1993, February 16). Throwing in a towel: Hyundai agrees to boycott Sports Illustrated's swimsuit issue. *Los Angeles Times*, p. D1. Retrieved July 31, 2006, from Proquest database.

Irving, L.M., DuPen, J. & Berel, S. (1998). A media literacy program for high school females. *Eating Disorders, 6*, 119–131.

Jones, K. (1997). Are rap videos more violent? Style differences and the prevalence of sex and violence in the age of MTV. *Howard Journal of Communication, 8*, 343–356.

Lamb, S. (2013). Toward a healthy sexuality for girls and young women: A critique of desire. In E. L. Zurbriggen & T.- A. Roberts (Eds.), *The sexualization of girls and girlhood: Causes, consequences, and resistance* (Chapter 14). New York: Oxford University Press.

Levine, M. P., & Murnen, S. K. (2009). Everybody knows that mass media are/are not [*pick one*] a cause of eating disorders: A critical review of evidence for a causal link between media, negative body image, and disordered eating in females. *Journal of Social and Clinical Psychology, 28*, 9–42.

Murnen, S. K., & Smolak, L. (2013). "I'd rather be a famous fashion model than a famous scientist": The rewards and costs of internalizing sexualization. In E. L. Zurbriggen & T.- A. Roberts (Eds.), *The sexualization of girls and girlhood: Causes, consequences, and resistance* (Chapter 12). New York: Oxford University Press.

Nathanson, A. I., Wilson, B. J., McGee, J., & Sebastian, M. (2002). Counteracting the effects of female stereotypes on television via active mediation. *Journal of Communication, 52*, 922–937.

Neumark-Sztainer, D., Story, M., Hannan, P. J., & Rex, J. (2003). New Moves: A school-based obesity prevention program for adolescent girls. *Preventive Medicine, 37*, 41–51.

Olweus, D. (1993). *Bullying at school: What we know and what we can do.* Oxford, UK: Blackwell.

Paul, P. (2005). *Pornified: How pornography is damaging our lives, our relationships, and our families.* New York: Henry Holt.

Petersen, J. L., & Hyde, J. S. (2013). Sexual harassment by peers. In E. L. Zurbriggen & T.- A. Roberts (Eds.), *The sexualization of girls and girlhood: Causes, consequences, and resistance* (Chapter 6). New York: Oxford University Press.

Purcell, N. J., & Zurbriggen, E. L. (2013). The sexualization of girls and gendered violence: Mapping the connections. In E. L. Zurbriggen & T.- A. Roberts (Eds.), *The sexualization of girls and girlhood: Causes, consequences, and resistance* (Chapter 8). New York: Oxford University Press.

Stone, M., & Couch, S. (2004). Peer sexual harassment among high school students: Teachers' attitudes, perceptions, and response. *The High school Journal, 88(1),* 1–13.

Stubbs, M. L., & Johnston-Robledo, I. (2013). Kiddy thongs and menstrual pads: The sexualization of girls and early menstrual life. In E. L. Zurbriggen & T.- A. Roberts (Eds.), *The sexualization of girls and girlhood: Causes, consequences, and resistance* (Chapter 11). New York: Oxford University Press.

Thompson, E. M. (2013). "If you're hot, i'm bi": Implications of sexualization for sexual-minority girls. In E. L. Zurbriggen & T.- A. Roberts (Eds.), *The sexualization of girls and girlhood: Causes, consequences, and resistance* (Chapter 7). New York: Oxford University Press.

Tiggemann, M. (2013). Teens, pre-teens, and body image. In E. L. Zurbriggen & T.- A. Roberts (Eds.), *The sexualization of girls and girlhood: Causes, consequences, and resistance* (Chapter 10). New York: Oxford University Press.

Tolman, D. L. (2013). It's bad for us too: How the sexualization of girls impacts the sexuality of boys, men, and women. In E. L. Zurbriggen & T.- A. Roberts (Eds.), *The sexualization of girls and girlhood: Causes, consequences, and resistance* (Chapter 5). New York: Oxford University Press.

Vooijs, M. W., & van der Voort, T. H. (1993). Learning about television violence: The impact of a critical viewing curriculum on children's attitudinal judgments of crime series. *Journal of Research and Development in Education, 26,* 133–142.

Ward, L. M., Rivadeneyra, R., Thomas, K., Day, K., & Epstein, M. (2013). A woman's worth: Analyzing the sexual objectification of black women in music videos. In E. L. Zurbriggen & T.- A. Roberts (Eds.), *The sexualization of girls and girlhood: Causes, consequences, and resistance* (Chapter 3). New York: Oxford University Press.

INDEX

Printed in the USA/Agawam, MA
August 31, 2018

682286.004